Evaluation for Health Policy and Health Care

Sara Miller McCune founded SAGE Publishing in 1965 to support the dissemination of usable knowledge and educate a global community. SAGE publishes more than 1000 journals and over 600 new books each year, spanning a wide range of subject areas. Our growing selection of library products includes archives, data, case studies and video. SAGE remains majority owned by our founder and after her lifetime will become owned by a charitable trust that secures the company's continued independence.

Los Angeles | London | New Delhi | Singapore | Washington DC | Melbourne

Evaluation for Health Policy and Health Care

A Contemporary Data-Driven Approach

Edited by

Steven Sheingold

Department of Health and Human Services

Anupa Bir

RTI International

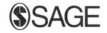

Los Angeles | London | New Delhi
Singapore | Washington DC | Melbourne

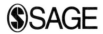

FOR INFORMATION:

SAGE Publications, Inc.
2455 Teller Road
Thousand Oaks, California 91320
E-mail: order@sagepub.com

SAGE Publications Ltd.
1 Oliver's Yard
55 City Road
London EC1Y 1SP
United Kingdom

SAGE Publications India Pvt. Ltd.
B 1/I 1 Mohan Cooperative Industrial Area
Mathura Road, New Delhi 110 044
India

SAGE Publications Asia-Pacific Pte. Ltd.
18 Cross Street #10-10/11/12
China Square Central
Singapore 048423

Printed in the United States of America

Library of Congress Cataloging-in-Publication Data

Names: Sheingold, Steven Howard, 1951- editor. | Bir, Anupa, editor.

Title: Evaluation for health policy and health care : a contemporary data-driven approach / Steven Sheingold, Department of Health and Human Services, Anupa Bir, RTI International.

Description: Los Angeles : SAGE, [2020] | Includes bibliographical references and index.

Identifiers: LCCN 2019013373 | ISBN 9781544333717 (paperback)

Subjects: LCSH: Medical policy–Evaluation–Statistical methods. | Medical care–Evaluation–Statistical methods.

Classification: LCC RA399.A1 S468 2020 | DDC 362.1072/7–dc23
LC record available at https://lccn.loc.gov/2019013373

This book is printed on acid-free paper.

Certified Chain of Custody
Promoting Sustainable Forestry
www.sfiprogram.org
SFI-01268

SFI label applies to text stock

Acquisitions Editor: Leah Fargotstein
Content Development Editor: Chelsea Neve
Editorial Assistant: Claire Laminen
Production Editor: Bennie Clark Allen
Copy Editor: Lana Todorovic-Arndt
Typesetter: C&M Digitals (P) Ltd.
Proofreader: Jen Grubba
Indexer: Jean Casalegno
Cover Designer: Ginkhan Siam
Marketing Manager: Shari Countryman

19 20 21 22 23 10 9 8 7 6 5 4 3 2 1

Brief Contents

Detailed Contents

List of Figures and Tables

Figures

Tables

Preface

This book offers the reader a window into a unique combination of program knowledge, evaluation experience, and methodological expertise that we hope will benefit the world of policy researchers, as well as those who aspire to become policy researchers. It is designed to provide real-world applications within health policy to make learning more accessible and relevant, and to highlight the remaining challenges for using evidence to develop policy. Developed through a combined effort of the U.S. Department of Health and Human Services (the Office of the Assistant Secretary for Planning and Evaluation and the Center for Medicare and Medicaid Innovation), RTI International, and an expert technical panel that agreed to serve as advisors, authors, and reviewers, the final product is a truly collaborative effort. It reflects a response from policymakers, academics, and policy researchers to the complexities of evaluating health care interventions in a timely, rigorous way with cutting-edge approaches.

As evidence-based policy gains momentum, this book will appeal to those studying, designing, and implementing or overseeing evaluations. It can be a resource for graduate programs in public policy or health policy, or for policymakers interested in newer guidance for evaluation applications. It offers two tracks: one for those who prefer an intuitive explanation, and one for those who prefer to see equations. Unique features of this book include the real-word examples throughout the text that keep the evaluation methods anchored within the health policy discourse; highlighting the utility of qualitative, quantitative, and meta-analytic methods separately and together for policy; and sharing an understanding that evaluation should be rapid, ongoing, and relevant as opposed to decade-long efforts that answer questions that had long dimmed from the policy radar. An additional benefit of this book is the focus on communicating evidence-based results to policymakers, including using interactive and visual methods.

To support the use of this book in the classroom, curated pedagogic materials are provided on the website and in the book. The textbook structure is easily extended by journal articles cited as examples and provided on the website. Additional pedagogic features are chapter-by-chapter learning objectives, discussion questions, real-world examples, sample code and data for practice, and ready-to-use teaching materials for instructors.

Our goal is to provide a new take on evaluation for health care policy, demystifying with real examples, understanding the importance of qualitative and quantitative approaches, and providing solutions to challenges faced by traditional evaluations that may be difficult to understand, deliver results too late to be useful, or ignore the interim information that an evaluation should provide to policymakers. Thus, the book not only extensively analyzes the modern methodological approaches to evaluation, but it adds several chapters on making evaluation results more accessible and useful to policymakers.

Resources for Instructors

Instructors have access to the companion website at
study.sagepub.com/sheingold1e

Password-protected instructor resources include the following:

- Editable, chapter-specific Microsoft® **PowerPoint® slides** offer you complete flexibility in easily creating a multimedia presentation for your course.

- **Lecture notes**, including Outline and Objectives, which may be used for lecture and/or student handouts.

- **Case studies** from SAGE Research Methods accompanied by critical thinking/discussion questions.

- **Tables and figures** from the printed book are available in an easily-downloadable format for use in papers, hand-outs, and presentations.

Resources for Students

Students have access to the companion website at
study.sagepub.com/sheingold1e

Open-access student resources include **case studies** from SAGE Research Methods accompanied by **critical thinking/discussion questions**.

Acknowledgments

As this endeavor began in 2012, the health care policy environment was shifting. We shared the momentous sense that we could contribute to improving the health care system by applying our core evaluation skill set to the anticipated wealth of questions and data. The topics we began to address raised many issues for discussion and continued to evolve long past the expected end of the process.

We were fortunate to share this adventure with the best company. A number of methodological experts agreed to collaborate with us, initially with the idea that each would address a separate issue in an independent chapter. Then through multiple rounds of discussion and review, the book became a product of the greater collaboration.

Our experts and their primary areas of contribution were Steve Asch (quality of care), Partha Deb (heterogeneity of impacts), Guido Imbens (randomization), Thomas Nolan (organizational change and statistical process control), Malcolm Maclure and Sebastian Schneeweiss (rapid-cycle decision making), Jeff Smith and Jeff Wooldridge (econometrics), and Alan Zaslavsky and John Orav (thoughtful interlocutors and reviewers of the entire volume).

There were a number of collaborators from Center for Medicare and Medicaid Innovation (CMMI), including Will Shrank (now with Humana), who began the discussions about the need for this book and led us in the initial stages, Jun Li (quality of care), and Rocco Perla and Bruce Finke (learning and diffusion). RTI experts include Jerry Cromwell (Medicare demonstration evaluations), Kevin Smith (propensity methods, heterogeneity, and meta-analysis), Martijn van Hasselt (Bayesian methods), Nikki Freeman (Bayesian methods and meta-analysis), Jim Derzon (meta-analysis), and Leila Kahwati and Heather Kane (qualitative comparative analysis).

From the Office of the Assistant Secretary for Planning and Evaluation, Department of Health and Human Services (ASPE) and RTI International, a number of people served multiple roles, made this work possible, and improved its quality. Susan Bogasky was the willing guide for the project, and her incredible skill in knowing how to get things done was invaluable. Rachael Zuckerman contributed in the last leg of the journey by filling a few key gaps in modeling.

From RTI, Kevin Smith, Nikki Freeman, Julia Cohen, Jim Derzon, Rob Chew, Lexie Grove, Ben Koethe, Terry Hall, Elliott Liebling, and Felicity Skidmore helped with thinking, writing, editing, creating figures, formatting, revising, and doing it all again. We appreciate your expertise and patience immensely.

Richard Frank (ASPE, Harvard) and Renee Mentnech (CMMI) made sure we stayed true to our mission of creating a supportive resource for evaluators and future evaluators facing a new set of policy questions with new twists and turns.

With our gratitude for your expert contributions and good humor,

Anupa and Steve

SAGE gratefully acknowledges the following reviewers for their kind assistance:

Alison K. Cohen, University of San Francisco

Nathan Hale, East Tennessee State University

Larry R. Hearld, University of Alabama at Birmingham

Lydia Kyei-Blankson, Illinois State University

Chad Murphy, Mississippi University for Women

E. John Orav, Harvard Medical School and Harvard TH Chan School of Public Health

John Paul, University of North Carolina at Chapel Hill

Sandra Schrouder, Barry University

Jiunn-Jye Sheu, University of Toledo

Brad Wright, University of Iowa

About the Editors

Steven H. Sheingold, Ph.D. is the Director of the Division of Health Financing Policy, Office of the Assistant Secretary for Planning and Evaluation (ASPE), Department of Health and Human Services. His areas of responsibility include economic and policy analysis of Medicare's payment systems, evaluation strategies, analysis of competition in insurance and provider markets, and economic issues related to health care and pharmaceutical markets. Prior to joining ASPE, Dr. Sheingold held several managerial and senior analyst positions within the Centers for Medicare and Medicaid Services and the Congressional Budget Office. As an adjunct, he has taught classes in health policy, health services research, and statistics at George Mason University and George Washington University. He has published articles concerning reimbursement systems; technology assessment and cost effectiveness analyses; value based purchasing programs; the use of evidence for health policymaking; and the impact of social risk factors on quality of care in journals such as *Health Affairs*, *New England Journal of Medicine*, *Medical Care*, and *the Journal of Health Policy*, *Politics and Law*. He holds a Ph.D. in Economics from the Pennsylvania State University.

Anupa Bir, ScD MPH is the Senior Director of the Center for Advanced Methods Development at RTI International. A health economist by training, much of her work has focused on the well-being of vulnerable populations and aligning incentives within various systems, including the welfare, child welfare, corrections, and health systems, to improve well-being. Dr. Bir currently leads several contracts to evaluate complex health and social policy interventions. These interventions include innovative workforce interventions to improve access to quality health care, interventions that offer financial incentives for asset development, and interventions that improve communication and family strength during stressful circumstances like incarceration and reentry. Within health care and health policy, she leads evaluations of State Innovation Models, efforts funded by the Centers for Medicare and Medicaid Innovation to accelerate the transition to value-based payment models in 11 states. She also leads meta-evaluation work to understand the lessons from state Medicaid demonstrations to improve service delivery for those with substance use disorders or serious mental illness. She holds an MPH from Yale University School of Public Health and a doctoral degree in international health economics from the Harvard TH Chan School of Public Health.

Setting Up for Evaluation

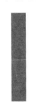

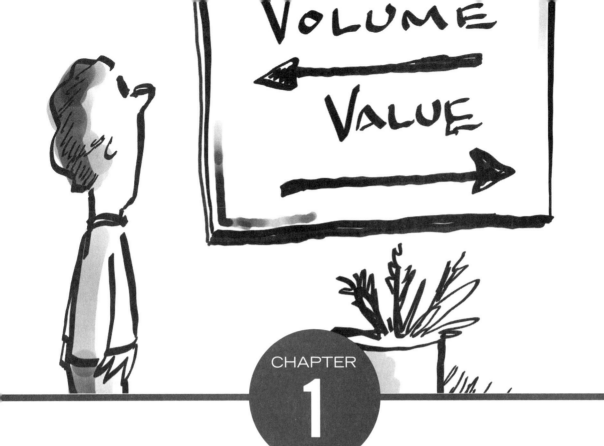

CHAPTER 1

Introduction

Steven Sheingold

William Shrank

Background: Challenges and Opportunities

A comprehensive and dynamic evaluation should be an integral part of developing and implementing all major programs and policies. Planned and conducted properly, evaluations can provide important benefits to program administrators, policymakers, and the public. Evaluations are essential to understand the effect of programs and policies on the populations they serve, providing crucial evidence for the diffusion of innovations into practice. High-quality evaluation can provide the objective information needed to support the optimal prioritization and allocation of resources among existing programs and proposed new initiatives in the face of budgetary constraints. Additionally, evaluations can provide monitoring and feedback components that allow for continuous assessment, quality improvement, and mid-course corrections.

Conducting and using rigorous evaluations presents challenges, however. Evaluations can be costly and time consuming, and they can yield conflicting or inconclusive results. For these and other reasons, program proponents can see them—particularly in evaluations where people who are eligible for the program are assigned to a group that does not receive services—as draining away scarce resources that "should" be used to serve the maximum number of clients. In addition to these organizational concerns, applying appropriate evaluation methodologies to address a program's unique objectives can be extremely complex. This is particularly true for impact evaluations, which are intended to answer two major and related questions with a known degree of scientific credibility:

- Did target outcomes for the program improve, for whom did they improve, and under what circumstances?

- Can the findings demonstrate in a scientifically credible manner that the program, as opposed to other environmental factors, contributed significantly to the observed improvement (known as internal validity)?

Answering these questions can be especially challenging in cases where the intervention/new initiative cannot be evaluated with a built-in randomized controlled trial (RCT) design. An RCT design is considered the gold standard for impact evaluations, because it virtually guarantees an unbiased control group. Often, it is not practicable, and sometimes, it is even impossible. In such cases, alternative methods of achieving internal validity are required.

Another important issue is that a program evaluation design that is not fully integrated into the program's initial development and implementation frequently leads to inappropriate research designs and/or a lack of needed evaluation data—preventing the evaluation from yielding the type of authoritative results that can credibly establish the program's effectiveness or lack thereof. In cases where the evaluation has been designed and implemented separately from initial implementation, the observed findings—whether positive, negative, or inconclusive—can raise the following difficult question: Were the methods and data insufficient to yield valid results—that is, to confidently establish whether the program was really effective or not?

While these challenges are very real, we believe that they can be minimized by a better understanding of evaluation methods and a clear vision of the utility of evaluation to promote learning, improvement, and rigorous outcome measurement. In our experience, obstacles to good evaluation, and the organizational concerns discussed above, arise from several factors: lack of understanding by program implementers of the variety of quasi-experimental and observational research designs that may be available when randomized trials are not possible; lack of understanding of the data flows required for implementing these methods; lack of understanding of relationships between monitoring, interim, or rapid formative evaluations and summative evaluation; and lack of familiarity with issues regarding translating evidence into practice or policy.

The age of "big data" also provides greatly expanded opportunities for overcoming past obstacles to evaluation. The increasing ability to collect, store, access, and analyze large quantities of data on a nearly real-time basis means that (1) multiple statistical methods may be available to improve the rigor of impact evaluations; (2) these methods can be applied on an ongoing basis; and (3) program monitoring can be seamlessly coordinated with the process and impact evaluation activities.

Evaluation and Health Care Delivery System Transformation

The delivery system transformation provisions of the Affordable Care Act (ACA) provided the impetus, indeed the necessity, of addressing the challenges and opportunities for strengthening the link between research and policy. ACA made the mandate clear—use innovation and experimentation to produce evidence that will help transform the health care system to deliver a higher quality of care at lower cost to Americans. Thus, developing methods to rigorously evaluate these programs and policies, and to do so expeditiously, has become critical.

The Center for Medicare and Medicaid Innovation (CMMI), which was authorized by the ACA, is charged with testing and evaluating innovative payment and service delivery models to reduce costs and improve quality of care in the broader, dynamic health care environment. The ACA provided $10 billion in CMMI funding from 2011 to 2019, combined with expanded authority to test innovative health care delivery system and payment models through Section 1115A of the Social Security Act (the Act).[1] The Act includes specific authority to expand program models if the evaluation finds, and the Centers for Medicare and Medicaid Services (CMS) Actuary certifies, that the model will either (1) reduce Medicare or Medicaid spending without reducing Medicare beneficiary access to care or (2) improve quality of care without increasing costs or reducing access. Once CMMI identifies the model, CMMI is responsible for development, implementation, and evaluation to determine the effectiveness and feasibility of initiative expansion or scaling[2] to national program policy. This broad authority makes ensuring rigorous impact evaluation a critical part of CMMI's responsibility to rapidly identify and test desirable innovations, and use the resulting information to drive delivery system change.

CMMI faces some unique methodological issues in fulfilling these responsibilities. The health care delivery environment is extremely dynamic, presenting providers and other stakeholders with multiple, potentially conflicting, and complementary incentives for achieving key objectives. A range of public and private efforts may target reduction in hospital readmissions, for example, or hospital-acquired conditions. Indeed, CMMI itself may have several initiatives that address the same target outcome through different programs and incentives. Thus, attributing changes in outcomes to a specific CMMI payment or service delivery model—as opposed to all the other factors in the different program environments that might potentially influence the same outcome—presents a formidable methodological challenge. For example, CMMI models may be based on voluntary participation—which raises important concerns about selection bias. Why do some providers choose to participate, and others do not? The reasons are very unlikely to be random. Some see more opportunity for profit than others; for example, some may simply have too small (or too large) a market share to find it interesting to participate. Since an RCT design is not possible in a voluntary situation, a comparison group design is required to minimize the effect of the voluntary decision environment.

Finally, implementing initiatives within reasonable timeframes may require tradeoffs between program goals and methodological rigor. For example, it may not be possible to establish data collection methods conducive to constructing optimal comparison groups. It then becomes critical to make the best choice possible from quasi-experimental, or if necessary observational designs, that are still feasible under the circumstances.

Beyond these challenges to rigorous evaluation, CMMI maintains a focus on providing meaningful feedback to providers about performance during the implementation phase of a model—known as a formative (as opposed to a summative) evaluation. Only by rapidly comparing one site's performance to its own historical performance—as well as to the performance of other sites participating in the model and comparison sites that are not—can CMMI support the real-time learning and improvement essential to engender success. Moreover, CMMI must also collect contextual qualitative information about the program structure, leadership, and implementation, to understand strategies and features associated with success. This enables identification, harvesting, and dissemination of effective approaches. Understanding how to deliver rapid feedback without compromising the rigor of the summative evaluation is a key evaluation challenge.

More recent legislation has further emphasized the importance of these evaluation methods. Section 101(e)(1) of the "Medicare Access and CHIP Reauthorization Act of 2015" (MACRA) establishes the Physician Focused Payment Model (PFPM)

Technical Advisory Committee (TAC). The TAC is to provide comments and recommendations to the secretary of Health and Human Services on PFPMs submitted by stakeholders. The Committee must review submitted models, prepare comments and recommendations regarding whether such models meet criteria established by the Secretary, and submit those comments and recommendations to the Secretary. In order for the Committee to conduct its work in a valid, evidence based, and credible manner, it needs to have information to better understand the effectiveness of alternative payment models (APMs) on health care utilization, expenditures, and quality of care. Thus, they need to understand evaluation, results of ongoing evaluation of CMMI models, and how the various methodologies would be used for the PFPMs they propose.

These tasks are immediate and critical for delivery system change in a complex world. Such direct links between evidence and immediate policy decisions have already spurred considerable thinking about a broad range of evaluation methods and ways to directly translate evidence into practice and policy. Health services researchers and evaluators who have long hoped for a stronger link between research and policy may now be in a "be careful what you wish for" moment. The window is open for demonstrating that methodologically rigorous and policy relevant results can be produced within a timeframe that makes them most useful to decision makers.

The Global Context for Considering Evaluation Methods and Evidence-Based Decision Making

The ACA and CMMI might be considered as precipitating events for the new emphasis on these topics because of the statutory link between evaluation results and policy decisions. But delivery system change is hardly the only evaluation game in town. There is a much broader and practical context for expanding our thinking and increasing our knowledge about creating high-quality evidence for policy decision making. Indeed, the current economic and budgetary climate has created a greater need for improving our evaluation capabilities and the ability to integrate the evidence they provide into decision-making processes at all levels of government.[3] Most importantly, fiscal pressures demand that public programs and policies yield greater value, requiring the use of more evidence for policymaking. Such evidence is critical for developing programs, implementing them, assessing their effectiveness, and making needed adjustments.

The Congress recognized the importance of evidence-based policymaking to making government more effective by passing two laws that will have a substantial effect on the evaluation community. The first was the Evidence-Based Policymaking Commission Act of 2016 (Public Law 114–140, March 30, 2016). The law reflected a bipartisan call to improve the evidence available for making decisions about government programs and policies. The Commission was established to develop a strategy for increasing the availability and use of data to build evidence about government programs, while protecting privacy and confidentiality. In September 2017, the Commission produced its final report and recommendations as required by the statute.[4]

In December 2018, the Congress passed Foundations for Evidence-Based Policymaking Act of 2017. The law will have substantial effects on government agencies with regard to formalizing evaluation planning and maintaining necessary data. It requires federal departments and agencies to submit annually to the Office of Management and Budget (OMB) and Congress a plan for identifying and addressing policy questions relevant to the programs, policies, and regulations of such departments and agencies. The plan must include (1) a list of policy-relevant questions for developing evidence to support policymaking, and (2) a list of data for facilitating the use of evidence in policymaking. The OMB shall consolidate such plans into a unified evidence-building plan.

The bill establishes an Interagency Council on Evaluation Policy to assist the OMB in supporting governmentwide evaluation activities and policies. The bill defines "evaluation" to mean an assessment using systematic data collection and analysis of one or more programs, policies, and organizations intended to assess their effectiveness and efficiency. Each department or agency shall designate a Chief Evaluation Officer to coordinate evidence-building activities and an official with statistical expertise to provide advice on statistical policy, techniques, and procedures. The OMB shall establish an Advisory Committee on Data for Evidence Building to advise on expanding access to and use of federal data for evidence building. Each agency shall (1) develop and maintain a comprehensive data inventory for all data assets created by or collected by the agency, and (2) designate a Chief Data Officer who shall be responsible for lifecycle data management and other specified functions.

These provisions do not, however, address how these data would be used to best inform the policymaking process. It will be necessary for program administrators and the research community to undertake the responsibility to develop rigorous evaluations pertinent to the unique questions raised by each program or policy area; conduct the evaluations in a timely manner; and learn how to translate the results in the most useful way to inform the decision makers in each situation.

This book will also be helpful to researchers in meeting these expanding responsibilities and to better understand the policy processes they hope to inform with their research. It will have particular value for readers who wish to concentrate on the most recent thinking on the methodological and translational issues *that are most key to informing program and policy decisions*. We recognize that a number of excellent primers and textbooks concerning evaluation are already available. In this text, we attempt to add to the knowledge base by comprehensively focusing on the translational and decision-making aspects of program evaluation, as well as providing a rigorous treatment of the methods issues. The evaluation, evidence, and decision-making topics discussed are applicable to most program and policy areas. Indeed, our illustrations and examples are drawn from a wide range of health care and non–health care policy areas. We make it a point to provide illustrations (with both existing studies and original data analyses) to show how rigorous evaluation supports data-informed decision making. In the health program/policy area, the foremost goals are to improve health care services and reduce costs, without restricting health care access. Other program/policy areas have analogous goals.

Book's Intent

This book is intended to comprehensively address these important evaluation issues in a way that is rigorous enough to be useful for evaluators, while being easy to access by program administrators and policy decision makers whose primary focus is not methodological. This is a complex task to accomplish. Several chapters, by their nature, address issues of methodology. These chapters, primarily Chapters 5 and 6, include formal mathematical derivations. These are clearly marked, and readers not primarily interested in the methodological details can skip them. A number of chapters clarify important issues that need to be understood by both evaluators and decision makers *as they work together* to translate evaluation evidence into policy. These include analyzing and using interim results, harnessing alternative methods for analyzing and presenting data, and applying decision-making frameworks to empirical results for policy decision making.

The intent is to provide useful information for two basic situations. For those with *programs already under way*, the book can inform choices of methods, given the constraints imposed by existing program structure and data availability. For those who are *planning programs* and wish to *prospectively build in evaluation components*, the primer does two things: It provides guidance in the design of new programs to ensure they can be rigorously evaluated, and it highlights the types of data that would have to be generated for evaluation use.

This book also breaks new ground by addressing "rapid-cycle" evaluation in terms of state of the art methodologies, integration with monitoring and feedback requirements, and seamless transition to final impact evaluation. One clear source of skepticism about rigorous evaluations is that results often become available only when the time has passed for them to be useful. Thus, while the emergence of the term *rapid cycle* is associated with CMMI's unique responsibilities and authorities, the ability to produce credible results on a more rapid and continuous basis will benefit evaluations across a range of program areas.

DISCUSSION QUESTIONS

1. How can evaluators convince skeptical program proponents that conducting evaluations is a necessary practice?

2. How can the nearly real-time availability of data, and sometimes big data, change the way that evaluations are conducted? How can this impact the implementation of programs being evaluated?

3. What are the advantages and disadvantages of basing policy on evidence?

NOTES

1. The Social Security Act, 42 U.S.C., § 1115A(c)(1).

2. Section 1115A(c)(2)&(3) of the Act requires the Chief Actuary of CMS to certify such expansion would reduce (or would not result in any increase in) net program spending under applicable titles, and the Secretary determines that such expansion would not deny or limit the coverage or provision of benefits under applicable title for applicable individuals. The Secretary shall focus on models and demonstration projects that improve the quality of patient care and reduce spending.

3. Liebman, Jeffrey B., "Building on Recent Advances in Evidence-Based Policymaking," a paper jointly released by the Hamilton Project at Brookings Institution and Results for America, April 2013.

4. Report of the Commission on Evidence-Based Policymaking, *The Promise of Evidence-Based Policymaking*, September 2017.

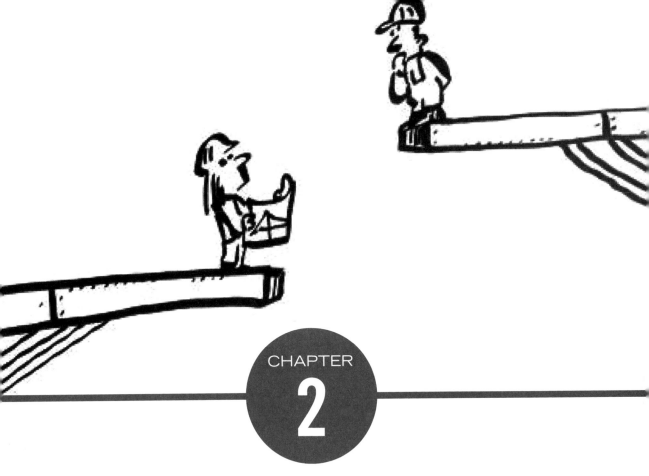

Setting the Stage

Anupa Bir

Steven Sheingold

Learning Objectives

This chapter presents an overview of three evaluation typologies: formative, summative, and process evaluations. It introduces logic models as the intermediary between program goals and evaluation design, guiding the type and timing of data collection. Many challenges complicate researchers' ability to properly evaluate

(Continued)

(Continued)

program impacts, and among these challenges is the question of when to plan and implement the evaluation. The timing of evaluation planning and implementation can substantially influence the rigor, statistical validity, and credibility of the evaluation findings. This chapter presents the idea of a prospectively planned and integrated program evaluation, offering a series of related evaluation-planning tools to help neutralize these evaluation limitations.

Distinguishing the many types of evaluation discussed in the literature is important to set the stage for the chapters that follow. This book primarily targets what is often called impact evaluation, but this is just one among many types of program evaluation. In this chapter, we describe and distinguish between the different types. While these are typically thought of as alternative evaluation designs, they can also be envisioned as successive stages in a comprehensive evaluation process.

Typology for Program Evaluation[1,2]

Most program evaluations can be classified as one of three types: formative, process, or summative. Although the vast literature on evaluation typology encompasses frameworks different from the three-legged framework we describe here, each has essentially the same purpose: to help researchers determine the best approach for answering their programmatic and intervention-related questions. We therefore frame the three types of evaluations presented in relation to the central research questions each serves to answer.

1.   **Formative Evaluation.** Generally, a formative evaluation gleans information that can contribute to further developing a program or intervention. It is most commonly used to answer questions that arise during program design and development, for example, "What components of the program should be included?"[3] Policymakers and program designers can find formative evaluation quite useful. Naturally this type of evaluation typically precedes implementation and as such, it has been termed *pretesting* or *developmental research*.[4] However, as discussed in later chapters, recent advances in both statistical methodologies and evaluative thinking have incorporated formative evaluation approaches into both rapid-cycle evaluation and theory-driven evaluation to aid in program improvement and in identifying what levers are central to change.

2.   **Process Evaluation.** Process evaluation, as its name suggests, "investigates the procedures that were used to implement a policy program"[5] or an intervention. To answer the *what* and *how* questions that may follow a formative evaluation,

a process evaluation is a good approach. One of the foundational findings in evaluation was that services are rarely implemented as planned (or not implemented at all) and that the clients served are often not those for whom the services are intended. Process evaluation describes what is being implemented, to what extent it is being implemented, and who is actually receiving the intervention. As such, process evaluations also assess the fidelity with which a program is implemented.

3.   **Summative Evaluation.** In contrast to formative evaluation, which precedes program implementation, summative evaluation answers questions about program outcomes and impacts. Research questions seeking to determine whether the program/intervention achieves the goal for which it was originally designed can be best answered by summative evaluation. This type of evaluation answers a fundamental research question: Is the program/intervention achieving the goals it is intended to achieve?[6] Even though summative evaluation requires data that are unavailable in full until program completions, the most complete and most efficient data collection requires even a summative evaluation to be planned prior to program implementation.

As in many areas related to evaluation and research, different individuals and groups can use different terminology to describe the same concept or method. For example, in this book, as in others, we use the term *impact evaluation* to describe evaluations that attempt to establish a causal link between a program and desired outcomes.[7] Such evaluations clearly fall under the general umbrella of summative evaluation. Often, these evaluations also separate outcomes and impacts, distinguished by timing and performance measures studied. Outcome evaluation measures program effects in the target population by assessing the progress in the outcomes or outcome objectives that the program is to achieve. It requires understanding of the kind of changes desired for participants, such as in learning, skills, behavior, and actions. Thus, evaluators must identify appropriate indicators that can measure these changes. Impacts are those effects consistent with the overall objectives of the intervention, such as measures of changes in health. For example, a program might train physicians in new ways to council patients on nutrition and weight loss. Outcome measures might be specific changes in physician practice, such as the number or content of counseling sessions, while impact might be measured by patient weight loss. As discussed in the chapters ahead, specifying the full range of performance measures for each stage in evaluation will be important. For the purposes of this book, we use the term *impact evaluation* in the general sense, that is, assessing all important program effects that might be associated with summative evaluation.

A modern, integrated, and comprehensive evaluation will draw on the lessons, practices, and principles of all three types of evaluation. For any given intervention, formative evaluation practices will inform program design; a process evaluation will assess if the design is implemented with fidelity and integrity; a summative evaluation will examine the program's success in achieving its goals. In rapid cycle evaluation, planned and unplanned variation can be documented by the process evaluation and combined with summative or impact evaluation findings to determine what components of the program or intervention are most significant in their contribution to particular outcomes. The quantitative and qualitative data collected in the observations required for process or diagnostic evaluation must be carefully selected, based on a theory of change that identifies the critical elements of a program and specifies their relation to proximal, intermediate, and long-term outcomes (as discussed later in this chapter). As programs are almost certainly adapted to local conditions when taken to scale, comprehensive integrated evaluations provide evidence on what are likely to be the core components of the intervention and which components are not associated with effectiveness—and can therefore be modified to better align, for example, with existing services.

After assessing the research questions, selecting the evaluation type will inform the steps that follow: timing of evaluation design, methods for actually conducting the evaluation (discussed in Part II), and measures involved in the ongoing monitoring required to conduct the evaluation (discussed in Part III), these measures being determinants of the data required to conduct the evaluation (as discussed in Chapter 3).

We emphasize again that although these are presented for simplicity as discrete forms of evaluation and may occur in isolation, an integrated comprehensive evaluation will draw on the lessons and practices of each, to create the evidence necessary for decision making that is maximally data informed. Integrating evaluation principles and practices into organizational practice will assist health care (and other service) providers to identify effective practices and the conditions necessary to support the implementation of those practices.

Planning an Evaluation: How Are the Changes Expected to Occur?

Programs and policies are implemented to achieve specific outcomes, generally by providing resources and incentives to change behaviors. Designing comprehensive evaluations therefore should begin by detailing the resources provided and exactly how the program is intended to change behaviors to achieve the desired outcomes. Such models of change are often called logic models or results chains.[8] They are typically a visual tool—usually represented as a flow diagram—intended to communicate the logic, or rationale, behind an effective program. These models detail a sequence of input, outputs, and activities that are expected to improve outcomes and final impacts. Essentially, the model should tell the story about what program resources are available to be used, how they are to be used by the program and participants, what short- or medium-term results are to be achieved, and the final outcomes.

A good logic model or results chain can serve several important purposes for developing and conducting the evaluation. First, it makes developing an evaluation plan much easier by making explicit your expected outcomes throughout the

Figure 2.1   Generic Logic Model

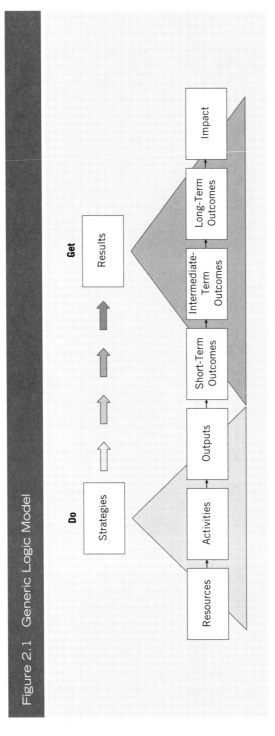

Source: The Logic Model Guidebook, Lisa Wyatt Knowlton and Cynthia C. Phillips, SAGE Publishing © 2013.

Figure 2.2 Program-Specific Model: Community Leadership Academy Program

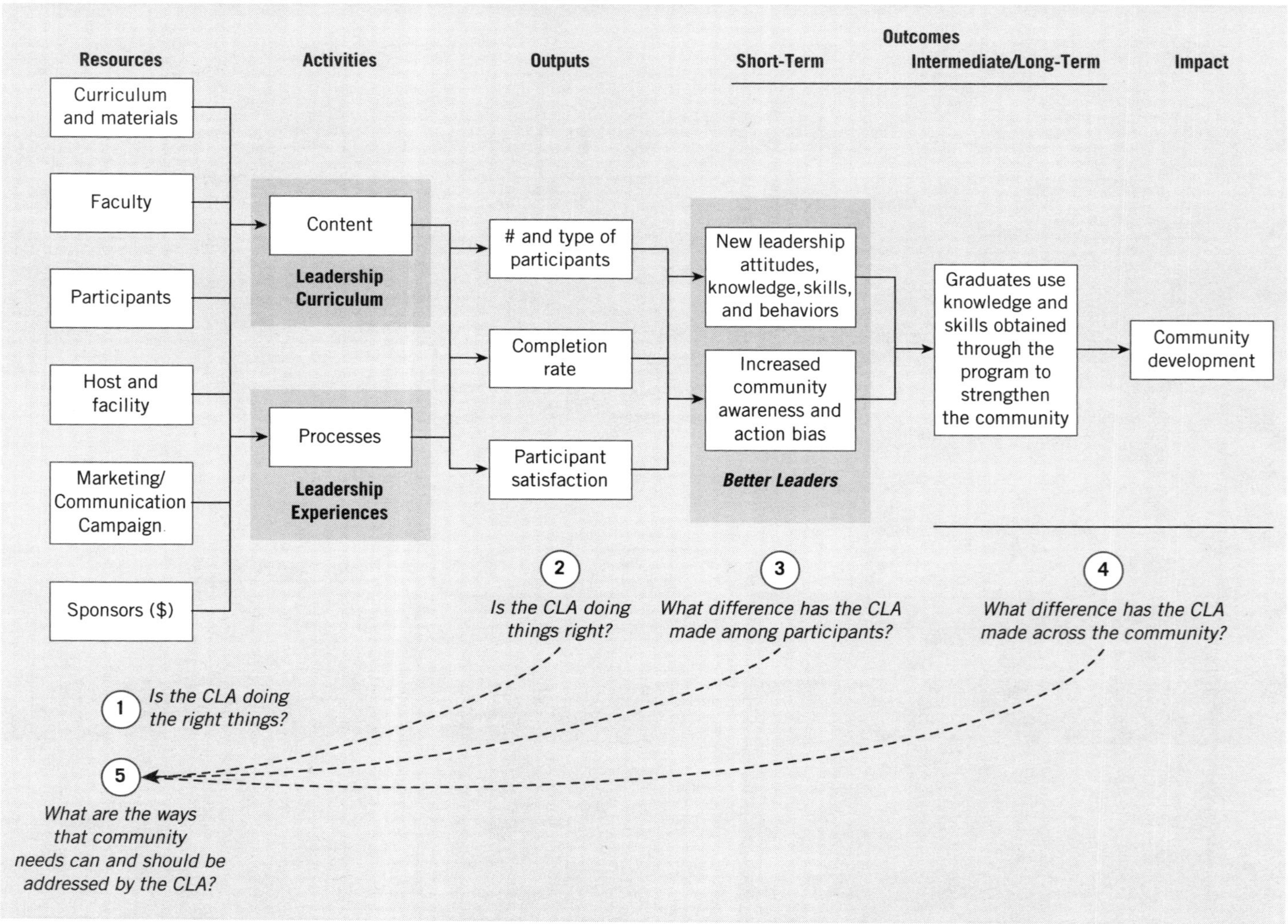

Resources
- Curriculum and materials
- Faculty
- Participants
- Host and facility
- Marketing/ Communication Campaign.
- Sponsors ($)

Activities
- Content — **Leadership Curriculum**
- Processes — **Leadership Experiences**

Outputs
- # and type of participants
- Completion rate
- Participant satisfaction

Outcomes

Short-Term
- New leadership attitudes, skills, and behaviors
- Increased community awareness and action bias

Better Leaders

Intermediate/Long-Term
- Graduates use knowledge and skills obtained through the program to strengthen the community

Impact
- Community development

1. Is the CLA doing the right things?
2. Is the CLA doing things right?
3. What difference has the CLA made among participants?
4. What difference has the CLA made across the community?
5. What are the ways that community needs can and should be addressed by the CLA?

Source: The Logic Model Guidebook, Lisa Wyatt Knowlton and Cynthia C. Phillips, SAGE Publishing © 2013.

course of the program, as well as the program elements that will lead to these outcomes. Thus, the model is critical in providing guidance for choosing performance indicators to be used for the various types of evaluation, from formative to impact. In addition, the model should set out reasonable expectations for the timeframes expected for successful results to be achieved. These purposes will become apparent for the planning steps detailed in the text that follows.

Figures 2.1 and 2.2 are examples of a generic logic model and then one developed for a specific program.[9] The generic model outlines the basic components of the model from the resources put into the program through the various levels of outcomes. The detailed model, based on the Community Leadership Academy (CLA), demonstrates the details that can be added from each component of the model.[10] In the following chapter, we describe using a logic model to organize evaluation measures.

Developing Evaluations: Some Preliminary Methodological Thoughts

Whether one of the evaluation types described at the beginning of this chapter is desired for any particular program or policy, or whether a comprehensive evaluation strategy incorporating all of them is desired, resolving basic design and data issues is essential. Each evaluation type requires measures of progress, success, or effectiveness to assess. These in turn require that appropriate data are available at critical time points for the program.

This is especially true for impact evaluation. As will be discussed in the later chapters, the research questions posed by impact evaluation require the establishment of a counterfactual, that is, what outcomes the intervention group would have experienced in the absence of the intervention. Establishing the counterfactual generally means a valid comparison group must be available. As will become apparent as the book proceeds, developing rigorous impact evaluations depends on four interrelated factors: how the program itself is designed and implemented; the research design for the evaluation; the availability of a comparison group; and the availability of necessary data. These factors are fully interdependent. For example, program design and data availability often determine whether a valid comparison group is available. The data and comparison group in turn determine what research design and statistical methods can be used to infer the attribution of the outcomes to the intervention.

As discussed in the following section, when evaluations are planned as part of program design and implementation, there are many choices over these factors. In other words, with this type of planning, program administrators and evaluators enhance their opportunities to ensure valid results. When evaluations are implemented retrospectively and separately from program design, these choices become much more limited.

Prospectively Planned and Integrated Program Evaluation

Program implementation and administration can be combined with evaluation in three basic ways. The first is to take a purely retrospective approach—the evaluation is planned and undertaken after the program has been implemented. This approach by definition limits the data available for analysis to secondary sources (e.g., administrative data, clinical records). The second is to plan the evaluation prospectively but still fail to integrate its design and data requirements into program implementation plans. This approach may likewise limit the evaluation to data available from secondary sources, which may not adequately address all the program-specific concerns administrators and other evaluation stakeholders may have. In both cases, an impact evaluation can face obstacles to construction of appropriate comparison groups and use of best available impact estimation methods, as well as potentially suffering from the absence of key data elements and/or less than optimal observation points. As a result, these evaluations may not allow us to answer whether the program achieved its goals and whether the program is likely responsible for the changes observed.

The third approach can be called prospectively planned and integrated evaluation (PPIPE), an example of which is presented in Chapter 9 and discussed further in Chapters 10–13. The PPIPE approach, which this book advocates, is a common-sense approach based on the editors' (Bir and Sheingold) many years of experience with research, evaluation, and policy issues. PPIPE integrates evaluation activities fully with program design and implementation from the very beginning. The PPIPE approach can be consistent with continuous monitoring of a program, feedback mechanisms, and methodologically credible rapid-cycle and final evaluations. It can be based on learning system approaches and continuous quality improvement. Indeed, the Institute of Medicine's report, "Rewarding Provider Performance,"[11] recommended that HHSs pay for performance programs be implemented within an active learning system that allowed monitoring, evaluation, and research:

> Monitoring, evaluation and research functions should not be divorced
> from program design and implementation or merely appended to pay
> for performance programs. Rather, their success depends on having
> a strong learning system that is intrinsic to the design and activities
> of the program. . . . Conversely, the absence of a scientifically valid,
> comprehensive, integrated, flexible system—one that facilitated learning
> from experience—would likely contribute to the failure of a pay for
> performance program.

The descriptors of most public programs could easily replace the words "pay for performance."

Taking a PPIPE approach can avoid some or all of the common evaluation obstacles. If implementing programs with truly experimental designs is thwarted for any of the many reasons already described, proper planning can enable program implementation in a way that allows for credible quasi-experimental designs. The PPIPE approach requires planning for comparison groups and statistical methods that are compatible, as well as ensuring all data flows are consistent with the chosen methods. The rest of this chapter provides planning tools for the PPIPE approach. Subsequent chapters address the methodologies that can be applied.

Evaluation Framework Elements: Suggested Planning Tools for the Prospectively Planned and Integrated Evaluation Approach

The logic model described above provides a theory of change for a program or policy from the program inputs, to changes in behaviors and finally desired impacts. A framework for establishing a PPIPE evaluation must include the following elements that should follow naturally from a good logic model or results chain:

1. **Clear Description of Program Objectives.** Framing the evaluation design requires a clear statement of program/intervention objectives. All the evaluation components described below will be based on these objectives. In particular, knowing what to measure, and therefore the choice of performance indicators, critically depends on program objectives. Choice of evaluation methods and comparison groups for impact evaluation should also depend on those objectives.

2. **Description of Target Population.** A clear description of the target population is needed to guide the choice of performance indicators and data sources for measurement and assessment at all stages of the evaluation process.

3. **Description of Measurable Performance.** One of the most important evaluation steps is to prospectively establish performance indicators that can demonstrate the impact of the program relative to the established objectives. These indicators, which are established in accordance with the stated objectives and target populations, are structured for use at different stages of the evaluation process. The three types of performance indicators are potentially useful to measure the short, intermediate, and long-term outcomes described in the logic model:

   a. *Measures for Process Evaluation.* These measures can be structured for the formative stages of an evaluation, as well as rapid and continuous monitoring of program progress. Rather than focusing on final or intermediate outcomes, process measures focus on the processes and infrastructure consistent with successful achievement of program objectives. Process measures may be related to recruitment, enrollment, changes in technology, and/or changes in organizational structure. Thus, whereas the outcome indicators discussed below are measured for the target population, process indicators are measured for those delivering the services or otherwise interacting with the target population.

b. *Measures for Outcomes Evaluation.* These measures would reflect changes in the target population that would be expected as a result of exposure to the intervention and that would be strongly related to changes in the final outcome measures. These measures may reflect changes in behaviors or in knowledge and abilities of the target population.

c. *Measures for Impact Evaluation.* The key measures that the program is ultimately intended to affect for the target population are the final outcome measures. They can include clinical, health, economic, or other performance outcomes that are most consistent with the program objectives.

Changes in many final outcome measures may occur slowly, and in some cases either very late in, or after, the program's period of performance. Thus, periodic monitoring of these measures will not necessarily provide useful information regarding the program progress or effectiveness. Where this is the case, intermediate outcome measures should be identified that allow demonstration of progress toward the outcomes desired. These intermediate measures chosen should be linkable to the final outcomes, preferably by a strong evidence base. For example, changes in the number of strokes that result from a blood pressure monitoring program would likely occur well in the future, but reductions in blood pressure readings that can be linked to strokes can be monitored on a timelier basis.

4. **Expectations for Trajectory of Changes in Performance Measures.** These should be based on the logic model and be clear and prospectively established to the extent possible. They should include expected timeframes for improvement in all performance indicators, expected rate of improvement, and mileposts for success or corrective action. While establishing the trajectory of expected improvement in outcomes is necessarily imprecise, it serves a useful purpose in guiding expectations and choosing intervals for data reporting, monitoring, and analysis. Of equal importance, these expectations guide the optimal timing for the program and the evaluation phases. For example, if it is a reasonable assumption that the program would affect the final outcome measures in 3 years, then the impact evaluation cannot be completed for some time beyond that period. If it is necessary for decisions to be made before that time, they would need to be based on the process or outcomes evaluation phases.

5. **Timeframes and Intervals for Data Reporting.** These should be established for the various performance indicators (see Item 3 above) to be consistent with monitoring and evaluation needs throughout the life of the program.

6. **Data Infrastructure and Flows.** This critical aspect of prospectively planned evaluation is to specify in advance and ensure that all data will be available consistent with the indicators specified in Item 3 and the timeframes established in Item 5. Most importantly, the planning must ensure appropriate data are available for implementing the research designs chosen (see Item 7), including data on both program participants and established comparison groups. Data planning should also establish the infrastructure needs to ensure efficient and timely data processing.

7. **Appropriate Research Designs.** Perhaps the most critical step is to determine and specify the research design to be used for the impact evaluation. As described above, decisions on the research design, data availability, and an appropriate comparison group are interdependent. This is why we advocate building evaluation into program design and implementation. In that way, more options available for such decisions improve the evaluation's ability to rigorously demonstrate the program's impact on specified outcomes. In other words, the design should answer the following questions: Did the outcomes improve? For whom? And can some or all improvement be attributed to the program operations themselves?

   The research design description should include an analysis and justification for the statistical methods to be used, data needs, and how comparison groups will be chosen. Any subgroup analyses that are anticipated should be specified in advance, with the rationale for their inclusion. It is important (as described in Chapter 7) to assess potentially differential outcomes across subgroups. For this analysis, an *ex ante* conceptual framework is important to provide a defense against concerns regarding *ex post* "fishing" for results.

8. **Monitoring and Feedback Mechanisms.** These mechanisms need to evaluate data on an ongoing basis and reflect policy changes as needed. Good program management will require systems in place, and staff responsibilities assigned, to enable the information flowing from the steps above to be readily processed and displayed in reports accessible to specific audiences. The ability to produce "dashboards" and other reports that can monitor what is working well and what is not is critical to support decision making about potential program changes. While early monitoring often focuses on process, as described below, adding early outcome results where feasible can be most valuable.

9. **Rapid-Cycle Evaluation.** The special responsibilities of CMMI, as noted, have given rise to a new approach known as rapid-cycle evaluation (RCE). RCE describes methods that provide interim information on a program's progress in both process and outcome measures. *Rapid* denotes frequent assessment of program model effectiveness. *Cycle* denotes real-time data monitoring and mixed methods approaches, to provide regular feedback to participating providers about their performance to support continuous quality improvement.

It is important to be clear that RCE and final impact evaluation should not be considered as alternatives, but rather as different phases within a comprehensive evaluation process—ideally using the same methods and measures in each phase. In this way, key outcome measures can also be assessed at regular intervals to provide interim results—for example, quarterly (rapid cycle) as well as at the end of a program period (outcome and/or impact).

10. **Stopping Rules and Evidence Thresholds.** Occasionally a PPIPE evaluation incorporating robust RCE methods yields strong enough evaluation findings (positive or negative) to argue for terminating the evaluation before its scheduled end date. There is a strong caveat to such a step, however. Critics are likely to assume, in the case of positive preliminary findings, that the program sponsors may be terminating the evaluation to prevent the possibility of negative findings later on. To guard against such criticism, it is critical that the rules for possible early termination—including how the strength of evidence will be determined and statistical rules applied to any such decision—are specified and justified when the original design decisions are made.

Following the general steps above will greatly increase the chances of obtaining robust results within a timeframe useful for decision makers. But no one should count on good and timely results by themselves to ensure that evaluation results will be enough to persuade program administrators, policymakers, and other decision makers to use them. Finding ways to present evaluation results and match them to meet the unique needs of the specific decision-making audiences is also essential. Later chapters address alternative ways of analyzing and presenting results to decision makers, as well as the types of decision-making frameworks real-world program stakeholders use.

SUMMARY

As presented in this chapter, evaluations can be formative, summative, or process evaluations, or any combination of the three. While many challenges may complicate researchers' ability to properly evaluate program impacts, many can be avoided through early planning and implementation of the evaluation. Incorporating evaluation planning and integrating evaluation activities fully with program design and implementation can determine the rigor, statistical validity, and credibility of the evaluation's findings and ensure that all elements necessary for the timely, accurate, and valid monitoring and assessment of program implementation and performance are achieved. A prospectively planned and integrated program evaluation (PPIPE) ensures the evaluation can provide an evidence- and experience-based learning system that supports the design, activities, and goals of the program.

The PPIPE framework provides a context for the later chapters, which contain detailed information and analyses related to its key components. When used in conjunction with the information this primer describes in later chapters, the PPIPE framework provides a useful planning tool/checklist for program managers and their evaluation partners to prospectively build effective evaluation into their program structures. In addition, the PPIPE framework can provide a benchmark for programs already under way that have yet to plan evaluations or that have planned them separately from the program implementation. Comparing what they have available to them in the way of evaluation design and data sources to the 10 points in the PPIPE framework can enable program managers to assess the opportunities they may still have available to improve the rigor and value of their evaluation.

DISCUSSION QUESTIONS

1. What steps need to be taken to ensure that an evaluation is properly prospectively planned and integrated?

2. Apply the PPIPE framework to the expansion of Medicaid coverage to low-income men.

3. Should program planning take into account evaluation design? Why, or why not? If so, how?

NOTES

1. R. Bruce Hutton, and Dennis L. McNeil, "The Impact of Program Evaluation Needs on Research Methodology," *Advances in Consumer Research* [serial online] 8, no. 1 (January 1981):547–52, http://www.acrwebsite.org/volumes/5856/volumes/v08/NA-08.

2. Huey-tsyh Chen, "A Comprehensive Typology for Program Evaluation," *American Journal of Evaluation*, 17, no. 2 (1996): 121–30.

3. Hutton and McNeill, 1981.

4. Ibid.

5. Ibid.

6. Ibid.

7. Paul J. Gertler, Sebastian Martinez, Patrick Premand, Laura B. Rawlings, and Christel M. J. Vermeersch, *Impact Evaluation in Practice* (Washington, DC: World Bank, 2011).

8. Ibid.; Centers for Disease Control, Division for Heart Disease and Stroke Prevention, *Evaluation Guide: Developing and Using Logic Models*, https://www.cdc.gov/eval/tools/logic_models/index.html.

9. Both figures are from Lisa Wyatt Knowlton and Cynthia C. Phillips, *The Logic Model Guidebook: Better Strategies for Great Results* (Thousand Oaks, CA: Sage Publications, 2013).

10. Ibid.

11. Institute of Medicine, *Rewarding Provider Performance: Aligning Incentives in Medicare* (Washington, DC: National Academies Press, 2007).

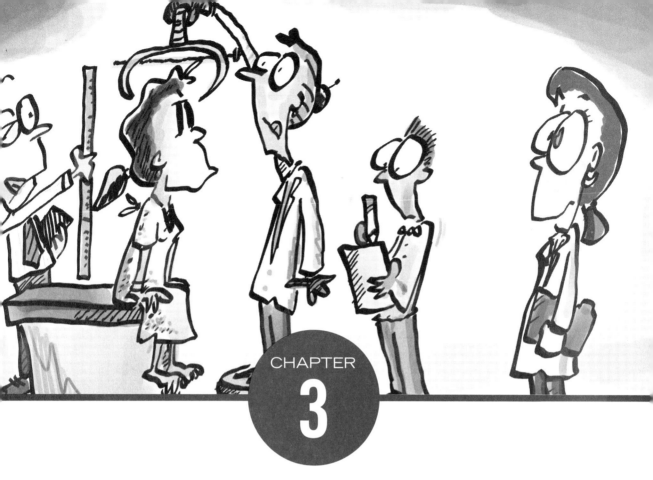

3

Measurement and Data

Steve Asch

Jun Li

Learning Objectives

This chapter provides a detailed introduction to selecting actual evaluation measures. Donabedian's model for quality measurement divides innovation or program evaluation measures into three domains: structural, process, and outcome measures. Measures of structure quantify the type and amount of fixed resources

(Continued)

(e.g., staff, supplies, beds, buildings) used by health delivery system (or other) programs and services. Structural tools are important for evaluations, as many programs specifically involve manipulations of structural elements. Process measures, by contrast, provide information about actions toward a desired goal and steps leading to an outcome. These are useful in informing trends and for strengthening observed process–outcome links. Outcome measures provide cumulative information on health (or other) endpoints resulting from various influences and inputs (examples of outcome measures in the health field span areas such as health, patient experience, or cost of care).

This chapter also provides background on the four general data sources from which health researchers most often get the data they use to construct their evaluation measures and addresses important considerations when selecting measures.

The literature on measuring health care performance, although stretching back to the early part of the 20th century, has exploded in recent years as the industry reorganizes. Diverse stakeholders—payers, patient advocates, provider and specialty groups, insurers, hospitals, and regulatory agencies—have put forward a plethora of measures from which evaluators can choose. Recent work has emphasized balanced measure portfolios that cover the major domains targeted by health care interventions. Efforts have also emphasized relating those domains to one another in a value ratio—with quality, access, and satisfaction in the numerator, and cost or utilization in the denominator.[1] This chapter outlines how to identify measures that match the innovation to be evaluated and discusses the benefits of choosing from a recommended measure set to facilitate cross-program comparisons.

Guiding Principles

A major purpose of evaluating innovations, as outlined in previous chapters, is to determine whether the populations or organizations exposed to an intervention achieved the stated goals to a greater degree than equivalent unexposed entities (after sufficient time has passed for outcome measurement). Evaluations can also collect information about whether an intervention was implemented as intended, identify intervention barriers and facilitators, and assess whether the intervention reached its intended targets (regardless of endpoint outcomes).

Organizing measures into a systematic framework is important to provide consistency in their structure and to focus the measurement strategy on linkages between key objectives and outcomes. Depending on the characteristics of the framework, linking the measurement strategy to established priorities can improve messaging across programs, assist in understanding the attributes of the measure, and facilitate alignment in health (or other) system improvement efforts.

An excellent example of well-defined priorities is the Institute of Medicine's value-based framework, which is organized around six specific quality improvement aims:[2,3]

- *Making care safer:* Reducing harm caused in the delivery of care

- *Person- and family-centered care:* Ensuring that each person and family is engaged as partners in their care

- *Effective communication and care coordination:* Promoting effective communication and coordination of care

- *Prevention and treatment of leading causes of mortality:* Promoting the most effective prevention and treatment practices for the leading causes of mortality, starting with cardiovascular disease

- *Health and well-being of communities:* Working with communities to promote wide use of best practices to enable healthy living

- *Making quality care more affordable:* Increasing affordability for individuals, families, employers, and governments by developing and spreading new health care delivery models

Linking outcomes and objectives is an important step in focusing the evaluator's measurement strategy. Well-defined key priorities can guide which measures are used and how measures are organized. The organizational framework for which we advocate in this primer is the logic model. The previous chapter described a generic logic model for guiding program implementation and evaluation strategies. The same model can be used to identify evaluation measures within a strong and explicit theory of change that links the specific change(s) being evaluated to the inputs and processes that define the program being tested. Such linkages have other names (e.g., driver diagrams, measures maps), but all follow a similar basic structure: *Given a specific set of **measurable** inputs, the program model says we can implement a specific set of **measurable** strategies and activities, to produce a specific set of **measurable** outputs, and accomplish specific and **measurable** intermediate and long-term outcomes.* Having a strong logic model facilitates identifying the measures that will be most useful for each evaluation and that ultimately document how the identified elements facilitated or inhibited program effectiveness. See Box 3.1 for further discussion of logic models.

Box 3.1
Logic Model Framework for Organizing Evaluation Measures

A basic logic model typically consists of an explicit diagramming of the logical hypothesis that undergirds an intervention or process. "A logic model is a plausible and sensible model of how a program will work under certain environmental conditions to solve identified problems."[4] According to McLaughlin and Jordan[5] the basic components are inputs, activities, outputs, and outcomes. Below, slightly modified, are their definitions:

- **Inputs** include the internal resources of a program, as well as the external antecedent factors theorized or believed to influence a programs' implementation or effectiveness. Inputs are essentially the contextual factors that are theorized to influence the potential success of an intervention. Key contextual factors that are external to the program and not under its control may influence its success either positively or negatively. They may include **input mediators** and/or **input moderators**. Mediators are those factors that directly influence the program (e.g., a downturn in resources eliminates some program activities), mediating program effectiveness or reducing the number of sessions. Moderators are those factors that influence the strength of the relationship between two other variables.

- **Resources** include human and financial resources, as well as other inputs required to support the program, such as partnerships. Information on the type and level of the problem addressed by the program is an essential resource for the program.

- **Antecedent factors** are the context the program starts out with, such as client characteristics, geographical variables, and economic factors. Typically, these are represented in different rows under the general Inputs column header.

- **Activities** are the essential action steps necessary to produce program outputs. This is what you do. These can be thought of as the intervention mediators—what you will do to affect change.

- **Outputs** are the products, goods, and services provided to the program's direct customers or program participants. For example, the reports generated for other researchers or the number of clients completing a workshop could be outputs of an activity. Customers or "reach" is sometimes put explicitly in the middle of the chain of logic. Many evaluators do not separate out activities and outputs in their models. However, activities typically represent what the program does, whereas outputs are what the program produces, and so we break the two out because this supports implementation evaluation. This can be a valuable distinction in that the intervention outputs quantify, or otherwise objectify, the implementation of the mediating activities. In other words, intervention outputs moderate the effectiveness of the assumed mediators of change.

- **Outcomes** are changes or benefits to people, organizations, or other program targets that are expected to result from their exposure to activities and outputs. Programs typically have multiple, sequential outcomes, sometimes collectively called the program's outcome structure.

- First, there are **short-term** (proximal) outcomes, the changes or benefits most closely associated with, or "caused" by, the program's outputs. These are the immediate effects of an intervention (e.g., to what extent did patients with diabetes learn the principals of effective self-management after being exposed to diabetes self-management education).

- Second are the intermediate outcomes, which are expected to result from the short-term outcomes (e.g., to what extent did those patients implement the practices of diabetes self-management).

- Long-term (distal) outcomes or program impacts are expected to follow from the benefits accrued through the intermediate outcomes (e.g., to what extent did implementing self-management practices improve their HbA1c (glaciated hemoglobin—a key indicator for diabetes)).

Note that there may be several outcome indicators of each phase of outcome, and they may be linked to specific inputs, activities, outputs, and outcomes (e.g., a person may be successful in adhering to his or her medications, but not adopting an effective diet or exercise strategy—resulting in better glycemic control, but no change in weight or fitness).

Beyond being organized, measures themselves should have specific characteristics. Different evaluation purposes have spawned distinct theoretical underpinnings and measurement sets, but most modern evaluations draw elements from each. Evaluation measures should have the following major characteristics:

- Be validated, concrete, and actionable, so future organizations adopting a similar innovation through their own efforts can demonstrate the desired change

- Be S.M.A.R.T., which is defined as follows: Specific (target specific area(s) for improvement); Measurable (quantify or otherwise precisely specify an indicator of progress capable of demonstrating change); Assignable (specify who will do it); Realistic (state what results can be achieved given available resources); and Time-related (specify when the result(s) can be achieved)

- Be robust to "gaming" or other forms of data manipulation

- Be standardized and comparable (instead of program specific) for better comparison of interventions. Greater comparability reduces measurement burden and fosters accountability, as well as serves a common goal of program or regulatory policymakers.

Measure Types

As noted at the start of this chapter, this discussion of measure types is based on Donabedian's model, which conceptualizes measurement into three domains: structure, process, and outcomes.[6] We modify Donabedian's quality measurement model to capture important health care features outside of the quality domain. For example, Donabedian's model does not address access to care or cost. Thus, we broaden and contextualize the definitions of structures, process, and outcome measures in the following way:

- **Structure** refers to the setting in which care is delivered, including adequate facilities and equipment, qualification of care providers, organizational characteristics, operations of programs, and payment factors.

- **Process** includes all aspects of health care delivery during a patient encounter. Such measures examine how care has been provided in terms of appropriateness, accessibility, acceptability, completeness, or competency. These measures also include technical aspects that address how care is provided and interpersonal processes.

- **Outcomes** take into account the net effect of health care on patients and populations. It refers to the endpoints of care, such as improvement in function, recovery or survival, and cost or satisfaction.

Appendix A, "The Primer Measure Set," is a detailed and very specific list of measures included in large publicly available datasets for use in health research, policy, and program analyses. The discussion below refers to some of these measures, by number, to help illustrate a particular point being made.

Measures of Structure

In the Donabedian framework, structural measures quantify the type and amount of relatively fixed resources (staff, supplies, costs, beds, buildings, etc.) used by a health system to deliver programs and services. Structural attributes can exist at the population (e.g., demographics), provider (e.g., training), and facility/system (e.g., telemedical infrastructure) level. Along with relevant external variables (e.g., features of the environment that may affect the organization, study participant access, or any aspect of the intervention being tested or its outcomes), these comprise the inputs in a typical logic model.

Structure measures are important for evaluation, because many of the interventions being evaluated deliberately manipulate elements of structure, and all interventions are bounded and affected by the setting's external, as well as internal, environment. For example, setting up telemedical consultation between cardiologists and primary care teams directly changes the structure of how cardiac care is provided. Many structure measures are concrete and have accessible data sources, making them relatively easy to assess. For example, it is relatively easy to determine the ratio of specialists to primary care physicians in an area, if a trauma center has a specialty physician available 24 hours a day, or the number of procedures performed in a year.

The main challenge to utilizing structure measures is that the association between structure and process and/or structure and outcome is often not well established.[7] The link between structure and process or outcome measures of quality is often very complex[8] and consequently weak.[9] *It is important not to make too many inferences from structural measures without balancing them with process or outcome measures.* For example, one can easily measure the number of board-certified cardiologists, but such a measure will not provide data on the quality of that specialty training or the extent to which the specialist uses that knowledge to coordinate care or reduce mortality or readmissions.

Measures of Process

Because measures of process provide assessment of actions and steps leading to an outcome, they provide useful and actionable information for rapid-cycle evaluations (RCEs).[10] Specifically, since process measures provide information about actions toward a desired goal, knowledge about individual processes can directly guide quality-improvement efforts in ways that structural and outcome measures cannot.[11]

Process measures, like measures of structure, can span the spectrum of health care delivery, ranging from patient to provider to system level. A process measure at the patient level might indicate whether the patient was able to make an appointment within a reasonable time or how often providers prescribe medications according to condition-specific guidelines represents a provider-level measure. An example of a delivery system process measure is examination of care transitions (referring to a patient's transfer between varying levels, locations, or providers during the trajectory of care). Recent research suggests a linkage between the coordination of care transitions and patients' health outcomes, prompting use of a variety of process measures (e.g., the "Three-Item Care Transition Measure," Measure 39 in appendix Table A.1) to gauge transitions and drive health delivery improvement.[12,13,14]

Process measures offer other benefits as well. They may be useful in informing trends and for strengthening observed process-outcome links. For example, if a study aims to improve diabetes outcomes, it may be useful to examine evidence-based measures of process, such as increased eye and foot exams (Measures 22 and 23 in appendix Table A.1). When activities and outputs estimated using process measures are consistent with the theory of change linking them to outcome measures, it is ensured that implementation of the intended intervention can plausibly produce the intended change.

When the true outcomes of interest are long term, requiring years to observe, measurements of the impact on the desired outcomes within a shorter time window, such as under RCE, can be difficult. Process measures may provide adequate information in that interim. For example, a program aiming to reduce preventable hospitalizations in children might use a measure such as the "Number of Well-Child

Visits in the First 15 Months of Life" (Measure 9, appendix Table A.1)[15] in lieu of obtaining long-term outcomes, such as hospitalizations and emergency room (ER) visits years after initial intervention.[16] How well these process (termed *proxy*) measures substitute for true outcomes is determined by their causal relation to the true outcome(s) of interest. If the proxy is fully deterministic of the outcome, of course, it can fully substitute for the outcome. The more other factors influence the outcome, the less adequate the proxy measures are substitutes for true outcome measures. If proxy measures are used as indicators of effectiveness, the knowledge claims of effectiveness should be appropriately tempered.

Their proximity to structural interventions is another advantage of process measures. The most direct effects of structural interventions will often be observed in the process of care, because structural effects may be diluted by unmeasured covariates as they filter through to outcomes. Thus, interim process results can be incorporated into feedback regarding the intervention progress, enabling mid-course changes.[17]

As a practical matter, certain health care processes are easier to measure through claims-based data systems than through structure and outcome measures. For example, measures that are service-based and have a reimbursement attribute may be more readily and accurately captured than intermediate or final health outcomes.[18]

A note of caution: Since the usefulness of a process measure as an outcome proxy depends on the relationship between the process and the outcome of interest, which is often relatively weak, it can be difficult to establish adequate evidence in support of the process–outcome relationship. Particularly among complex outcome measures such as hospital readmissions, it can be challenging to isolate individual process components enough to build a widely convincing linkage because of a variety of potential nonintervention influences attributable to both clinical and nonclinical care.

Measures of Outcomes

Outcome measures provide cumulative information on health endpoints resulting from various influences and inputs. For this discussion, we break outcome measures into three major groups: health outcomes, patient experience outcomes (such as satisfaction), and cost.

Health Outcomes

Perhaps the most compelling reason to use health outcome measures is that they represent precisely what medical care aims to achieve. The purpose of health care is to improve health, reduce morbidity, and prolong life. Health outcomes can be universal and integrative, such as mortality (Measures 48–51, appendix Table A.1) or condition specific, such as lower-extremity amputation (Measure 15, appendix

Table A.1). Even short of these ultimate endpoints, intermediate outcomes, such as blood pressure control (Measure 33, appendix Table A.1), represent measurable clinical parameters that strongly predict morbidity, mortality, and quality of life.

Because health outcomes are the final link in the chain leading through structure and process, patients, providers, and payers are affected by and care about such measures. However, because outcome measures reflect processes rather than inputs, there are fewer opportunities to measure change. This can be a significant disadvantage if study participants have limited resources or capacity to internally identify and monitor processes. This is further complicated by a plethora of influences beyond health care that may impact observable outcomes. Environmental and socioeconomic factors, for example, are strongly associated with key health services outcomes (such as hospital readmissions or mortality), as is preexisting clinical severity.[19] These inputs are difficult to fully account for in the outcome measure, and as a result, can generate resistance from providers (who fear being held at risk for outcomes they know are not totally under their control).[20]

Most relevant to RCE is the ability to obtain meaningful outcome measures when the analytic period is shortened.[21] Analysis of certain outcome measures for evaluation purposes can be slow and require long data collection periods to meet criteria such as minimum sample sizes and outcome maturation.[22] Therefore, to meet the frequency required under RCE, certain outcome measures need to be examined carefully. For example, individual safety concerns such as pressure ulcers may be more appropriately combined into the composite safety measure "Patient Safety for Selected Indicators" (Measure 58, appendix Table 2.1), given the relatively few occurrences of an individual safety concern at the provider-level within the short analytic window of RCE.[23]

Evaluators may have to rely on proxy measures for other reasons as well, as when obtaining health outcome measurement is not feasible due to data constraints. For example, a commonly used proxy to measure quality and access to care is ER use. However, identifying avoidable and preventable ER utilization in a credible manner is always a challenge, which is made even more complex by the need to separate inappropriate use from other confounding factors affecting ER use, such as lack of alternative sources of care.

Patient Experience

Patient experience, the second major category of outcome measures,[24] includes feedback and input from patients on the health care processes they receive. Patient experience measures are truly patient centered and provide information that cannot be obtained through other means. Patient experience provides useful information on potential intervention achievements and unintended consequences, which may not be apparent through traditional health care measures. However, because patient experience measures are subjective and possibly influenced by non–health care inputs (e.g., parking or other amenities), evaluating quality based on patient experience has received some criticism.[25] Critics argue that patient satisfaction measures have limited ability to holistically measure health service delivery and that instead, they capture only specific aspects of care, such as provider–patient communication. Critics also argue that patient experience measures reflect patient expectations rather than clinical appropriateness. Despite such disadvantages, studies have found that well-designed patient experience instruments do provide important indications of care quality and health, particularly when used in conjunction with other types of measures.[26,27] For all these reasons, making sure an evaluation uses scientifically sound instruments to measure patient experience is very important to mitigate the challenges inherent in its measurement.

Cost

Central to measuring cost in evaluations is how to gain an understanding of cost and value—measurement of which depends on the particular perspective taken. Here we focus on provider and payer costs, while recognizing that patient and societal perspectives are also important to gain a complete cost picture for public policy decision making.[28]

Examinations of costs and productivity that focus on hospitals and physicians as the primary sources of health care spending have been extensive. But other health sectors have sector-specific cost measures that vary by the payment or utilization measure (e.g., hospital outpatient, ER visit). Cost and productivity exhibit a dual relationship: the greater the productivity of inputs (output per unit input), the lower the cost for an unchanged set of factor input (unit) costs. Efficiency usually is expressed using a cost metric ratio such as cost per hospital discharge, while productivity measures remain a distinct concept directly affecting efficiency—with higher input per unit of output resulting in greater efficiency for a fixed set of input costs. An efficient producer is one that produces a given level of output at minimum cost, either in total or per unit.

Cross-sectional comparisons of producer costs and efficiency (e.g., acute hospitals, skilled nursing facilities) are complicated by differences in input unit costs and unequal value added in services provided. One provider may appear more efficient (lower cost) than another only because it faces lower input costs (e.g., lower nursing wages). Another provider may appear more efficient based on an adjusted count of output (e.g., discharges) but is in fact adding less value than another, seemingly more costly, provider. Teaching hospitals, for example, may appear less efficient and less productive because they treat a more severe patient case mix, requiring a case mix adjustment to enable a proper accounting for the improvement in health status between admission and discharge for teaching vs. nonteaching hospitals.

Certain cost analyses may call for more disaggregated cost and productivity measures. It is possible, for example, to disaggregate hospital cost per discharge into the product of

(1) Cost per input (e.g., RN hourly wage)

(2) Inputs per service (e.g., RN hours per day)

(3) Services per discharge (length of inpatient stay)

Disaggregating costs in this fashion allows researchers to isolate the intensity of services—captured in elements (1) and (3)—from factor costs and case mix.

Episode-based cost measures examine resource use within a predefined episode. Episodes can be initiated by diagnoses or by an event such as a hospitalization, as in "Medicare Spending per Beneficiary" (Measure 70, appendix Table A.1). When the evaluation interest is in detecting unintended consequences of an intervention—such as provider shifting of services and costs either before or after a stay—measuring efficiency on an episode basis is more appropriate than measuring individual service costs. The reason is that it avoids biasing the cost and efficiency estimates in favor of one category of providers (say hospitals) that manage to shift more costs to other providers (say nursing homes). A "window" of costs, such as 30 days post discharge, captures readmission and other costs necessary to complete an episode of care. Costs also need to be adjusted for input costs and case mix (as noted), and possibly other factors.

Patient- or population-based cost measures examine costs associated with a set of services to care for a patient population. A population-based denominator for cost (efficiency) captures "unnecessary" usage at a population level, to provide an overall indication of resource use. These measures are often direct costs associated with specific categories of services or settings, such as inpatient costs, physician costs, and pharmacy costs. An example of costs across care settings and service types being included and adjusted to reflect a provider's efficiency at managing the patient population is Measure 71, "Total Cost of Care Population-Based PMPM Index" (appendix Table A.1). Condition- or disease-specific cost measures further delineate a specific patient type associated with a disease or condition to assess these patients' resource use. Measures of condition-specific direct costs include, for example, health care costs associated with asthma, cardiovascular conditions, diabetes, and chronic obstructive pulmonary disease (Measures 72–75, appendix Table A.1).

Other common ways to examine costs include setting-specific costs (e.g., inpatient, nursing facility) and service-specific costs (e.g., physician). Physician costs, efficiency, and productivity can be evaluated either individually (e.g., surgeons) or in groups (e.g., medical homes). Physician costs can also be limited to their physicians' practice-level services or extended to other services they either directly command (e.g., inpatient nursing, computerized tomography scans) or indirectly influence (e.g., hospital readmissions). For true comparisons across physicians, caseloads must be risk-adjusted based on forecasts. This is usually done using age, gender, and lists of preexisting diagnoses and chronic conditions (e.g., diabetes, heart failure, depression, cancer).

Selecting Appropriate Measures

Evaluation design and analysis methods will guide measure selection and will depend on evaluation questions to be answered, how well the intervention is understood, time and resources available, and stakeholder expectations. Widely used standards adopted by the National Quality Forum (NQF), a national consensus-based entity, indicate that a measure should be assessed for several key attributes that fall into three broad conceptual areas:

(1) Importance

(2) Scientific soundness

(3) Feasibility

Importance of the Measure

- *Relevance:* The topic area of the measure should be of interest to stakeholders.

- *Health importance*: Measuring what matters is more important than measuring what is convenient. A health care problem is important if it (1) contributes significantly to morbidity and mortality, (2) is associated with high rates of utilization, or (3) is costly to treat.[29]

- *Allows for useful comparison*: The measure should be usable for subgroup analysis among diverse patient populations, to evaluate potential disparities among groups.

- *Potential for improvement*: An evidence base should identify poor quality or variations in quality among populations or organizations that indicate a need for the measure.

- *Actionable*: Results of the measure should identify factors amenable to improvements in performance. Measures should relate to interventions that are under the control of those providers whose performance is being measured.

Scientific Soundness: Clinical Logic

- *Explicitness of evidence*: Evidence underlying the measure should be clinically detailed and explicitly stated.

- *Strength of evidence*: The topic area addressed by the measure should be strongly supported by evidence. When evaluating scientific strength, the number of studies conducted, methods used, and consistency of findings should all be considered.

Scientific Soundness: Measure Properties

- *Reliability*: The measurement, when repeatedly applied to the same population in the same way, should yield the same result in a statistically high proportion of the time.

- *Validity*: The measurement should actually measure what it is supposed to measure.

- *Adequacy of case mix adjustment:* The measure of case mix (severity of illness) adjustment should allow for comparability of heterogeneous populations. It levels the playing field by accounting for health status differences so that results reflect differences in care provided and resources used for a given patient. Use of demographic factors, such as race and ethnicity, for case mix adjustment should be carefully weighed, since case mix adjustment removes the ability to identify and eliminate disparities by controlling for population differences directly.

- *Price standardization*: Analyses requiring measurement of cost variables should use price standardization to adjust for payment system variation that is not driven by utilization.

- *Interpretability*: The measure should generate information that is comprehensible and easy to use by end-users and stakeholders.

Feasibility

- *Explicit specification of numerator and denominator*: The measure should have explicit and detailed numerator and denominator specification.

- *Data availability*: The data source needed to implement the measure should be available and accessible within the required timeframe. The four data types most commonly used for quality assessment are enrollment, administrative, clinical, and survey data.

- *Burden*: The burden of providing and collecting required data elements for both evaluators and those providing the data should be carefully assessed.

Selecting the appropriate measures for inclusion in a measure set is complex and time consuming. Despite best efforts to choose high-quality measures, it is important to consider how other contextual factors, latent or not easily amenable to measurement, may influence outcomes. Measure sets should also include measures that can capture potential unintended consequences of the intervention or policy being evaluated. Finally, it is important to periodically reevaluate the set after its creation. Some measures may need to be retired due to clinical or technological advances or significant restriction in variance (floor/ceiling effects). Conversely, advances or changes to the health system may call for new measures to be included.

Data Sources

Selection of measures is often driven by the availability and quality of accessible data. A number of different data sources are available to evaluators, each with their own advantages and disadvantages. Four general types of data source—clinical databases, administrative databases, surveys, and health system databases—are commonly available for health care evaluation.

Medical records contain the richest source of clinical data on diagnoses, treatments, and clinical outcomes, but they are costly and difficult to obtain. Medical records are also often limited to care provided within specific settings, which poses challenges for longitudinal assessment. For all clinical data not routinely collected through an existing data collection infrastructure, obtaining comparison group data may not be feasible, limiting their usefulness in evaluations.

For publicly available clinical data, a number of national quality reporting programs can serve as useful tools. The Hospital Inpatient Quality Reporting Program and Nursing Home Quality Initiative are examples of quality reporting programs where clinical quality metrics (such as process and outcome measures) are reported across providers in a standardized format. These quality reporting programs were created with the intent to inform consumers. Quality programs include information gathered from patient reports, claims, and clinical assessments. In addition to examining topical relevancy present in the quality programs, evaluators should also be aware of each program's requirements and characteristics (such as provider participation rates and any associated incentives).

Other potential sources of publicly available clinical data include population and disease- or condition-specific databases (such as the Surveillance, Epidemiology, and End Results [SEER] Medicare linked databases). The SEER–Medicare database provides a linkage between two major population-based sources of cancer statistics that uniquely combines clinical registry information with Medicare claims, allowing for a variety of analyses not otherwise feasible. While the database files are complex, researchers have the benefit of being able to risk-adjust for beneficiary health status beyond claims data and to examine for patterns of care longitudinally across the cancer control continuum.[30]

Administrative databases (enrollment and reimbursement data) are another major source of measure data. Enrollment data are gathered by payer or insurance plan to track provider enrollment and beneficiary entitlement. Commonly collected patient-level information includes patient identifiers, patient demographics, enrollment periods, third-party buy-in, and enrollment into other benefit programs, such as managed care. The provider information gathered reflects similar information (such as provider identifiers, provider demographics, facility size, and staffing). Because of the nature of the data collected through enrollment (*not* service receipt), whether such data can be used for the purpose intended has to be carefully considered.

Reimbursement databases contain information used by insurers to make payments to eligible providers for covered services delivered to eligible beneficiaries.

Claims data offer utilization-based information that can be used to construct process and outcome measures. Interpreting claims data should be done with caution, however. Since they are service based, they only include individuals who seek health care. In addition, certain services that are not specifically reimbursed cannot be obtained for measurement purposes. The benefit of reimbursement data is coverage across all eligible covered populations, putting minimal data collection burden on study subjects—a great benefit for evaluations in obtaining comparison group data.

A major family of health care databases established through a multistakeholder partnership is the Healthcare Cost and Utilization Project.[31] These databases are built from hospital administrative data and provide patient, facility/provider, and utilization information on demographics, comorbidities, diagnoses, procedures, length of stay, and service charges. Encounter-level information is captured in six databases and covers a variety of hospital settings (e.g., ER, inpatient, and ambulatory surgical sites).

Surveys can provide information on patient experiences (e.g., communication with providers), patient activation, health status and outcomes, and patient perceptions that cannot be obtained through other data sources. Similarly, surveys can be used to obtain data on provider experience, including disruption, workflow, organizational culture, leadership style, and other intervention and organizational features that are otherwise difficult to capture. Disadvantages of survey data include potential bias, data collection burden on study subjects, and cost. The good news is that a number of existing survey sources can be used, particularly to obtain patient-level information. Examples include the Health and Retirement Study (HRS)[32] and the Consumer Assessment of Healthcare Providers and Systems (CAHPS).[33] HRS collects self-reported information on socioeconomic status, function, and health care utilization every 2 years, and it can be used to examine the impact of system-level interventions on the aged. In particular, the data can be helpful for assessing national trends and understanding contextual changes across populations over time. CAHPS is a survey provided in the public domain that focuses on answering questions about quality of care from the health care consumer's perspective. For example, it asks questions related to provider communication and health care service accessibility.

Contextual, health system level information can be found in a variety of systems-level databases. Data offerings such as the Area Resource File[34] developed by the Health Resources and Services Administration provide county, state, and national files on economic activity, demographic characteristics, workforce, and health care resources. These data, combined with quality and cost information from other data sources, can provide valuable information for measurement and analyses.

Methodology Note: Each of the measures and measure resources discussed in this chapter assume the constructs of interest are well specified and understood *in advance of an evaluation*. In recognition of the limitations of human imagination, many evaluations now adopt mixed method approaches, which include qualitative methods (e.g., observation and free text responses, key informant interviews, focus group data) in their assessments. Analyzing such data often reveals relevant themes for an evaluation that have not been anticipated at the beginning of the study. With direction and magnitude, or variation over time or across sites, these unanticipated consequences can be standardized into metrics that can then be included in quantitative analysis. Direct quotes and summaries from such data can also be used in evaluation reports to illustrate analysis findings in a way that engages the reader.

Looking Ahead

With rapid growth in health care costs and an urgent need to improve health care quality, local and national efforts are actively testing different approaches to identify promising innovations in health care payment and delivery. To properly understand the impact of these changes, methodologically sound measures and comprehensive data infrastructure supportive of RCE are particularly crucial in the health reform area.

Efforts across private and public sectors have begun to bridge gaps in key measurement domains.[35] In response to the Affordable Care Act[36] and the National Quality Strategy,[37] multistakeholder collaborations, such as the Measures Application Partnership and Buying Value Initiative, have convened to identify and prioritize needs and align measures to promote better care, better health, and lower costs, while minimizing measurement burden.

In areas of population health, entities such as the NQF are developing measures that bridge the health care system with that of population health. As health system goals[38] and provider accountability broaden in scope, spurred by large-scale initiatives and recognition of the importance of nontraditional health care inputs, measurement tools that enable the assessment of a health care system's ability to positively affect population well-being will be increasing.[39]

Scientifically proven measures of health care efficiency that adequately account for both health outcomes and costs are not yet readily available. While measures that integrate resource use and quality remain underdeveloped, the work is already underway in the development, and endorsement of resource measures[40] to facilitate the understanding of efficiency will go a long way to support the evolution of efficiency measurement within the health care system.

Interest in the development and use of patient-reported outcomes has grown as the health care system focuses on achieving more patient-centered care and a better quality.[41] The National Institutes of Health's Patient Reported Outcomes Measurement Information System has demonstrated that patient-reported outcomes can be scientifically sound and provide meaningful information on quality. However, barriers in methodological and data accessibility must still be overcome before patient-reported outcomes can be fully incorporated in a variety of health care reform evaluations.[42] For some drugs, diseases, and conditions, crowd-sourced information (like the website PatientsLikeMe.com) offers data on patient experiences with their disease and with health care interventions.

SUMMARY

Measures provide the building blocks for evaluation and research and are the foundation for assessment. Measures should be selected based on a strong theory of change; be validated, concrete, and actionable; be S.M.A.R.T (Specific, Measurable, Assignable, Realistic, Time-related); be robust to gaming and manipulation; and be comparable with measures used in other evaluations. Donabedian divides innovation or program evaluation measures into three domains: structural measures (which quantify the type and amount of fixed resources), process measures (which provide information about actions toward a desired goal and steps leading to an outcome), and outcome measures (which may be near-, intermediate-, or long-term, and which provide cumulative information on health [or other] endpoints resulting from various influences and inputs). Measures should be selected based on (1) their importance to all evaluation stakeholders and their capacity to answer evaluation questions; (2) the scientific soundness of the measure (i.e., whether the measure is statistically reliable, measures what it intends to measure, and is logical from the standpoint of the particular program); and (3) the feasibility of collecting the necessary data to construct the measure. In addition to collecting observational data, four general sources of data—clinical databases, administrative databases, surveys, and health system databases—are commonly available for health care evaluation.

DISCUSSION QUESTIONS

1. When is it a useful practice to substitute a proxy process measure for an outcome measure?

2. When are each of the four general sources of data (clinical databases, administrative databases, surveys, and health system databases) best used, and how can they be combined to improve evaluation?

3. Describe the ideal data source(s) for evaluating a handwashing intervention in intensive care units.

4. Are there any other characteristics of measures beyond the ones mentioned in this chapter that you see as important?

NOTES

1. McClellan, M., A. N. McKethan, J. L. Lewis, J. Roski, and E. S. Fisher, "A National Strategy to Put Accountable Care Into Practice," *Health Affairs* 29, no. 5 (2010): 982–90.

2. Institute of Medicine, *Crossing the Quality Chasm: A New Health System for the 21st Century* (Washington, DC: National Academies Press, 2001).

3. The National Quality Strategy framework—guided by the three aims of better care, healthy people and healthy communities, and affordable care—is another example. Accessed July 2015, http://www.ahrq.gov/workingforquality/.

4. Bickman, L., "The Functions of Program Theory." In L. Bickman (ed.), *Using Program Theory in Evaluation. New Directions for Program Evaluation*, no. 33 (1987), San Francisco: Jossey-Bass.

5. McLaughlin J. A., and G. B. Jordan, "Logic Models: A Tool for Telling Your Program's

Performance Story," *Evaluation and Program Planning* 22, no. 1 (February 1999).

6. Avedis Donabedian, *Explorations in Quality Assessment and Monitoring, Volume 1: The Definition of Quality and Approaches to Its Assessment* (Ann Arbor, MI: Health Administration Press, 1980).

7. "Evaluating the Quality of Healthcare," e-Source, Behavioral and Social Sciences Research, accessed July 2015, http://www.esourceresearch.org/Default.aspx?TabId=816.

8. Landon B. E., I. B. Wilson, and P. D. Cleary, "A Conceptual Model of the Effects of Health Care Organizations on the Quality of Medical Care," *Journal of the American Medical Association,* 279, no. 17 (1998): 1377–82. doi:10.1001/jama.279.17.1377.

9. Landon, B. E., A. M. Zaslavsky, N. D. Beaulieu, J. A. Shaul, and P. D. Cleary, "Health Plan Characteristics and Consumers' Assessments of Quality," *Health Affairs* 20, no. 2 (2001): 274–86.

10. Shrank, William, "The Center For Medicare and Medicaid Innovation's Blueprint for Rapid-Cycle Evaluation of New Care and Payment Models," *Health Affairs* 32, no. 4 (2013): 807–12. doi:10.1377/hlthaff.2013.0216.

11. McGlynn, E. A., S. M. Asch, J. Adams, J. Keesey, J. Hicks, A. DeCristofaro, and E. A. Kerr, "The Quality of Health Care Delivered to Adults in the United States," *New England Journal of Medicine* 348 (2003): 2635–45. doi: 10.1056/NEJMsa022615.

12. Kim, Christopher S., and Scott A. Flanders, "Transitions of Care," *Annals of Internal Medicine* 158 no. 5 part 1 (2013): ITC3–1. doi:10.7326/0003-4819-158-5-20130305-01003.

13. Oduyebo, Ibironke, C. U. Lehmann, C. E. Pollack, N. Durkin, J. D. Miller, S. Mandell, M. Ardolino, A. Deutschendorf, and D. J. Brotman, "Association of Self-Reported Hospital Discharge Handoffs with 30-Day Readmissions," *JAMA Internal Medicine* 173, no. 8 (2013): 624–9. doi:10.1001/jamainternmed.2013.3746.

14. "NQF Endorses Care Coordination Measures," *National Quality Forum*, August 10, 2012. http://www.qualityforum.org/News_And_Resources/Press_Releases/2012/NQF_Endorses_Care_Coordination_Measures.aspx.

15. National Committee for Quality Assurance (2009). Well-Child Visits in the First 15 Months of Life (W15). Accessed September 21, 2015, from www.ncqa.org.

16. Rosemarie B. Hakim, and Barry V. Bye, "Effectiveness of Compliance with Pediatric Preventive Care Guidelines among Medicaid Beneficiaries," *Pediatrics* 108 (2001): 90–97.

17. L. Solberg, G. Mosser, and S. McDonald, "The Three Faces of Performance Improvement: Improvement, Accountability and Research," *Joint Commission Journal on Quality Improvement* 23, no. 3 (March 1997): 135–47.

18. McGlynn et al., 2003.

19. Arbaje, A. I., J. L. Wolff, Q. Yu, N. R. Powe, G. F. Anderson, and C. Boult, "Post Discharge Environmental and Socioeconomic Factors and the Likelihood of Early Hospital Readmission among Community-Dwelling Medicare Beneficiaries," *The Gerontologist* 48, no. 4 (2008): 495–504.

20. Joynt, K. E., and A. K. Jha, "A Path Forward on Medicare Readmissions," *New England Journal of Medicine*, 368, no. 13 (2013): 1175–7.

21. Shrank, 2013.

22. Solberg et al., 1997.

23. Patient Safety for Selected: Indicators: Technical Specifications, Patient Safety Indicators 90 (PSI #90) *AHRQ Quality Indicators*, Version 4.5, May 2013. Available at http://www.qualityindicators.ahrq.gov.

24. Patient experience may also be structural measures or process measures, depending on the types of information requested.

25. Manary, M. P., W. Boulding, S. W. Glickman, and R. Staelin, "The Patient Experience and Health Outcomes," *New England Journal of Medicine* 368, no. 3 (2013): 201–3.

26. Glickman, S. W., W. Boulding, M. Manary, R. Staelin, M. T. Roe, R. J. Wolosin, E. M. Ohman, E. D. Peterson, and K. A. Schulman, "Patient Satisfaction and Its Relationship with Clinical Quality and Inpatient Mortality in Acute Myocardial Infarction" *Circulation: Cardiovascular Quality and Outcomes* 3, no. 2 (2010): 188–95.

27. Boulding, W., S. W. Glickman, M. P. Manary, K. A. Schulman, and R. Staelin, "Relationship between Patient Satisfaction with Inpatient Care and Hospital Readmission Within 30 Days," *The American Journal of Managed Care* 17, no. 1 (2011): 41–8.

28. McGlynn, E. A., Identifying, Categorizing, and Evaluating Health Care Efficiency Measures. Final Report (prepared by the Southern California Evidence-Based Practice Center—RAND Corporation, under Contract No. 282-00-0005-21), AHRQ Publication No. 08-0030, Rockville, MD: Agency for Healthcare Research and Quality (2008).

29. McGlynn, E. A., and S. M. Asch. "Developing a Clinical Performance Measure." *American Journal of Preventive Medicine* 14, Suppl. 3 (1998): 14–21.

30. National Cancer Institute, National Institutes of Health, "Brief Description of the SEER-MHOS Database," (updated May 2015). Available at http://healthcaredelivery.cancer.gov/seer-mhos/overview/.

31. Healthcare Cost and Utilization Project (HCUP), Agency for Healthcare Research and Quality, "HCUP Overview," (June 2015), Rockville, MD. Available at http://www.hcup-us.ahrq.gov/overview.jsp.

32. Institute for Social Research, University of Michigan, "Growing Older in America: The Health and Retirement Study." Available at http://hrsonline.isr.umich.edu/.

33. Agency for Healthcare Research and Quality, "CAHPS: Surveys and Tools to Advance Patient-Centered Care." Available at https://cahps.ahrq.gov/.

34. Health Resources and Services Administration, U.S. Department of Health and Human Services, "Area Health Resources Files (AHRF): National, State and County Health Resources Information Database." Available at http://ahrf.hrsa.gov/.

35. U.S. Department of Health and Human Services, "2013 Annual Progress Report to Congress: National Strategy for Quality Improvement in Health Care" (July 2013): Figure 3. Available at http://www.ahrq.gov/workingforquality/nqs/nqs2013annlrpt.htm#fig3.

36. Patient Protection and Affordable Care Act, 42 U.S.C. § 18001 et seq. (2010). Department of Health and Human Services, accessed September 18, 2015, from http://www.hhs.gov/healthcare/rights/law/.

37. Patient Protection and Affordable Care Act, 42 U.S.C. § 18001 et seq, Sec. 3011. (2010), pp. 682–88. Available from Department of Health and Human Services, accessed September 18, 2015, from http://www.hhs.gov/healthcare/rights/law/.

38. U.S. Department of Health and Human Services (2013). 2013 Annual Progress Report to Congress: National Strategy for Quality Improvement in Health Care, accessed September 18, 2015, from http://www.ahrq.gov/workingforquality/nqs/nqs2013annlrpt.htm.

39. Schoen, C., S. Guterman, A. Shih, J. Lau, S. Kasimow, A. Gauthier, and K. Davis, "Bending the Curve: Options for Achieving Savings and Improving Value in US Health Spending," *The Commonwealth Fund* (December 2007).

40. National Quality Forum (2012). National Voluntary Consensus Standards for Cost and Resource Use: Final Report, accessed September 18, 2015, from http://www.qualityforum.org/.

41. National Quality Forum (2013). Patient Reported Outcomes (PROs) in Performance Measurement. Accessed September 18, 2015, from http://www.qualityforum.org/.

42. Ibid.

Evaluation Methods

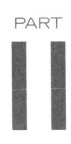

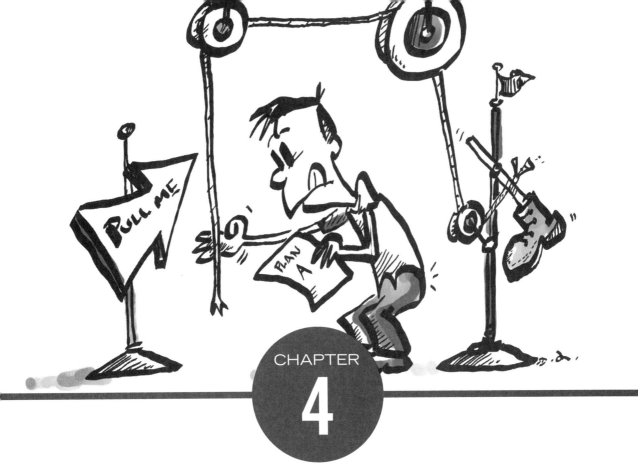

Causality and Real-World Evaluation

Anupa Bir

Nikki Freeman

Jeffrey Wooldridge

Learning Objectives

This chapter begins to tackle the fundamental issue in rigorous program evaluation, that is, how to measure what would have happened to the treatment group

(Continued)

if, all other things equal, it had not been exposed to the program. Without a good measure of this, the counterfactual situation, it is impossible to isolate the program effect from the many other influences on outcomes.

With a reasonable counterfactual, treatment effects can be estimated using statistical inference. Three kinds of treatment effects are covered in this chapter:

1. The average treatment effect is the average effect on the population.

2. Because not all study participants in the treatment group receive treatment in some studies, the average treatment effect on the treated looks at only the treatment effect on the subgroup of the treatment population who actually receives the intervention.

3. The intent-to-treat effect examines the difference in average intervention effects between those eligible for treatment (some of whom may not have received the treatment) and those ineligible for treatment.

The theoretical framework from which we begin this chapter must be understood in the context of real program evaluation. Thoughtful evaluation planning and design are key tools for mitigating threats to the validity and generalizability of evaluation findings.

In Chapter 2, we discussed the full range of activities and methods that might be part of a comprehensive evaluation of a program or policy.[1] Chapter 3 described the important issue of performance measures. The remainder of this book focuses on the methods and results related to impact or outcome evaluation.

A primary goal in an evaluation is determining the causal impact of an intervention. We will want to know how big the impact is, whether it is significant, and how trustworthy the evaluation findings are. This chapter begins our discussion of causal impacts, a conversation that continues through the next four chapters. Here we lay out the framework for causal inference and impact estimation, provide the statistical ideas that are used throughout the remainder of the text, and put these ideas in the context of real-world evaluations.

We begin this chapter by defining causality, building a formal vocabulary to precisely describe causal effects. We will see that how causality is estimated is strongly related to the design of the intervention, whether treatment units (patients, hospitals, etc.) are assigned randomly to treatment or not. Three treatment effects are defined: the average treatment effect, the average treatment effect on the treated, and the intent-to-treat effect. The determination of which treatment effect to estimate depends on the study design and the questions being asked in the evaluation.

Statistical inference is an essential element of impact estimation. Although not a comprehensive guide to statistics, we present a few key ideas from statistics, such as hypotheses tests and confidence intervals that are necessary to understand evaluation findings.

Finally, we address evaluation in the real world. While formal causal and statistical theories are useful for conceptualizing and quantifying impacts, they must be reconciled with demonstrations and evaluations that take place in reality. Poor planning and execution of an evaluation threaten the validity of findings. We highlight threats to validity and provide advice on how to avoid those failures.

Altogether, the topics in this chapter lay the foundation for the technical details of how to estimate treatment effects in Chapters 5 and 6.

Evaluating Program/Policy Effectiveness: The Basics of Inferring Causality

Impact evaluation strives to determine with scientific credibility that particular measures of program effectiveness differ between those subject to the program/policy (treated) and those not subject to the program/policy—all else the same.[2] Such a determination is one that establishes with some confidence causality between the program and the desired effects. It is the "all else the same" issue that poses the substantial methodological challenges that evaluators can face.

The optimal but impossible way of establishing causality is to observe the desired outcomes for individuals under both the treated and nontreated scenarios. For example, if we want to know the impact of a particular job training program on earnings, it would be optimal to observe individuals who received the training and their subsequent earnings streams. Once we were satisfied we had observed earning for a sufficient period, we would turn back the clock and observe the earnings for the same individuals, but this time without having them receive the training. Of course, unless you are in the Star Trek universe or at Hogwarts, it is impossible to turn back the clock in this manner. This is known as the fundamental problem of establishing causality.[3]

Thus, researchers have developed a framework and methods to overcome this fundamental problem. We generally use control or comparison groups to establish what is known as the *counterfactual*. The counterfactual is what would have happened to the treated units had they not been exposed to the treatment. Program/policy effects can then be estimated as the difference in outcomes between the treated and comparison group. If we are confident that the comparison group established a valid counterfactual, we can infer causality between the treatment and the observed effects. A valid counterfactual, however, means we are very confident that our comparison group is identical to the treated group in all measured and unmeasured characteristics that might influence the outcome; or that we can apply statistical methods to remove the influence of any differences in these characteristics. Factors other than the treatment itself that can affect the outcomes of interest are often called confounders or confounding factors. When we can successfully remove the influence of confounders, we can choose study designs that are appropriate under the assumption of "unconfoundedness."

As we will detail, the gold standard for establishing the counterfactual is to use a truly experimental approach—one which randomly selects participants to the treatment or the comparison. If participants are assigned to treatment or comparison groups based on the flip of a coin, one would not expect any systematic differences between the groups. While these studies are common to clinical trials of drugs for Food and Drug Administration (FDA) approval and many National Institutes of Health (NIH) clinical studies, they are not feasible or ethical in all situations. Fortunately, there are a number of quasi-experimental study designs and accompanying statistical methods that can be used as reasonable alternatives to the randomized trial. The remainder of this and several following chapters are devoted to a more rigorous description of these issues, and the variety of methods frequently used for evaluation.

Defining Causality

To motivate our discussion of the analytic framework of causality,[4] we begin with an example. Let us imagine a single patient with hypertension who is contemplating whether to take a new medication to manage his or her condition. The outcome of interest is whether the patient's blood pressure meets a lower threshold after taking the medication for 2 weeks. Before the patient makes a decision, there are two potential outcomes: the outcome if the patient takes the medication, *Y(medication)*, and the outcome if the patient does not take the medication, *Y(no medication)*. The causal effect is the comparison between these two potential outcomes. That is, the causal effect is the comparison between what happens if the patient takes the medication, and what happens if we go back in time and observe what happens to the patient's blood pressure if he or she did not take the medication.

Two things are important to note. First, a causal effect is not a comparison in outcomes at different time points (before and after), but rather a comparison of potential outcomes for a particular individual at a particular time after the treatment has taken place. Second, both potential outcomes cannot be observed; at most one will be observed. This means that we will need a way to represent what would have happened in the absence of the treatment, the counterfactual. Without a reliable measure of the counterfactual, isolating the effect of the intervention is impossible. To develop a counterfactual, we will need to observe multiple units and utilize inferential techniques to estimate causal effects. The remainder of this chapter develops the counterfactual framework and the measures used to estimate causal effects, but first we introduce formal notation that we will use throughout our ensuing discussion.

Scaling up from our single patient in the hypertension medication example, we consider: $i = 1, \ldots, N$ individuals who either receive or do not receive the treatment.

We assume that treatment has one level (you either get the treatment or not), and we represent treatment with the binary indicator W_i, where $W_i = 1$ if treatment is received, and $W_i = 0$ if treatment is not received. We denote the outcome of interest by Y_i.

The causal framework begins by thinking about what are the possible outcomes *before the treatment* takes place. In the example, the patient can either take the blood pressure medication for 2 weeks and see what happens, or he or she can forgo it for 2 weeks and see what happens. Expressing this formally, each individual has two potential outcomes:

$$\text{potential outcome} = \begin{cases} Y_i(0) & \text{if } W_i = 0 \\ Y_i(1) & \text{if } W_i = 1. \end{cases} \qquad (4.1)$$

$Y_i(0)$ is the potential outcome if treatment is not received, and $Y_i(1)$ is the potential outcome if treatment is received. If we could observe both outcomes (remember, we cannot), then the causal effect of treatment for the i-th individual could be calculated by taking the difference $Y_i(1) - Y_i(0)$.

What we can observe is the effect *after the treatment* takes place or does not take place. Specifically, we can know

- whether the individual received the treatment, and

- either $Y_i(0)$ if treatment was not received or $Y_i(1)$ if treatment was received.

Table 4.1 shows these unobserved and observed outcomes.

To estimate causal effects, we only have the observed outcomes available, and as a result, estimation necessarily involves observing outcomes on multiple individuals

Table 4.1 Potential, Observed, and Unobserved Outcomes

	Unobserved			Observed (after treatment)	
i	Potential Outcomes		Causal Effect	Treatment Status	Observed Outcome
1	$Y_1(0)$	$Y_1(1)$	$Y_1(1) - Y_1(0)$	Received	$Y_1(1)$
2	$Y_2(0)$	$Y_2(1)$	$Y_2(1) - Y_2(0)$	Not received	$Y_2(0)$
3	$Y_3(0)$	$Y_3(1)$	$Y_3(1) - Y_3(0)$	Not received	$Y_3(0)$
4	$Y_4(0)$	$Y_4(1)$	$Y_4(1) - Y_4(0)$	Received	$Y_4(1)$
5	$Y_5(0)$	$Y_5(1)$	$Y_5(1) - Y_5(0)$	Not received	$Y_5(0)$

and using inference to compare the observed outcomes. At first glance, it may seem obvious to compare the average difference in outcomes for those that were assigned to the treatment and those that were not:

$$\text{average observed difference in outcomes} = E\,[Y_t(1)] - E\,[Y_c(0)], \qquad (4.2)$$

where $E\,[Y_c(0)]$ is the average outcome for those in the comparison group (did not receive treatment), and $E\,[Y_t(1)]$ is the average outcome for those in the treatment group. Two problems immediately emerge. First, assignment to treatment does not necessarily imply receipt of treatment. In some cases, treatment may be completely voluntary. We will need to account for this in our estimation approach. Second, the average observed difference in outcomes may not be an unbiased estimate of the average treatment effect; this bias is called selection bias. Selection bias occurs when those in the treatment group are systematically different from those in the comparison group. This may occur when the decision to receive treatment is left to the patient to decide. Those who choose treatment may be sicker (or healthier) or more (or less) likely to utilize health services than those that elect to not receive the treatment. Thus, any differences observed between treatment recipients and those in the comparison group may be due to the treatment, but they may also be due to the underlying dissimilarities between the two groups. In our task of teasing out the causal effect, we will seek to minimize selection bias since it may be so large in magnitude that it completely obscures the treatment effect.

Assignment Mechanisms

Selection bias is associated with the assignment mechanism, that is, the mechanism by which individuals are assigned to the treatment or comparison group. There are two broad classes of assignment mechanisms: random assignment mechanisms and nonrandom assignment mechanisms. These mechanisms are a fundamental part of program design. We emphasize the importance of the assignment mechanism because whether assignment is random or not is intrinsically linked to the best method for estimating treatment effects.

   With a random assignment mechanism, the decision whether an individual is assigned to treatment or not (assignment to the control group) is completely random, that is, it is equivalent to a simple coin toss. Under random assignment, other sources of variation—except the manipuland (the thing being tested, also known as the stimulus, independent variable, treatment, or intervention[5]) are held constant across conditions. In the language of causal inference, we say that assignment to treatment is unconfounded under random assignment, that is, assignment to treatment is independent of any underlying characteristics of the individuals being assigned to treatment. Box 4.1 describes the 2008 Medicaid expansion in Oregon that was studied using a randomized evaluation design.[6]

Box 4.1
Medicaid Expansion in Oregon

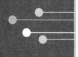

In 2008, Medicaid was expanded in Oregon. Because the demand for coverage was expected to be greater than the number of funded slots available, the expansion benefits were allocated by a lottery. Approximately 2 years after the lottery, Blaicker, Finkestein, et al. obtained data for 6,387 adults who were randomly selected to apply for Medicaid and 5,842 adults who were not. They collected clinical measures (e.g., blood pressure, cholesterol levels) as well as health status, health care utilization, and out-of-pocket spending measures.)

For their analysis, the individuals who lost the lottery provided the counterfactual (what would have happened if Medicaid enrollment was not offered). Because of randomization, the researchers did not need to worry about temporal trends because the control group would experience the same trends. Similarly, prior health status and other subject characteristics were also not systematically different between the control group and Medicaid group; they were balanced by randomization. (It is worth noting that randomization does not ensure covariate balance, each covariate having the same distribution for the treatment and control groups.)

This randomized controlled trial showed that Medicaid coverage generated no significant improvements in measured physical health outcomes in the first 2 years of implementation. However, it increased health care service utilization, rates of diabetes detection and management, lowered rates of depression, and reduced financial strain.

Nonrandom assignment mechanisms can occur when treatment is voluntary or when only eligibility can be randomized. That is, we allow for the possibility of nontreatment and noncompliance in the eligible treatment group. Nonrandom assignment is a common feature in the Centers for Medicare and Medicaid Services' (CMS) demonstrations where individuals, physicians, or practices may choose to participate in the demonstration or where all Medicare and/or Medicaid beneficiaries are eligible to participate. Under nonrandom assignment, estimating the treatment effect is more difficult—those who do not receive the treatment do not necessarily represent the counterfactual and minimizing selection bias will be of great importance.

The study design used when estimating causal effects under nonrandom assignment is called quasi-experimental design. Estimation begins with identification of a comparison group that is similar to the treatment group in terms of observable, pre-intervention characteristics. Unconfoundedness in the context of quasi-experimental designs means that statistical controls, the aforementioned observable, preintervention characteristics, can be used to minimize the impact of nonrandom selection. As a result, the outcomes of the comparison

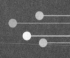

Although evidence from observational studies have shown that the use of surgical safety checklists improves surgical outcomes, the effect of mandatory surgical checklists is unclear. In Ontario, Canada, a policy was introduced in 2010, which encouraged the universal implementation of surgical checklists by requiring all hospitals to publicly report their adherence to surgical safety checklists. Rapid adoption soon followed, providing a natural experiment to test the effectiveness of mandatory surgical checklists.

In this situation, the randomization of patients (or hospitals) was not possible by design. To overcome this, Urbach et al., surveyed all acute care hospitals in Ontario to find out when surgical safety checklists were adopted. They then collected administrative data for patients in these hospitals for the 3 months before and after surgical checklists were adopted. The 3 months prior to the implementation of the surgical checklists provided the counterfactual for the first 3 months of surgical safety checklist utilization. The measures collected include operative mortality, surgical complication rates, length of stay, readmissions, and postdischarge emergency department visits. After analyzing the data, the researchers found that the mandatory implementation of surgical safety checklists in Ontario was not associated with significant reductions in surgical mortality or complications.

group approximate the counterfactual, and the treatment effect can be estimated. Defining the comparison group and estimating treatment effects in quasi-experimental designs is the focus of the next two chapters. Box 4.2 describes a quasi-experimental design about surgical safety checklists that took advantage of a policy change in Ontario, Canada.[7]

Three Key Treatment Effects

To this point, we have been deliberately vague about defining the actual treatment effects that might be estimated in the counterfactual framework. We now turn to this topic and define three treatment effects of interest to policymakers.

Average Treatment Effect

The average treatment effect (ATE) is the average treatment effect conditioned on *assignment* to the treatment. In terms of the formal notation we have established, the ATE, τ_{ATE}, is given by

$$\tau_{ATE} = E\,[Y_i\,(1) - Y_i\,(0)]. \tag{4.3}$$

The ATE is also known as the average causal effect; it is the population-averaged value of the unit-level causal effect from treatment. The ATE has "external validity" or generalizability. That means that it informs us about the average effect of the treatment on a unit drawn randomly from the population.

Average Treatment Effect on the Treated

The average treatment effect on the treated (ATT), τ_{ATT}, is the average treatment effect conditioned on *receiving* the treatment:

$$\tau_{ATT} = E\,[Y_i(1) - Y_i(0) \,|\, W_i = 1]. \tag{4.4}$$

In some studies, the effect of the intervention on individuals actually treated (that is, individuals with positive dosages) is a more interesting parameter than the overall average effect. For example, when participation in a program will always be voluntary, the average treatment effect on the treated may be the most relevant statistic. In such cases, we do not wish to extrapolate to the entire population because many will not accept treatment. Most CMS demonstrations, for example, are voluntary for both providers and beneficiaries, and within any demonstration, not all units actually receive intervention services. Were CMS to scale up to a voluntary national program, and only be interested in effects on the voluntary participants, the ATT might be the appropriate measure of demonstration performance.

Alternatively, consider research to document if a certain treatment is efficacious when delivered in full and assume that, because of implementation problems, only a subset of those receiving the treatment receive a full dose. In this case, limiting the analysis to only those who received the full treatment may be warranted. The estimate of the ATT would then be an estimate of the capacity of the treatment to produce an effect. But the interpretation of the result must be limited by the understanding that not everyone exposed to the treatment was included in the analysis. That limitation must be reported clearly by the evaluator along with the evidence of efficacy.

Intent-to-Treat Effect

Finally, the intent-to-treat effect (ITT), τ_{ITT}, is the average treatment effect conditioned on *eligibility* for treatment. This is the case when treatment is not mandatory, but depends on voluntary take-up. Letting Z_i be an indicator of eligibility with $Z_i = 1$ for those who are eligible for the treatment, and $Z_i = 0$ for those who are not eligible, we have

$$\tau_{ITT} = E[Y_i(1) \,|\, Z_i = 1] - E[Y_i(0) \,|\, Z_i = 1]. \tag{4.5}$$

Randomized "mandatory" treatment assignment is impossible when individuals are free to choose (either by law or by evaluation decision), not to take up the treatment (i.e., not to be part of the treatment group). This applies in particular to the statutorily voluntary CMS demonstrations. Randomizing eligibility is comparatively relatively easy; however, it is subject to addressing ethical concerns that arise in any evaluation that involves giving some units access to a program, while excluding others.

Statistical and Real-World Considerations for Estimating Treatment Effects

The next chapter discusses the mechanics of estimating these treatment effects under random assignment. We examine treatment effect estimation in the simplest randomized design—the randomized controlled trial—and then discuss more complicated randomized studies. Because study design and the methods for evaluating treatment effects are closely linked, we discuss quasi-experimental designs, the development of comparison groups, and the estimation of treatment effects under nonrandom assignment extensively in Chapter 6. Whether randomized or not, the estimation of treatment effects requires statistical inference. So, before turning our attention to specific evaluation designs, we conclude this chapter by considering some key statistical ideas that are important for understanding treatment effect estimation and discuss estimation in the real world.

Statistical Toolbox

Statistical inference begins with a question about a population. Ideally, data would be available for every individual in the population, and the question could be answered directly. However, this is generally not the case. Instead we must use a sample from the population to make inferences about the population as a whole; this process is statistical inference. Statistical inference usually focuses on two related tasks:

1. *Estimation.* For example, we may want to know the ATE for a population, but only have access to a subset of the population—the sample. Using the sample to estimate the ATE for the population is statistical estimation. Statistical estimation may provide a point estimate or a range of plausible values (an interval estimate).

2. *Testing Hypotheses.* We may also want to test a hypothesis about the population based on the available sample. Hypothesis tests provide a way to weigh the evidence for or against a given hypothesis.

Estimation

The language of statistical inference begins with populations and samples. Populations are what we want to make inferences about (a population may be composed of people, objects, or events). Samples are a subset of the population on which those inferences are based. Population characteristics, such as age, have distributions that can be described by parameters such as the mean and variance.[8] Sample characteristics also have distributions, and they are described by statistics. Point estimates are statistics generated from sample data that function as a "best guess" for an unknown population parameter. For example, if we want to know about the population mean, a best guess (point estimate) might be the sample mean. The sample mean, in general, will not coincide with the population mean because of sampling error. Because of the imprecision associated with the sample mean, we may want to instead provide a range of estimates—a confidence interval—that are a good guess of the parameter. Usually, three components make up a confidence interval: a point estimate, a margin of error, and a confidence level:

$$\text{confidence interval} = \text{point estimate} \pm \text{margin of error}.$$

The margin of error determines how wide the confidence interval is. It is a function of the standard error and the confidence level. The magnitude of the standard error relates to the precision or imprecision of the point estimate. Large standard errors indicate greater uncertainty than small standard errors (of course, large and small are relative terms, and what may be considered large or small depends on the nature of the data at hand). The confidence level is the probability that this method of constructing the confidence interval captured the true value of the population parameter. Notably, it is not the probability that the true value of the parameter is in the confidence interval, and theoretically, one cannot guarantee that the true parameter value lies in the interval.

Hypothesis Tests

Tests of significance, or hypothesis tests, assess evidence from the sample in favor of or against a claim about the population. The null hypothesis, H_0, represents the default position. The alternative hypothesis, H_A, represents what the test is trying to establish. For example, the null hypothesis might be that there is no change in per beneficiary savings after 1 year of a program and the alternative might be that savings are not zero.[9] In the parlance of statistics, this is a two-sided test. Using typical statistical notation, we can write this as

$$H_0 : \mu = 0,$$
$$H_A : \mu \neq 0,$$

where μ represents per beneficiary savings after 1 year. To assess the hypotheses, we might use the sample mean. The sample mean, $\bar{x}$, in general, will not be equal to the population mean (because of random sampling error) but should be a reasonable approximation. Intuitively, observing a sample mean "very different" from 0 would be evidence against the null hypothesis, and we would reject the null hypothesis in favor of the alternative. Observing a sample mean "close" to 0 would not be convincing evidence against the null, and we would fail to reject the null hypothesis. This begs the questions: How much is "very different," and what is "close"? To answer this, the researcher computes the p-value. The p-value is the probability of observing a sample statistic (such as the sample mean) equal to or more extreme than the one observed assuming that the null hypothesis is true. Small p-values are evidence against the null—it would be unlikely to observe a sample mean that far away from the population mean if the null hypothesis was true. The p-value is compared to the significance level, represented by α, which is a threshold probability set by the researcher before the test is conducted. A p-value less than α leads to the decision to reject the null hypothesis; a p-value greater than α leads to the decision to fail to reject the null hypothesis.

Tests of significance are not infallible. The researcher cannot know whether the null hypothesis is true or false; he or she can only know the conclusion of the test. Because of this, four outcomes are possible and shown in Table 4.2:

Table 4.2 Possible Outcomes From a Hypothesis Test		
	Reject the Null Hypothesis	Fail to Reject the Null Hypothesis
Null hypothesis is true.	Type I error	Correct inference
Null hypothesis is false.	Correct inference	Type II error

Two outcomes lead to correct inferences: either the null is true and the test fails to reject the null, or the null is false and the test rejects the null. Two outcomes lead to errors. The first is called a Type I error and sometimes a false positive. In a test of significance, the probability of a Type I error is the significance. Recall that the significance is also the threshold for the test decision. In essence, the significance level in a hypothesis test is the researcher's tolerance for making a Type I error; to reject the null, the researcher must observe evidence different enough from the null that probability of the difference being noise and not due to the intervention is α. The second error, a Type II error, is sometimes called a false negative and represented by β. A trade-off exists between the likelihoods of Type I and Type II errors, and without changing the sample size, minimizing the likelihood of one increases the likelihood of the other.

Statistical power is the probability of rejecting the null hypothesis when the null hypothesis is false; it is the probability of correctly having a significant result. It is also equal to 1: probability of a Type II error. Statistical power can be increased by increasing α, which is undesirable, or by increasing the sample size.

Finally, we address the difference between practical and statistical significance. The statistical strategies used in program evaluation must be understood in

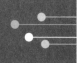

"It is essential not to confuse the statistical usage of 'significance' with the everyday usage . . . in which 'significant' means 'of practical importance,' or simply 'important.'" Indeed, study findings may provide great practical meaning in the policy realm, even if they fail to meet the traditional criterion of an $\alpha = .05$ significance level. Ziliak and McCloskey highlight with several real-world examples of study findings that, although lacking a low observed standard error, a study can still have meaningful implications for potentially life-saving policy decisions. For example, if deciding whether or not to implement stricter penalties for dangerous driving based on a 1% significance level instead of a 5% significance level, a UK simulation found that policymakers would *not* implement these penalties, despite the fact that doing so would save approximately 100,000 lives over a 10-year period. Statistical significance is effectively an arbitrary label based on an arbitrarily determined cut-off point. The 5% rule indicates how different an observed estimate must be from the null hypothesis in order for it to be "significant." A smaller significance level, say 0.01, simply moves the bar for significance farther away from the null hypothesis. A study may have large effect sizes that are somewhat imprecise—findings that may have practical implications for human services policymakers looking to target limited public resources most efficiently. Conversely, studies are routinely published if they have statistically significant results, even when those results yield limited information (if any) for use in calibrating the allocation-limited public resources. Also worth considering is that the policy research community may often derive greater benefit from demonstrations with insignificant findings—which may be worth repeating for that reason. Moreover, the methods may, in themselves, provide useful insight to related future endeavors.

the greater context in which evaluation findings are used. Beginning the discussion in Box 4.3, this is an idea we return to in later chapters when we discuss using evaluation findings for decision making in the real world.[10,11]

Validity and Evaluation in the Real World

A primary goal in evaluation is determining if the intervention caused a change in an outcome of interest (health status, total cost of care, etc.). However, poor planning, poor execution, and poor luck—in other words, the real world—can threaten the trustworthiness of a causal impact. In the language of experimental design, validity is the extent to which an inference is accurate. Taking the steps necessary to ensure validity to the greatest extent possible and assessing validity during and after an evaluation is an important task. To assess validity, it is easiest to consider four broad types of validity:[12] construct validity, statistical validity, internal validity, and external validity. We consider each of these in turn, as well as the real-world threats they face.

Construct validity is the extent to which a measure captures what it is supposed to be measuring. Evaluation planning is an essential step maximizing construct validity; this involves ensuring that measures are linked to target outcomes, that the relevant data are available, and that the collection of those data is a part of the intervention's implementation. Starting to plan an evaluation after an intervention has already begun means that the data necessary to answer the primary evaluation questions may not be available or severely limited. Other properties of robust, valid measures are discussed in Chapters 2 and 3.

Statistical validity refers to the validity of inferences about the relationship between the treatment and the outcome. This involves verifying that the statistical procedures and tests used are appropriate. Among the many things that jeopardize statistical validity, two stand out as particularly important for evaluations of health care demonstrations. First, low statistical power may hinder the ability of a significant relationship between the treatment and the outcome being detected. Given the time, cost, and effort of an evaluation, it is worthwhile to plan upfront on having an adequately powered demonstration. In Chapter 5, we discuss two randomized study designs, adaptive and factorial, that can maximize statistical power. For those as well as other designs (random or otherwise), power can be increased by using larger sample sizes. This means planning demonstrations to have enough participants that it is likely to detect an effect if one is present. Statistical methods exist for computing the number of participants needed to achieve a particular level of statistical power (80% power is a common threshold in scientific studies). Along with low statistical power, heterogeneity between the units being tested can obscure treatment effects. With greater variation between outcomes, teasing out a relationship between the intervention and the outcome becomes harder. This is especially pertinent in contemporary health care demonstrations. For example, in pay-for-performance demonstrations, participating practices receive financial incentives to lower costs while meeting health care quality standards. How the participating practices do so is open ended and can lead to a wide mix of outcomes, and in this, the evaluator must determine which, if any, models work and by how much. Chapters 7, 8, and 12 deal with ways to assess and quantify program and outcome heterogeneity.

Internal validity is concerned with causation. Did the treatment really cause the outcome, or is there some other reason that can explain the outcome? The evaluator must ensure internal validity to the greatest extent possible; it involves methodically ruling out other possible reasons for the outcomes that are observed. Selection, systematic differences in the baseline characteristics of those receiving the treatment and those not receiving the treatment, is a key threat to internal validity. Randomized controlled trials, in which the treatment is unrelated to participant characteristics by design, is considered the gold standard in program evaluation design. Frequent critiques of nonexperimental evaluations relate to the problem of the self-selection of participants into treatment, especially based on unobservable elements like motivation. For example, those who seek to participate in an employment intervention may be more motivated that the nonintervention group if assignment to treatment is not random.

Although random assignment to treatment or control status is not always feasible, it should always be considered. Nonexperimental evaluation designs generally seek to mimic the features of true experiments to the greatest extent possible by using statistical techniques and available data to make those in the comparison group as similar as possible to those receiving the treatment. Again, evaluation planning is key here. Being able to access preintervention and postintervention data for both the treatment group and comparison group will allow for the best evaluation design to go forward.

Temporal trends, exogenous contemporaneous events, and changes in the implementation of the treatment over time events are also threats to internal validity. Sometimes they can be controlled for statistically, but being aware of them and identifying them are key tasks for the evaluator. Attrition from a study can also affect internal validity if it is correlated with treatment outcomes. Box 4.4 describes a study affected by attrition.[13]

Box 4.4
Individual Random Assignment at Program Entry

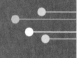

One arrangement that often lends itself to randomized designs is the Cooperative Agreement, in which multiple sites have agreed to follow a standardized research protocol. Clinical staff participating in these studies often has experience implementing complex research designs. One example of this is CMS' Cancer Prevention and Treatment Demonstration (CPTD). In this four-arm experiment, Medicare beneficiaries receiving services at four major medical centers were first screened for eligibility, placed in either the prevention services or diagnosed cancer treatment arm, and then randomly assigned to either a Patient Navigation intervention group or to the control group. The group assignment for each patient was determined by contacting a project website that randomly allocated patients to groups. Designed and operated by a separate contractor, the website relieved the sites of the need to develop and monitor their own assignment protocols. The website approach also helped to ensure cross-site uniformity in the randomization protocol. Analyses of baseline clinical and self-report measures confirmed that the intervention and control groups were similar prior to the start of intervention activities. Significant differential attrition over the intervention period was an issue, however. Final analyses compared the treatment effects generated through random assignment to treatment and control groups with those generated using quasi-experimental matched comparison groups. In this case, however, because of the extent of attrition, the nonexperimental results were more robust.

External validity is the extent to which conclusions can be generalized. An important aspect of external validity is whether the intervention participants represent the composition of the population to which one wants to generalize. Threats to external validity include interactions between the setting (e.g., academic medical center versus a rural hospital) and the causal relationship being tested and interactions of different components of models being tested. Failure to articulate and classify program components and characteristics pose a serious threat to the greater usability of evaluation findings. Results may be valid for the intervention being tested, but those results may not be useful to decision makers who must decide whether to expand a program or not. Chapters 7 and 8 discuss the methods for assessing these contextual program factors and how to incorporate them into evaluation findings.

SUMMARY

Ascertaining causal effects begins with the counterfactual framework, comparing what happened with treatment to what would have happened without. Randomization yields a natural control group from which to infer treatment effects. Nonrandomized designs generally rely upon the acquisition of comparison group data to make the comparison.

The choice of evaluation design is essentially an assessment of trade-offs in each particular case. Emerging best practice is to begin with the most analytically defensible treatment assignment rule that is feasible; then consider the likely magnitude of its impact in determining

the size of the study, data collection timing, and approach; and follow this by allowing for different analytic approaches that can demonstrate empirically whether the benefits of random assignment outweigh other research and implementation concerns.

Failing to consider the real world in evaluation design threatens the validity of evaluation findings. Planning and integrating evaluation activities with program implementation can greatly improve the likelihood of having the right information and enough information to answer decision maker questions.

DISCUSSION QUESTIONS

1. How do random and nonrandom assignment mechanisms differ? Describe a situation for which nonrandom assignment may be better suited.

2. Are there certain situations in which a researcher would have a higher tolerance

for Type I error than Type II error? How about the reverse?

3. Should policymakers take statistically insignificant results into consideration? Why, or why not?

NOTES

1. Note that most evaluations relate to the effects of particular programs and policies. As we begin to discuss methodological issues for evaluations, programs and policies are often referred to as treatments or interventions. Unless otherwise noted, these terms are used interchangeably.

2. In practice, evaluations need not be treated vs. nontreated—comparisons might be made among individuals or groups subject to different treatments or ways of implementing a program.

3. Rubin, Donald B., "Causal Inference Using Potential Outcomes: Design, Modeling, Decisions," *Journal of the American Statistical Association* 100, no. 469 (2005): 322–30.

4. Much of our discussion is drawn from Imbens, Guido, and Donald B. Rubin. *Causal Inference for Statistics, Social, and Biomedical Sciences: An Introduction* (New York: Cambridge University Press, 2015).

5. We use *treatment* and *intervention* interchangeably in the discussion that follows.

6. Baicker, Katherine, Amy Finkelstein, Jae Song, and Sarah Taubman, "The Impact of Medicaid on Labor Market Activity and Program Participation: Evidence from the Oregon Health Insurance Experiment," *American Economic Review: Papers and Proceedings* 104, no. 55 (May 2015): 322–8.

7. Urbach, D. R., A. Govindarajan, R. Saskin, A. S. Wilton, and N. N. Baxter," Introduction of Surgical Safety Checklists in Ontario, Canada. *New England Journal of Medicine* 370 (2014): 1029–38. doi: 10.1056/NEJMsa1308261.

8. We focus our discussion on continuous variables. However, descriptives such as frequencies or proportions may be used to characterize populations. Sample proportions can be used as estimators of population proportions, and confidence intervals can be computed.

9. Again, we focus on the continuous case; however, tests of statistical significance exist for categorical data.

10. Wallis, Allen W., and Harry, V. Roberts. *Statistics: A New Approach* (Glencoe, Illinois: The Free Press, 1956).

11. Arnold, Wilfred Niels. *The Cult of Statistical Significance*, edited by Stephen T. Ziliak and Deirdre N. McCloskey (Ann Arbor: University of Michigan Press, 2008).

12. Shadish, W. R., T. D. Cook, and D. T. Campbell. *Experimental and Quasi-experimental Designs for Generalized Causal Inference* (Boston, MA: Houghton Mifflin, 2002).

13. Mitchell, J., A. Bir, S. Hoover, et al. *Evaluation of the Cancer Prevention and Treatment Demonstration Report to Congress*. Prepared for the Centers for Medicare & Medicaid Services, March 2012.

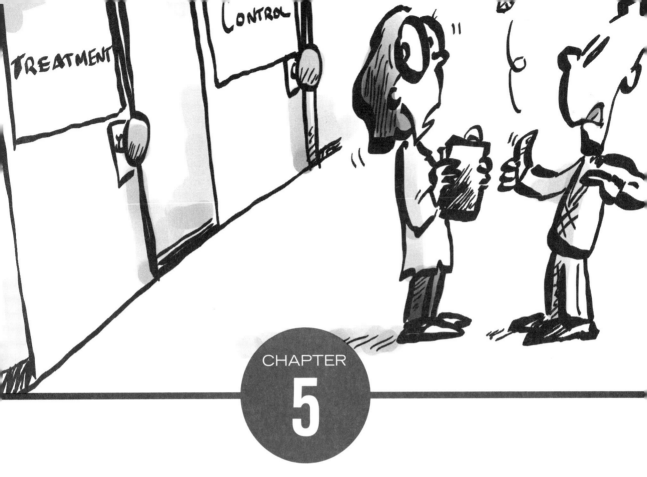

Randomized Designs

Jeff Wooldridge

Guido Imbens

Nikki Freeman

Rachael Zuckerman

Learning Objectives

Random assignment—the essence of the experimental design or the randomized clinical trial—guarantees a theoretically perfect counterfactual. With the control

(Continued)

group established, treatment effects can be estimated readily, and we describe the relevant estimation techniques in this chapter. We also describe estimation strategies for stratified randomized and group randomized trials.

Chapter 5 also describes two study designs that utilize randomized assignment and are particularly pertinent to health care interventions. Factorial design is well suited for estimating the effects of individual intervention components. Adaptive design assumes rolling assignment and uses the previous performance of the treatments to allocate individuals so that treatment effects can be estimated with increased precision.

This chapter addresses the issue of how to represent *what would have happened in the absence of the intervention*—the counterfactual. Without a reliable measure of the counterfactual, isolating the effect of the intervention from the effect of nontreatment factors is impossible. A randomized controlled trial (RCT) is generally considered the gold standard of modern program evaluation. Pure random assignment—allocating program eligible beneficiaries to the treatment or control group by a method basically equivalent to a simple coin toss—is often not feasible. Nonetheless, it is a good starting point as preparation for the more complex methods of developing the counterfactual that we go on to discuss in Chapters 6 and 7.

In a well-designed randomized experiment with only one treatment, the outcomes observed in the control group act as an estimate of the observed, and more importantly the unobservable, outcomes for the treatment group that would occur in the absence of treatment. *A powerful feature of the counterfactual approach is that different measures of the treatment effect can be measured directly by definition.* This approach is flexible and can be generalized to multiple treatment arms within the same experiment. Deep understanding of the counterfactual approach is critical for understanding cutting-edge evaluation methods.

Using random assignment as a benchmark, we then consider estimation of program effects (i.e., the difference between outcomes for the treatment group and the group representing the counterfactual). Afterward, we consider situations when treatment is voluntary and only eligibility can be randomized.[1] That is, we allow for the possibility of nontreatment and noncompliance in the eligible treatment group. Finally, we consider two randomized study designs, factorial and adaptive, that can be useful in evaluating health care interventions.

Randomized Controlled Trials

We begin with the simplest randomized design—the RCT. In its simplest form, the researcher has specified the population prior to randomization, drawn a representative sample from it,[2] and assigned one of the two randomized groups to the treatment, which may be a policy intervention (health care examples include a novel payment arrangement or process of care change) and the other randomized group to the control (i.e., nontreatment) condition.[3]

In much of the literature on estimating causal effects, samples are assumed to be random and drawn from a very large population. One implication of this random sampling assumption is that the treatment of one particular individual has no effect on any other individuals.[4] Yet, many health care interventions that improve health outcomes can have positive spillover effects on family and community members. One way to capture spillover effects is to aggregate outcomes across individuals, which includes interaction effects among them. Unfortunately, with some interventions, particularly health interventions, the appropriate level of aggregation is not clear.[5] The next section begins by assuming random sampling from the population with no interactions or spillovers; it then covers the case where treatment assignment occurs at a larger group level.

Our discussion is general and does not assume that randomization is at a particular level (individual, physician, practice, etc.); we will use the term *unit* as a stand in for whatever is the unit of randomization. Special care must be taken when estimating treatment effects at the group level; we discuss this later in the chapter.

Average Treatment Effect in Randomized Controlled Trials

Random assignment of the treatment implies that eligible individuals have no choice of whether to be in the treatment or the control group. That means individuals who may benefit more from treatment cannot decide to join the treatment group. If the policy under consideration would eventually expose all units to the treatment, the average treatment effect (ATE), τ_{ATE}, is the most relevant quantity. For example, if a change in the delivery of health care is under consideration for universal adoption, one would want to know its expected effect on a randomly drawn unit from the population. This parameter is best in such a situation because it would reflect the average of individuals who responded to the treatment and those who did not.

Box 5.1 provides a formal derivation of the ATE. Readers not interested methodologically are encouraged to skip the formal derivation of Box 5.1.

To illustrate the ATE, we consider Lalonde's work regarding the effects of job training. In addition to exemplifying the ATE, this example utilizes covariates to estimate the ATE. Covariates are not necessary to obtain an unbiased estimate of the ATE; however, they can be used to make estimates more precise.

Box 5.1

Formal Derivation of the ATE

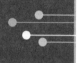

Using the notation we developed in Chapter 4, we write the ATE in terms of an expected value:

$$ATE = \tau_{ATE} = E\left[Y_i(1) - Y_i(0)\right] \tag{5.1}$$

The ATE is obtained by averaging the difference between $Y_i(1)$ and $Y_i(0)$ across the population of interest. Recall that the potential outcomes, $Y_i(1)$ and $Y_i(0)$, cannot both be observed; either the patient receives the treatment or not. Under the strong assumption of random assignment, estimation of the intervention effect is straightforward because the assignment of treatment or control conditions is independent of how units might respond to the intervention. It follows that an unbiased and consistent estimator of $E\left[Y_i(0)\right]$ is obtained by averaging Y_i over the observations with $W_i = 0$ and $E\left[Y_i(1)\right]$ by averaging Y_i over observations with $W_i = 1$. This leads to the standard difference-in-means estimator for τ_{ATE} that is familiar from introductory statistics.[6] This estimator is easily obtained in a simple regression of Y_i on a treatment group indicator across all observations:

$$Y_i = a + \tau_{ATE}W_i + \varepsilon_i \tag{5.2}$$

where ε_i equals the variation in outcomes unexplained by treatment. In a randomized experiment, additional covariates are not required to obtain an unbiased estimate of the overall intervention effect because their effects cancel out between treatment and control groups. However, including covariates can improve statistical precision of the estimated average treatment effect.[7]

Lalonde used data from an experimental job training study, administered in 1976 and 1977, in his evaluation of nonexperimental estimators.[8] Participation was randomized. There are data for 445 men in the dataset and 260 controls. Of the 445 men, 185 participated in the job training program. The data on labor market outcomes were from 1978, and any heterogeneity in the treatment effects was not systematically different in the control and treatment groups.

We consider two outcome (response) variables to job training. The first is a binary variable, unem78, indicating whether a man was unemployed at any time in 1978; the other is his labor market earnings in 1978, re78, which was zero for a nontrivial fraction of unemployed workers. Neither of unem78 nor re78 has a normal distribution in the population, and so we rely on large-sample approximations in obtaining t-tests and confidence intervals.

The estimated unemployment rate in the control group was .354 compared with .243 for the participating group. Therefore, $\tau_{ATE} = -0.111$. The t statistic (robust to different variances) was t = –2.55, with a 95% confidence interval (CI) of (–.196, –.025). The effect is statistically significant at approximately the 1% significance level against a two-sided alternative. The magnitude of the difference is also meaningful for policymakers, given that the unemployment rate was approximately 11 percentage points lower for those participating in the training program.

The average earnings for the control and treatment groups are $4,555 (with 35% unemployment) and $6,349 (with 24% unemployment), respectively. The t statistic for the difference was t = 2.67, with the 95% CI (476, 3113). Again, we find a statistically significant and practically important effect.

The dataset includes preprogram labor market outcomes in 1974 and 1975, as well as some demographic variables. We can test for whether the randomization was successful by estimating a simple binary logit model that includes the training indicator, the two prior unemployment dummies, and the two earnings variables, along with age, education, and binary indicators for marital status, being black, and being Hispanic. The test of joint significance gives a *p*-value = .231, providing little evidence against randomization.

Average Treatment Effect on the Treated in Randomized Controlled Trials

The average treatment effect on the treated (ATT) is similar to the ATE, except it is conditioned on the individual actually receiving the treatment. Reasons individuals might not be treated include that they were not contacted (either intentionally or because they were unreachable) or that they refused to participate in the intervention. In terms of estimation, most estimators that work for estimating the ATE also work in estimating the ATT[9] (modifying them so that the estimate is computed on the treated). Perhaps of more interest is comparing the ATE and the ATT. The difference between the ATE and the ATT can be substantial if the original intervention population is not carefully targeted. Certain interventions may have a positive effect on those who actually received the treatment while having a zero (or even negative) effect on those who did not participate, possibly leading to a situation where τ_{ATE} is much smaller than τ_{ATT}, and possibly zero. Box 5.2 compares the ATT and ATE. Readers who are not interested in the methodological details are encouraged to skip Box 5.2.

Intention-to-Treat in Randomized Controlled Trials

When eligibility for treatment differs from assignment to treatment, the appropriate counterfactual framework is an intention-to-treat (ITT) evaluation. Box 5.3 presents the formal derivation for the ITT. Readers not interested in methodology are encouraged to skip the formal derivation.

Although large randomized experiments in policy evaluation are considered to be the gold standard, they can be difficult to conduct in health care settings where withholding treatment is not feasible. The evaluation of Medicare's Health Support Disease–Management Pilot Program carried out from 2005 to 2009 provides examples of the possible strategies researchers can use to implement random assignment within disease management demonstrations.

The Medicare Modernization Act of 2003 provided funding for Centers for Medicare and Medicaid Services (CMS) to test the effectiveness of the commercial

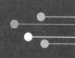

Rigorously, we can write the ATT as

$$\tau_{ATT} = E\left[Y_i(1) - Y_i(0)|W_i = 1\right]$$

(5.3)

For interpreting estimates of τ_{ate} and τ_{att} in applications, a useful relationship is

$$\tau_{ATE} = (1-\rho)\tau_{ATU} + \rho\tau_{ATT}$$

(5.4)

where $\rho = P(W_i = 1)$ is the probability that a randomly drawn unit from the population receives the treatment, and τ_{ATU} is the average treatment effect (without spillovers) for the untreated segment of those assigned to the intervention group. It is often assumed that τ_{ATU} equals zero, in which case $\tau_{ATE} = \rho\tau_{ATT}$. Of course, if the treatment effect affects all units equally regardless of dosage, then $\tau_{ATE} = \tau_{ATT}$.

Box 5.3
Formal Derivation of the ITT

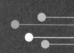

For ITT analyses, we have an indicator of eligibility, Z_i, along with the indicator of the treatment received W_i. Generally, the potential outcomes are written as $Y_i(z,w)$, with one of three combinations: $(0,0)$ = not eligible, that is, no treatment within the control group; $(1,0)$ = eligible but without treatment in an intervention subgroup, which almost always occurs in a real-world evaluation; and $(1,1)$ = eligible with treatment.

Rather than compute the difference in means based on actual treatment received, one estimates an ITT effect by differencing the average outcomes for the eligible beneficiaries assigned to the treatment group and noneligible beneficiaries assigned to the control group. Equivalently, one can obtain the ITT effect by regressing the outcome on the eligible indicator alone:

$$Y_i = \mu_0 + \tau_{ITT}Z_i + \varepsilon_i$$

(5.5)

The ITT regression produces an estimate of the gross effect of introducing a new program to the entire population, regardless of how many units actually choose to participate. However, the regression does not allow us to estimate the average effect on participants alone, because the effect is diluted by the null effect on nonparticipants in the treatment group.[10,11]

disease-management model, which relies primarily on remote nurse-based call centers, in the Medicare fee-for-service program. Eight companies participated in this pilot program and were paid a monthly fee per participant by CMS to provide commercial disease-management access to a randomly selected pool of Medicare beneficiaries. The size of the fee received by each company was tied to clinical quality, beneficiary satisfaction, and a reduction in Medicare expenditures by at least the amount of the initial fee.

The sample was selected using a population-based strategy with several strata. Roughly 240,000 beneficiaries were identified with equal numbers in eight separate geographic areas. There were two criteria for admission into the sample: a history of heart failure or diabetes, and a Hierarchical Condition Category (HCC) risk score of 1.35. Beneficiaries were stratified according to type and presence of chronic disease, Medicaid eligibility, and HCC risk score, and assigned with a 2:1 ratio to intervention or control groups. Observation weights were used to account for the stratified sampling design.

The random assignment approach raised concerns. The disease management companies found it difficult to convince randomly assigned beneficiaries in the intervention group to participate in the program. Since convincing beneficiaries to participate would be part of any such intervention, the evaluation might be better off thinking of this as a case for an ITT evaluation method rather than as an evaluation problem that needed to be fixed.

Out of the 40 evidence-based process-of-care tests (eight firms, five process rates), 14 were statistically significant, all in a positive direction. However, the absolute level of change was small. The interventions had little effect on reducing all-cause hospital admissions and ER visits. Four of eight firms exhibited slower (negative) cost growth, that is, gross savings, in their intervention group, but none of the differences was statistically significant. Given the large sample sizes, detectable savings were as small as \$50–\$60 per beneficiary per month, or 3%–4% of average comparison group costs. Analysis of covariance (ANCOVA) regressions produced very similar null findings for savings with detectable differences as low as 2.5% after controlling for beneficiary characteristics. The relatively low participation rates in some interventions, coupled with the generally limited number of (and remote) contacts with beneficiaries, were given as reasons for the lack of pilot success.

Multilevel Treatments

Sometimes there are multiple levels of a program or treatment. In some cases, the values chosen for the treatment levels have ordinal (describes rank or position, e.g., "more" or "less" treatment), or more rarely, cardinal (describes magnitude or quantity, e.g., "10 sessions") meaning. For example, a person may participate in a training program part time or full time or does not participate. In other cases, the treatment values may be nominal, acting merely as group identifiers, such as when the treatments are two different new health plans and the control group stays with

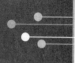

Box 5.4

Statistical Detail on Multilevel Treatments

With $G+1$ treatment levels (including control group), we have $G+1$ potential responses for each unit, $Y_i(g)$, with g ranging from zero to G. As in the binary treatment case, for each g, we define the mean potential outcomes as $\mu_g = E\left[Y_i(g)\right]$. If higher values of g represent an increase in treatment intensity, then we likely are interested in the change in the intervention's effect when treatment intensity increases from $g-1$ to g.

the current plan. In this situation, we relate the desired outcome measure to the changes in treatment intensity.

For methodologically interested readers, Box 5.4 details the statistical derivation. Other readers are encouraged to skip Box 5.5.

Stratified Randomization

Pure random assignment means that individual units (e.g., persons, medical homes) are randomly assigned to the control or the treatment group and that everyone in the population has an equal probability of assignment. Sometimes, however, the probability of assignment is not equal because different groups (strata) in the population being assigned are present in different proportions. When the probability of assignment is unequal, two-stage randomization is used to identify each stratum (typically based on geography or some other easily observable characteristic such as age), and then units are randomized within each stratum. This might, for example, be done to ensure proportionate representation from key segments of the population and thus enhance the generalizability of the final results. After stratified randomization, the ATE can be obtained by taking a weighted average. Readers not interested in the details of the statistical derivation are encouraged to skip Box 5.6.

Group Randomized Trials

Assignment to the control or treatment is often done at the group rather than individual level. One reason is that group-level randomization is often easier to implement. For example, the use of bar codes to improve patient-sample tracking is easier to test by comparing all patients in one hospital wing who received bar codes to those in another wing who did not, than by allocating barcodes on an individual patient basis. As long as treatment and comparison groups are separated by time or space, group

Box 5.5
Formal Detail on Stratified Random Assignment

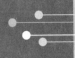

Suppose the population is divided into G strata or blocks (e.g., medical homes). Under random assignment within each stratum, we can use

$$ATE_g = \tau_g = \left[Y_{g1} - Y_{g0} \right] \tag{5.6}$$

as the unbiased, consistent estimator of the average treatment effect, where Y_{gw} denotes the sample average within stratum g of treatment group w. Assuming we have enough observations per stratum, the τ_g estimators have normal distribution properties.

In general, the overall treatment effect can be written as a weighted average of the within-group effects:

$$ATE = \tau_{ATE} = a_1\tau_1 + \ldots + a_G\tau_G \tag{5.7}$$

where the a_g is the population shares of the different strata. For example, if treatment effects are estimated for small, medium, and large hospitals in a state with a new reimbursement system, then the overall effect of the policy change statewide is the sum of the effects of the three hospital sizes weighted by the average number of admissions. This approach treats individual patients as the unit of observation, and the overall average effect is what one would expect if a patient were drawn at random from the total set of admitted patients. By contrast, if we put equal weight on each stratum, then $a_g = 1/G$ for all g, the resulting overall treatment effect would ignore differences in hospital size. Note that this may be appropriate in some policy contexts—for example, if regulators want to treat all hospitals as equals in terms of, say, avoidable readmission rates.

Inference on the overall treatment effect is easily carried out by setting the problem up as a regression equation. Let B_{ig} be a binary indicator equal to one if observation i belongs to block g, and let W_i be the treatment assignment, as usual. Then the τ_g are obtained from the heteroscedasticity-robust regression on a set of block indicators and interactions of block indicators and the treatment indicator using the entire set of data. The fitted equation looks like

$$y_i = \mu_{10}B_{i1} + \ldots + \mu_{G0}B_{iG} + \tau_1 B_{i1}W_i + \ldots + \tau_g B_{iG}W_i + \varepsilon_i \tag{5.8}$$

Given the constants a_g, it is easy to obtain the standard error for linear combinations of the τ_g estimates: $a_1\tau_1 + \ldots + a_G\tau_G$. (Both SAS and Stata provide software routines for a joint test of the combined standard error for the group-specific effects.) If we want the a_g to represent population shares, we can often get that information from other sources, such as the census.

randomization is immune to contamination from untreated individuals changing behavior because they observe what other group members receiving the treatment are doing and follow suit. Also, it is often economical to sample units within preselected larger groups (such as medical homes or hospitals). In settings with randomization at the group level, one possibility is to use group-level averages and then treat the group as the unit of observation. Provided we can assume that groups are independently sampled from a population of groups (such as medical practices), the group-level aggregates can be analyzed much as we analyze individual-level data.

A disadvantage of group randomization is loss of precision in estimation. For example, even though we have patient-level data, convenience or cost may lead us to assign treatment at the practice rather than the individual patient level. In statistical terms, the effect is to greatly reduce degrees of freedom and raise standard errors.[12] But if we choose to use individual-level responses in this instance, we must be sure not to act as if we have independent responses across all individuals, because the selection of people into groups almost certainly introduces an unobserved group effect (referred to as a cluster effect) into the outcomes.[13,14] That is, individuals within groups are often more similar to each other than they are to those in other groups. For example, patients within the same practice may have unobserved attributes that are similar. In addition, unmeasured characteristics of the practice

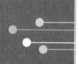

Box 5.6
Formal Modeling of Group Effects

Mathematically, common group effects can be modeled as fixed effects:

$$Y_{gi} = \mu_0 + \tau W_g + \beta C_g + \varepsilon_{gi} \tag{5.9}$$

where Y_{gi} is the observed outcome for unit i in group g. The term C_g is the cluster effect, captured by a set of 0,1 cluster indicators, and the ε_{gi} reflects unobservable variation in Y specific to unit i in cluster g. The treatment indicator, W_g, has a g subscript, because assignment is at the group level (i.e., all units in a group have the same 0,1 designation). If we estimate Equation 5.9 using pooled ordinary least squares (OLS) on the individual units without the C_g group indicators, the usual OLS standard error on τ (even using the heteroscedasticity-robust version) is generally not valid. The presence of C_g in the error term (instead of in the set of covariates) means that every two units within cluster g are positively correlated to some unknown degree. The usual OLS standard errors assume no correlation (independence) and can suffer from severe downward bias. In effect, standard OLS inference acts as if we have more independent sources of information (data) than we actually do; consequently, it is too optimistic. Fortunately, many statistical packages have options to allow for cluster sampling when choosing standard errors. For example, in Stata, the command would be *reg yw, cluster(groupid)*, where "groupid" is the group identifier. The resulting standard errors and inference allow any kind of within-cluster correlation as well as heteroscedasticity as a function of treatment or control group, W_i. An example of the effects of adjusting for clustering in a study of student incentive payments follows.

are likely to have an effect on each patient's outcome, further confounding our ability to attribute all differences observed to the tested treatment.

For methodologically interested readers, Box 5.6 gives the mathematical derivation of this discussion. Other readers are encouraged to proceed directly to the example in Box 5.7 that follows the formal derivation.

Angrist and Lavy[15] studied the effects of an experiment where a set of Israeli schools with low-performing students were randomized, so students at the treatment schools would receive incentive payments for obtaining the Bagrut certificate that allowed them to attend college. In a design using matched pairs of schools, 40 schools were chosen for the study: 20 treatment and 20 control. Treatment was randomized between school pairs. Based on 2001 data, the number of students per school ranged from 9 to almost 250 (yielding a total number of students in the thousands). Approximately 24.3% of students earned the Bagrut certification in schools without incentive payments.

The dependent variable is a binary indicator equal to unity if the student obtains the Bagrut certificate. Does the randomization by school yield an unbiased estimator of the treatment effect? Running the simple regression in Equation 5.9 without cluster indicators shows that the incentive raised the probability of receiving the Bagrut by 4.7 percentage points; using the unclustered standard error gives a statistically significant effect at the usual significance levels, with $t = 3.42$. But the cluster-robust t statistic shows this is much too optimistic. The valid t statistic is $t = .99$, indicating substantial clustering within schools.

When the students are disaggregated by gender, the effect for boys is small (.010) and very insignificant ($t = .19$). By contrast, the effect for girls is large (.109) and significant against a two-sided alternative at the 10% level ($t = 1.73$, p-value = .093). The degrees of freedom in the t distribution used to compute the p-values is 32, the number of groups with available data minus two for the parameters in text Equation 5.12.

The structure of this example raises an important point. The cluster-robust inference is known to perform poorly when the number of groups is, say, less than 10. For a small number of groups (fewer than 10), the more observations within a group, the worse is the cluster approximation.

Randomized Designs for Health Care

Up to this point, we have discussed estimating the effect of an entire intervention under random assignment. However, the programs being evaluated by CMS may have several different program components that are being simultaneously implemented. In this case, assessing the effect of individual components and the interactions of those components may be as informative or more informative to policymakers than assessing the success of the intervention as a whole. Although several study designs can be used to evaluate individual program components, we highlight the factorial design because it is particularly suitable for evaluating individual program components.

Factorial Design[16]

We begin our discussion of factorial design with a simple, hypothetical example. Suppose that an intervention is aimed at individuals with multiple chronic diseases. The intervention is implemented at the practice level and has three components: (1) care coordination, (2) patient portals, and (3) patient education. For simplicity, we assume that for each component, there are two levels (high and low) at which the component can be implemented:

1. Care coordination is the intentional organization of patient care between multiple participants to facilitate the delivery of health care services. For this example, the high level of care coordination means that the practice will hire or train staff to provide 40 hours of care coordination per week, while the low level of care coordination means that the practice will hire or train staff to provide 20 hours of care coordination per week.

2. Patient portals in this example will be the adoption of online patient portals where patients can access their personal health records and communicate with their health care provider. The high level involves utilizing this technology while the low level means not adopting the technology.

3. Patient education is the provision of educational services by health care staff to help patients understand their health care status and to build the skills necessary to manage their health problems. For this example, a high level of patient education means prescribing online disease management classes to patients, while the low level of patient education means not providing online education tools.

For this hypothetical example, the factorial experiment has eight experimental conditions, the eight possible combinations of the three factors (see Table 5.1). To implement the experiment, participating practices are randomly assigned to be in exactly one of the eight conditions. Ideally, the factorial design will have the balance property: each experimental condition will have the same amount of subjects, and the level of each factor appears the same number of times with each level of the other factors.

Data from a factorial experiment can be used to estimate two types of effects: main effects and interactions. Main effects are the effects that a factor has averaged over all of the different levels of the other factors. Interactions occur when the size of the effect of one factor changes given the level of another factor. Both of these effects are estimated using a linear modeling technique called the analysis of variance. Intuitively, the estimates for component main effects are computed on unique groupings of conditions. For example, to estimate the effect of high levels of care coordination to low levels of care coordination, outcomes for experimental Conditions 1 through 4 would be compared to outcomes for experimental Conditions 5 through 8. To compare utilizing patient portals to not utilizing them

Table 5.1 Experimental Conditions of Our Factorial Design Example

Experimental Condition	Care Coordination	Patient Portals	Patient Education
1	High	High	High
2	High	High	Low
3	High	Low	High
4	High	Low	Low
5	Low	High	High
6	Low	High	Low
7	Low	Low	High
8	Low	Low	Low

would compare Conditions 1, 2, 5, and 6 to experimental Conditions 3, 4, 7, and 8. Interaction effects can be estimated using a linear model in statistical packages such as R, SAS, or STATA.

An important aspect of factorial designs is that the estimates obtained are for individual factors and not comparisons between factors, although it can also be used to estimate effects for combinations of factors. Expanding analysis to factors with more than two levels is straightforward. In terms of estimation properties, effect estimates are estimated using the entire sample, thereby the statistical power of the estimate is not based on the sample size of each experimental condition. This means that factorial experiments can be adequately powered even if the number of experimental units assigned to each experimental condition is small. Furthermore, factorial designs make efficient use of experimental subjects; essentially the same number of subjects it would take to estimate the effect of only one component can be used to estimate the effect of many components. Of course, the trade-off is that as the number of components increases, the number of experimental conditions that need to be implemented also increases. When implementation is a barrier, fractional factorial and multiple factorial experiments are possible alternatives. Statistically, adding factors also increases the risk of a Type I statistical error due to multiple hypothesis testing.

Adaptive Design[17]

A final study design that utilizes random assignment that we will discuss is an adaptive design. An adaptive design has one control condition, one or more treatment conditions, and assignment to the different experimental conditions occurs on a rolling basis. Initially, experimental units are assigned randomly to the different experimental conditions with equal probability. The probability of being assigned to a particular experimental condition is called the random assignment ratio. Data are collected on outcomes once it seems feasible to expect impacts, and the relative effects of the treatments is estimated as are the effects on specific subgroups. Given the impact estimates, the random assignment ratios are updated for the next round of assignment. Higher random assignment ratios (higher probabilities) are given to those treatments that are found to be more effective and lower ratios are given to those found to be less effective (in fact, treatments that are uniformly ineffective may be terminated). Thus, in the second round of assignment, experimental units are more likely to be assigned to treatments that are more effective for subjects with their specific characteristics. After this round of assignment, data are collected, and the random assignment ratios are adjusted based on those results.

By updating the random assignment ratios, subjects are still randomly assigned to treatment (or one of the treatments) or the control, avoiding the problems associated with selection bias, but the proportion of subjects in the most effective treatment is increasing. This means that for the more effective treatments, the impact estimates are more precise, and the ability to detect even a small effect is enhanced. An adaptive study design is also fairer to participants that enroll in the later assignment rounds; they have a higher likelihood of receiving the treatment that would be the most effective. Nonetheless, implementing an adaptive design may be challenging. Some outcomes take a long time to observe, meaning long periods of time between each assignment round and measurement round. Measurement is also a particular challenge; outcome measurement and impact estimates, both of which can be difficult and time consuming in health care interventions, would need to be done efficiently and with enough time to make decisions about how to best calibrate the study for the next round of assignment.

SUMMARY

Because the same group cannot simultaneously be exposed and not be exposed to an intervention, the fundamental issue in rigorous outcome evaluation is how to estimate what would have happened to the treatment group if, all other things equal, they have not been exposed to the program. Accurately estimating the counterfactual situation makes it possible to isolate the program effect from the many other influences on outcomes; failure to appropriately estimate the counterfactual risks selection bias. In a well-designed randomized experiment with only one treatment, the outcomes observed in the control group act as an estimate of the observed and unobservable outcomes for the treatment group that would occur in the absence of treatment, the counterfactual.

With a method for estimating the counterfactual, three treatment effects were introduced in this chapter and the methods for estimating them were discussed. The average treatment effect (ATE) estimates the average effect on the population. In contrast, the average treatment effect on the treated (ATT) looks at the treatment effect on those who actually receive the intervention (because, in some studies, not all participants in the treatment group receive treatment). Finally, the intent-to-treat effect (ITT) estimates the treatment effects on those eligible for treatment. Which treatment effect is appropriate depends on what conclusions are to be drawn from the evaluation.

Finally, two randomized study designs were presented. Factorial and adaptive designs are attractive options for analyzing complex health care demonstrations and reaping the benefits of a random assignment mechanism. A factorial design is well-equipped for assessing interventions with multiple components. An adaptive design exploits rolling admission so that the most promising programs are likely to have the statistical power to detect even modest effects.

DISCUSSION QUESTIONS

1. Why is an RCT considered the gold standard in evaluation?

2. How important is it to consider contamination between intervention and control participants? At what point is it necessary to randomize at the group instead of individual level?

3. Describe real-world examples of ATE, ATT, and ITT in an evaluation of an intervention

to make the flu shot available to everyone in a state Medicaid program.

4. Find an example of the use of adaptive design in health care in the media. Share with your classmates to determine the conditions under which this approach is considered optimal.

NOTES

1. The simplest form of random assignment is not a typical feature of health-related evaluations and is not possible in most CMS demonstrations.

2. The discussion in this section draws on Imbens, G., and J. M. Wooldridge, "New developments in econometrics," Lecture Notes, CEMMAP, UCL2009b (2009), and describes what is widely referred to as the "Rubin Causal Model" after Rubin (1974). A recent, comprehensive treatment is in the book by Imbens and Rubin (2015). Imbens, G. W., and D. B. Rubin, *Causal Inference in Statistics, Social, and Biomedical Sciences* (New York: Cambridge University Press, 2015).

3. It is important in real-world research to understand, however, that what the control group receives cannot be assumed to be nothing. There are many other influences out there that need to be identified and measured by process research, so they can be netted out to identify the net treatment effect.

4. In the statistics literature, this assumption is referred to as the Stable-Unit-Treatment-Value Assumption, or SUTVA. Rubin, D. B., "Discussion of 'Randomization Analysis of Experimental Data in the Fisher Randomization Test' by Basu," *The Journal of the American Statistical Association* 75, no. 371 (1980): 591–93.

5. Imbens, G., and J. M. Wooldridge, "New developments in econometrics," Lecture Notes, CEMMAP, UCL2009b (2009). The notes include lists of studies that have modeled the spillover or interactive effects.

6. Rosner, B. *The Fundamentals of Biostatistics* (Pacific Grove, CA: Thomson-Brooks/Cole, 2006).

7. In the real world, of course, this counterfactual would not be literally randomly selected from the eligible population, although, as explained in this chapter, it can often come close.

8. LaLonde, R. J. "Evaluating the Econometric Evaluations of Training Programs with Experimental Data." *The American Economic Review* (1986): 604–20.

9. National Bureau of Economic Research Summer Institute (with Guido Imbens), "What's New in Econometrics?" Cambridge, MA. July/August 2007. Retrieved from http://www.nber.org/minicourse3.html.

10. If we assume, as shown in this chapter, that eligibility has no direct effect on the outcomes, then we can still index the potential outcomes as Y(W) for w = 0,1. The idea is that Z_i only influences Y(W) through its effect on participation, W_i.

11. There is, in principle, a fourth combination: (0,1) = not eligible, but with treatment in a contaminated control group. CMS takes special precautions to avoid contaminated control groups; when it does occur, the treatment effect is correspondingly weakened and becomes an underestimate of the "true" impact of the intervention.

Note that τ_{ATE} is not an appropriate measure in the case of nonconstant (heterogeneous) treatment effects, which can be very different among subgroups.

12. For example, an intervention in Rhode Island may involve 20 medical homes, each with 500 Medicare beneficiaries in a given year. With 10,000 beneficiaries, variances in costs at the patient level could be adjusted by the square root of 10,000 (i.e., 100) rather than the square root of 20 (i.e., 4.5).

13. Bloom, H. *Learning More from Social Experiments* (New York: Russell Sage Foundation, 2005), Chapter 4.

14. Greene, William H. *Econometric Analysis*. 7th ed. (Boston: Prentice Hall, 2012).

15. Angrist, Joshua, and Victor Lavy, "The Effects of High Stakes High School Achievement Awards: Evidence from a Randomized Trial," *The American Economic Review*, 99, no. 4 (2009): 1384–414.

16. Our discussion is drawn from American Institutes for Research (AIR), MDRC, MEF Associates, and Child Trends, *Head Start Professional Development: Design Options and Considerations for an Evaluation of Head Start Coaching*, eds. E. C. Howard, and K. V. Drummond. (Washington, DC: U.S. Department of Health and Human Services, Administration for Children and Families, Office of Planning, Research and Evaluation, 2014).

17. Ibid.

CHAPTER 6

Quasi-experimental Methods

Propensity Score Techniques

Jeff Wooldridge

Guido Imbens

Nikki Freeman

Rachael Zuckerman

Learning Objectives

We turn our attention to evaluation methods for observational, or quasi-experimental, designs. Because participants are not randomized into the treatment group(s) and comparison group, we cannot assume upfront that those receiving the treatment(s) and those who are not have similar baseline characteristics. This chapter discusses methods for constructing a group comparable to the treatment group for evaluation. Once a comparison group has been created, numerous treatment effect estimation techniques are available to the evaluator. We pay special attention to the types of data often encountered in health care program evaluations and the corresponding estimation strategies that are appropriate for those data structures.

As in Chapter 5, our goal in this chapter is to estimate causal effects, the difference between what happened with treatment and what would have happened without treatment. Unlike Chapter 5, we will assume that our data are observational rather than data from a randomized study. Two issues often arise when estimating treatment effects with observational data: selection bias and statistical nonindependence. We will deal with each issue in turn. This chapter addresses ways to approximate randomization by creating comparison groups. Then we move on to a discussion of unconfounded models where we think we have accounted for group differences, and confounded models, where we have not been able to approximate what would have happened without treatment. Finally, we address ways to treat data that have some underlying structures limiting independence, like geographic or provider-level clustering.

Selection bias occurs when systemic differences exist between those receiving treatment and those who are not. Consequently, differences between the treatment and nontreatment groups due to the intervention will be muddled with the underlying differences between the two groups. To address selection bias, we will first discuss unconfoundedness, the assumption that observable covariates can model the selection process. Comparison group construction, propensity score (PS) computation, and regression techniques will be our primary tools producing an unconfounded design.

We discuss methods for estimating treatment effect when it is not realistic to assume that observable covariates can control for confoundedness. If treatment assignment is thought to depend on unobserved factors that affect potential outcomes, instrumental variables can be applied. In other cases, the intervention's structure warrants a regression discontinuity design. In both cases, the kind of treatment effect that can be estimated is usually limited unless we are willing to make strong functional form and homogeneity restrictions.

Statistical dependence means that knowing something about one observation helps predict the outcome for a different observation—a problem frequently encountered with observational data. This may occur when a program or policy is implemented at the group level rather than at the individual level. For example, a program implemented at the hospital level may yield outcomes for each patient.

In this case, outcomes could be evaluated for each patient, yet the hospital a patient is admitted to is likely to affect the outcome. Dependencies may arise from geographic factors (e.g., clinics that are located near each other) or hierarchical groupings (e.g., patients within participating practices).

A special case of dependent data are longitudinal data in which multiple observations are taken on the same units over time. Depending on the number of time points available, either an interrupted time series design or difference-in-difference design may be appropriate.

Dealing With Selection Bias

Well-conducted randomization creates covariate balanced groups differing only in their receipt or nonreceipt of the treatment being tested. Even with randomization, covariate balance should be checked. This is especially true in studies with multiple time periods, where variable rates of attrition (or participants leaving the study) can have consequences for unconfoundedness assumptions. For example, if more participants assigned to the comparison leave the study because they feel they are not receiving a treatment of value, covariate balance is jeopardized. Without a random assignment mechanism, the researcher must *assume* that sufficient covariates are available to render assignment independent of the counterfactual outcomes.[1] The researcher is making the case that the available data permit modeling of the selection process, and after adjustment, that the assignment process is unaffected by preexisting covariates. This is the basis of an unconfounded design and our first method for dealing with selection bias.

Unconfounded Design

Unconfoundedness under a nonrandom assignment mechanism is a powerful but controversial assumption. It assumes that there are sufficient statistical controls to overcome any omitted variables that may be correlated with intervention participation or could bias treatment effects.[2] Accordingly, estimates of the average treatment effect (ATE) and average treatment effect on the treated (ATT) will be defined conditionally on a set of preprogram covariates such as age, income, preprogram health status, preprogram health insurance coverage, and zip code residence. To achieve unconfoundedness, the covariates must meet the following criteria.

Key Assumptions Justifying Unconfoundedness

Observed (measured) covariates: Unconfoundedness holds when nonrandom selection into treatment is explained by observable, measured, and available characteristics. If the assignment process relies on unobserved, unmeasured differences between treatment and comparison groups (e.g., the motivation to voluntarily participate in treatment), then unconfoundedness cannot be assumed.

Complete accounting of controls: Unconfoundedness can hold for a large set of controls but fail when the set of controls is reduced. For example, if eligibility for

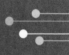
Suppose we are evaluating a job training program. Some people are assigned to participate, and others are not. Workers were randomized into the control or treatment group depending on low, medium, or high preprogram labor market earnings. Confoundedness arises because the probability of receiving treatment will generally differ across the three earnings classes, with those in the low-earnings group having a higher chance of being jobless and therefore treated, and those in the high-earnings group having a higher chance of being employed and lower chance of being treated. Defining X to be a measure of preprogram earnings, we can assert that treatment assignment is unconfounded conditional on X. That is, we can produce an unbiased estimate of average treatment effects, as long as we adjust for the nonrandom proportions of low and high earners who received treatment.

a job training program is determined by the prior 2 years of labor market history, but we condition only on the most recent year, unconfoundedness will generally fail. See Box 6.1 for an example of possible confoundedness in a job training program and how to deal with it.

Control variables are uninfluenced by treatment: Unconfoundedness can fail if we control for "too much" or "the wrong" variables. If the adjustment includes a postintervention measure that is also influenced by the treatment, then unconfoundedness generally fails. For example, in explaining *postprogram* annual health care costs for an individual, it is inappropriate to include postprogram health outcomes as a covariate. The treatment affects health outcomes which, in turn, affects health care costs. Including postprogram health status as a covariate reduces (biases downwards) the estimated treatment effect. By contrast, we should include *preprogram* health measures, because those are predictive of both future health costs and (probably) program participation.

Comparison Group Formation and Propensity Scores

Producing a convincing unconfounded design begins with construction of a comparison group. It is helpful to use the following steps:

- Describe the ideal (or target) population based on eventual scale of the program, and choose the group that will be used to develop the counterfactual (comparison) sample.

- Obtain the best data possible on both groups from the target population.

- For the two groups, assess the overlap in covariate distributions and calculate the PSs.

- Improve overlap by adjusting the sample.

- Assess, to the extent possible, the validity of the unconfoundedness assumption.[3]

In the sections that follow, we describe each of these steps in greater detail. Further methodological and statistical details can be found in Appendix B.

Describing the Target Population and Choosing Eligible Comparators

The first step in comparison group selection is identifying the population for which results are intended to generalize. This involves describing the ideal (or target) population *based on the eventual scale* of the program. For instance, if a new health payment system is aimed at essentially *all* medical practices, then the comparison population for estimating the ATE is *all* medical practices not participating in the new payment system. However, if a new insurance program is targeted at low-income families, then we are interested only in the program's potential impact on low-income families not participating in the evaluation. A representative sample of similarly low-income nonparticipants should comprise the comparison group.

Selecting the population of those eligible to be in the comparison group *based on the targeting* of the program increases the chances of an unconfounded design. Some early program evaluation studies were designed with the misperception that the relevant comparison population is somehow immutable. For example, it was believed that the comparison sample should be given to the researcher externally, perhaps defined by geography. Such a view can lead to unconvincing and unstable estimates of treatment effects. See Box 6.2 for a job training example.

Obtaining Data for the Treatment and Comparison Groups[4]

The hallmark of an unconfounded design is the assumption that, once we condition on (control for) an observed set of covariates, treatment assignment is unrelated to any pretreatment status or condition that would influence uptake or receipt of treatment. While it may seem obvious, obtaining the best data on each group is essential; without baseline data for the comparison and treatment groups, conducting an unconfounded design cannot go forward. A rich dataset of preintervention characteristics for both groups also allows us to develop effects for key baseline subgroups. For example, if it is reasonable to expect the treatment effect to differ among subgroups (say, men and women), separate ATEs and ATTs can be estimated.

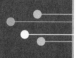

Box 6.2

Comparators Unlike Target Population in Job Training Evaluation

Consider an influential study in program evaluation by Lalonde who compared estimates from a randomized job training experiment with estimates obtained from nonexperimental data. Lalonde found that using the randomized experimental data on 450 men gave large, positive, and statistically significant estimates of job training on earnings. By contrast, depending on the particular estimation technique, the nonexperimental data produced a wide range of estimates. The initial reaction to Lalonde's finding was that applying econometric methods—regression or otherwise—to observational data, assuming selection on observables, was unlikely to produce good estimates of causal effects.

Reevaluating Lalonde's work reveals that the lack of overlap in the nonexperimental data is the source of the problem. Lalonde "constructed" the nonexperimental data in one case by taking a random sample of participants from the Panel Study of Income Dynamics (PSID) and using them as the control group for the treated group in the job training experiment. (The men drawn from the PSID were assumed to not have participated in job training during the relevant period.) But the male population represented by the PSID was very different from the population targeted by the job training study. For example, the average pretraining labor market earnings in the experimental sample, in 1978 dollars, was about $1,500, with a maximum of approximately $25,000. In the PSID sample, the average earnings were approximately $19,000 with a maximum of over $150,000. Using a random sample from the PSID and linear regression, LaLonde was essentially assuming that the target population was well represented by the PSID as a whole, whereas only a very small segment of that population actually "looked like" the job training participants.

Assessing Overlap and Creating the Propensity Score

Covariate balance means that the treatment group and comparison groups look the same across baseline characteristics. For example, if the treatment group is primarily older adults, then a comparison group of primarily younger adults would not be balanced on the covariate age. However, if the age distributions for the treatment group and comparison groups are similar, then there is balance between the groups on the age covariate. Of course, age is only one covariate that may bias treatment assignment. We will want to model treatment assignment as being unconfounded conditional on a rich set of control variables. Hence, we will need to ensure balance across all of the covariates.

Initial efforts to achieve group similarity focused on serially matching units in the treatment group with units in the comparison group on variables of interest. Serial matching designs, however, quickly become unwieldly with matching breaking down after only a few variables are considered. An alternative, the PS, combines all matching variables in a single common metric. It was identified in

1983 when Paul Rosenbaum and Donald Rubin demonstrated that when certain assumptions were met, adjustment for the scalar PS was sufficient to remove bias due to all observed covariates.[5] That is, rather than controlling for each covariate, the researcher can control for just the PS. Specifically, the PS is an estimate of the likelihood of treatment after controlling for baseline characteristics (for example, low income, uninsured, etc.). Throughout the rest of this chapter, we will write the PS as $e(x)$. Box 6.3 gives a technical description of the PS. Readers not interested in methodology are encouraged to skip Box 6.4.

Use the PS to ensure covariate balance in an iterative process. Treatment and comparison cases are matched on the proximity of scores to each other. Once they have been matched, covariate balance is assessed, and further adjusting may be required. The following three steps may be repeated several times to refine the comparison group before proceeding with treatment effect estimation.

Step 1: Choose variables to include in PS.

Step 2: Ensure that PS is balanced across treatment and comparison groups.

Step 3: Ensure that covariates are balanced across treatment and comparison groups within blocks of the PS.

Step 1. Choose the variables to include PS. The best data are the observable characteristics that *completely adjust* for treatment-comparison differences at baseline such that no material selection bias remains (see Box 6.5 for an example of control variables identified for the Medicare Multipayer Advanced Primary Care Practice [MAPCP] Demonstration). No set number or universal set of control variables will be appropriate for all analyses. The best data will include variables

Box 6.3
Rigorous Definition of the Propensity Score

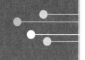

The PS is the conditional probability, $e(x)$, of an observation (e.g., patient, hospital, medical home) receiving treatment, W, conditional on the covariates, X:

$$e(x) = \text{Pb}[W = 1 \mid X = x] \qquad (6.1)$$

It is calculated using logistic regression with the treatment group (coded as 0 or 1) as the dependent variable. A probability (ranging from 0 to 1) is calculated for each case in the treatment and comparison groups.

theoretically related to treatment and outcome, available and easy to collect, and correlated with unmeasured confounders. There are also variables to avoid. These include variables that may be affected by the treatment and variables that predict the treatment status perfectly.

Step 2. Balance the propensity score across treatment and comparison groups. For every possible covariate outcome, it is necessary that each unit in the defined population has some chance of being treated and some chance of not being treated (see Box 6.4 for the rigorous expression of this condition). For example, if an insurance program targets people with chronic conditions, the probability that individuals with a chronic condition will participate in the program is much greater than the probability that those without a chronic condition will participate. Unless one makes the implausible assumption that health status at baseline is unrelated to health status and costs at outcome, including substantial numbers of persons without a chronic condition in the comparison— but not the treatment group—will not create an average treatment effect generalizable to persons without chronic conditions. It may also bias the results of the evaluation.

To assess the balance of the PSs, it is common to first study the full distributions of the PS scores in the treatment and comparison groups. A histogram can be used and generated with statistical software (see Figure 6.1 for a graphical example of a smoothed histogram). We should see sufficient overlap in the histograms of the estimated PSs to justify continuing the analysis of treatment effects. Intervention group subjects will often have higher PSs than those in the comparison pool, which is not surprising because they are, by design, in the treatment group to begin with. But, there has to be overlap; one can infer causal effects only for regions of overlap in the scores.

Box 6.4
Overlap Restriction of the PS

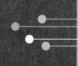

Technically, balance for the PS means that for all possible outcomes *x* of *X*, it is necessary that each unit in the defined population has some chance of being treated and some chance of not being treated, $0 < e(x) < 1$. The overlap restriction on the PS ensures that the possible values of the conditional distribution of X_i given $W_i = 1$ (treatment group) overlap completely with those of the conditional distribution of X_i given $W_i = 0$ (comparison group). Analyzing the overlap assumption and changing the sample, if necessary, to achieve "good overlap," have become important steps in any program evaluation that assumes unconfounded assignment.

Medicare participated in the Medicare Multipayer Advanced Primary Care Practice (MAPCP) Demonstration currently taking place in eight states (2012–2015). Hundreds of certified medical homes (PCMHs) are receiving monthly fees to provide added care management services to non-Medicare and Medicare beneficiaries. Research Triangle Institute (RTI) is conducting an impact evaluation of the demonstration on Medicare beneficiaries based on a range of quality, satisfaction, and cost outcomes. Comparison groups were formed for each state with nonparticipating medical homes taken either from within or proximate to each state. Once comparable PCMHs were identified, beneficiaries in them were screened using demonstration inclusion and exclusion criteria. Those meeting the criteria were eligible to form a comparison pool of beneficiaries. The next step was to balance the comparison and intervention groups using PSs.

PS are the probabilities that sampling units belong to the intervention group, conditional on a set of observable characteristics. In the MAPCP evaluation, the PS is the probability that a beneficiary is assigned to a MAPCP intervention practice. PSs were estimated from a series of logistic regression models that relate group status (MAPCP Demonstration or comparison group) to a set of beneficiary-, practice-, and region-level characteristics. The values of the beneficiary-level covariates were taken from the period prior to the start of a state's pilot activities. Practice- and region-level variables come from the demonstration period:

Beneficiary-level variables: age, sex, Hierarchical Condition Categories score, Charlson morbidity score, and indicators for white, disability status, Medicaid, end-stage renal disease status, and being institutionalized.

Practice- and region-level variables: median household income (in $10,000s), indicators for urbanity (rural, micropolitan, metropolitan), indicators for practice size (by number of physicians: solo, small [2–5], medium [6–10], large [>10]), and indicators for primary-care-only practices, multispecialty practices, federally qualified health centers, critical access hospitals, and rural health centers.

Step 3: Balance covariates within blocks of the propensity score. Creating PS balance is an iterative process of model construction, testing, refinement, and retesting until the best possible balance is achieved. Ideally, for every unique treated individual's PS, there is an exactly matched PS for an individual in the comparison group. Because the PS is a continuous measure, an exact match is generally not possible. The goal, therefore, is to create the closest balance possible, given the data available. This is done by checking the balance of each observed covariate within blocks of the PS. Some imbalance between the groups

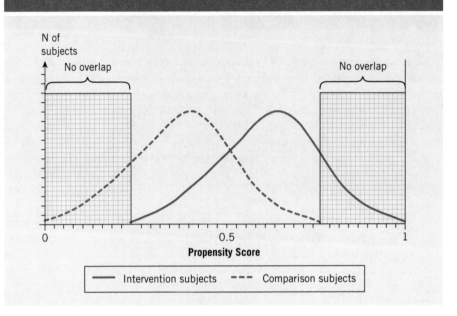

Figure 6.1   Hypothetical Distribution of Propensity Scores by Group, Showing Regions in Which Scores Do Not Overlap

is to be expected. When imbalance is detected, it is appropriate to reconsider the variables included in the propensity model. Variables that are theoretically the most important for predicting assignment to treatment are the most important to include. Consider interactions between covariates and discard variables that are less theoretically important or highly correlated with theoretically important variables. It may help to re-categorize variables, include higher-order terms, or use splines of variables. Box 6.6 discusses the calculations used for assessing covariate balance.

The net result of these procedures is a propensity-to-be-treated value attached to each unit in the treatment group, which aligns closely with a propensity-to-be-treated value for some unit(s) in the comparison groups. Before moving to how this score can be incorporated in analysis, it is worth recalling that PSs only balance measured confounders. This does not indicate balance in any unmeasured variables that may still bias treatment effect estimates in several settings. When using PSs, it is appropriate always to consider the potential of unmeasured variables biasing the treatment effect estimates. In fact, Judea Pearl has argued that hidden bias may actually increase because matching on observed variables may unleash bias due to dormant unobserved confounders and proposes a simple graphical test, called the "back-door criterion" to detect the presence of confounding variables.[6]

Box 6.6
How to Assess Covariate Balance

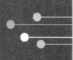

Assessing the balance between groups involves estimating the standardized difference between the groups for each variable in your analysis. For continuous variables the formula is

$$d = \frac{\left(\bar{x}_{treatment} - \bar{x}_{comparison}\right)}{\sqrt{\dfrac{s^2_{treatment} + s^2_{comparison}}{2}}}$$

while for dichotomous variables the formula is

$$d = \frac{\left(\hat{p}_{treatment} - \hat{p}_{comparison}\right)}{\sqrt{\dfrac{\hat{p}_{treatment}\left(1 - \hat{p}_{treatment}\right) + \hat{p}_{comparison}\left(1 - \hat{p}_{comparison}\right)}{2}}}$$

Large standardized differences (>10) could indicate a problem with covariate balance and the need for model refinement. Ideally, the standardized differences for each covariate will be near 0.

Comparison Group Refinement

Once the PSs are calculated and covariate balance has been refined, the PSs are used to refine the comparison group and sometimes directly incorporated into treatment effect analyses. Several strategies for refining the comparison group exist, and unfortunately, none are optimal in every instance. The choice of strategy typically involves a tradeoff between the quality of the match and the quantity of data available for analysis. Matching strategies reduce bias at the expense of sample size. Weighting reduces bias and retains the bulk of the sample that is sensitive to individuals with extreme PSs. Which strategy is best can only be assessed by examining the covariate balance using each method and selecting the one that has the best balance and still meets the analytical goal. The principal strategies are stratification, nearest neighbor, caliper or radius matching, kernel and local linear matching, and inverse probability of treatment weighting. Each is introduced briefly below.

Stratification

Stratification on the PS offers the simplest approach. Units are first ranked according to their estimated PS and then, using previously defined thresholds of the estimated PS, stratified into mutually exclusive subsets. Five groups is generally sufficient to eliminate approximately 90% of the bias due to measured confounders when estimating a linear treatment effect. The effect of treatment on outcomes is then estimated within each stratum, and the overall treatment effect is the weighted average of the within strata results. When the strata are equally sized, weighting by the inverse of the number of strata provides an estimate of the ATE. Weighting by the proportion of treated subjects that lie within each stratum allow one to estimate the ATT.[7] The principal advantage of stratification is its simplicity. The principal disadvantage is that it discards observations in blocks where either treated or control units are absent.

Nearest Neighbor Matching

In nearest neighbor matching, all treated units are listed, and the comparison unit with the closest matching PS is paired with each treated patient. Once all treated units are matched, the unmatched comparison units are deleted. Several variations on this method are available, including matching with or without replacement and optimal versus "greedy" matching. In optimal matching, pairs are formed to minimize the total within-pair difference of the PS. In greedy matching, a treatment unit is selected at random, and the untreated unit whose PS is closest is chosen for matching without replacement—even if a later treated unit's PS is closer to the comparison unit's score. This is repeated until all treatment units are matched. The principal advantage of the nearest neighbor approach is that all treated units are included in the analysis. The principal disadvantages are that information is lost from the unmatched units in the comparison group, potentially restricting the variance in the analysis, and that the nearest match in the comparison group may have a very different PS, resulting in increased bias.

Caliper Matching

A variation on nearest neighbor matching is caliper or radius matching. In this approach, a maximum permissible difference ("caliper") is selected (often .2 standard deviation of the logit of the PS is used) that will be used to define the match. These methods consider PS matches that fall within the specified caliper. In caliper matching, only one comparison unit closest to the treated unit is selected; in radius matching, all comparison units within the caliper are included in the sample. If no within-caliper match is found, individuals from both treatment and comparison groups are dropped from the sample. The principal advantage of the radius matching approach is that there is often less bias in the analysis as the comparability of groups is improved. The principal disadvantage is that observations are lost from both the treatment and comparison groups.

Kernel and Local-Linear Matching

Kernel and local-linear matching are nonparametric matching estimators that compare the outcome of each treated person to a weighted average of the outcomes of all the untreated persons, with the highest weight being placed on those with scores closest to the treated individual. Kernel matching can be seen as a weighted regression of the counterfactual outcome on an intercept with weights given by the kernel weights and is appropriate when the kernel is symmetric, nonnegative, and unimodal. If the comparison group observations are distributed asymmetrically around the treated observation, or when there are gaps in the PS distribution, then the local-linear approach is preferred. One major advantage of these approaches is the lower variance, which is achieved because more information is used. A drawback of these methods is that some of the observations used may be poor matches. Hence, the proper imposition of the common-support condition is of major importance for these approaches.[8] These approaches provide an average treatment effect.

Propensity Score Weighting

Many matching algorithms limit the generalizability of findings by omitting a significant proportion of the population when comparison groups are being constructed, and they may result in units in the treatment and comparison groups being clinically indistinguishable. An approach that makes fewer distributional assumptions about the underlying data is inverse probability of treatment weighting (IPTW). Using the IPTW approach, units in the treatment group are assigned a weight of 1/PS, while each unit in the comparison group receives a weight of 1/(1–PS). This approach has the advantage of including all the data (unless weights are set to 0); however, it has the disadvantage of being sensitive to extreme propensity values such as when a unit with a low probability of being treated is included in the treatment group. For example, a PS = .05 in the treatment group would have a weight of [1–.05]/.05[1–.05] = 20, while a PS = .95 would have a weight of .05/.0475 = 1.053. Thus, estimates of the ATE with IPTW can be sensitive to the estimated PSs; when estimating mean performance of the treated group, treated observations with PSs close to zero receive substantial weight as do comparison observations with PS close to unity. Constraining observations to those with PS between 10% and 90% makes the ATE estimate using PS weighting much less sensitive to changes in specification of the PS.[9] An example of IPTW is provided in Box 6.7.

Assessing the Comparison Group

Multiple checks are necessary to assess balance in sample-matched or weighted PS models. Keep evaluating the standardized differences in the matched sample and visually inspecting distributions using histograms and graphs of covariate balance. For unweighted continuous variables, the covariate mean in the treated group is

Box 6.7

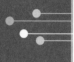

Constructing Propensity Score Regression Weights in
the Medicare Multipayer Advanced Primary Care
Practice Demonstration

Box 6.5 provided a general description of the Medicare Multipayer Advanced Primary Care Practice (MAPCP) Demonstration, how the propensity scores (PSs) were estimated, and how they were used for selecting a comparison group. In this example, we show how outcomes were weighted by beneficiaries' likelihood of participating in the multivariate analyses of intervention effects. The weights for beneficiaries assigned to comparison practices incorporate the "normalized odds"

$$\frac{PS}{1-PS} \div mean\left(\frac{PS}{1-PS}\right)$$

The first term, $\frac{PS}{1-PS}$, is the odds ratio, and the second term, $mean\left(\frac{PS}{1-PS}\right)$, is a normalizing constant calculated by taking the mean over beneficiaries in the comparison group.

Considering only the weight, that is, the odds ratio part, and ignoring the normalizing constant, if a comparison beneficiary had a PS equal to 0.75, he or she is fairly similar to the typical demonstration beneficiary, and the PS weight would be $\frac{0.75}{0.25}=3.0$. Alternatively, a score of 0.25 would result in propensity odds of $\frac{0.25}{0.75}=\frac{1}{3}$, which is low because this person does not "look like" the average demonstration beneficiary.

The weighted comparison group is more similar to beneficiaries in the MAPCP Demonstration group in terms of the characteristics (covariates) that determine the PS. As such, the effect of weighting is similar to the effect of randomization in experimental designs by effectively "creating" more beneficiaries in the comparison group who are typical of intervention beneficiaries.

dot-plotted against the covariate mean in the comparison group. For weighted continuous variables, density plots are created for each group and compared. Finally, the ratio of the variances both before and after matching or weighting should also be checked to confirm it is near 1. Values less than ½ or greater than 2 should be considered extreme. Combined, the satisfactory results from these multiple tests increase the likelihood that covariates are balanced across treatment and comparison groups and analysis of the treatment effects can begin. Keep in mind, however, that the results of analyses using propensity matching or weighting hold only for the region of common support, that is, for the range of covariate values shared by the treatment and comparison groups. Confirming the overlap and recognizing the region of common support between treatment and comparison group is central to interpreting findings. Confirming the existence of potential

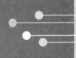

Box 6.8
Propensity Score Performance

The primary problem with nonrandomized designs is the potential for selection bias—that is, that a nonrandomized comparison group may not provide an accurate estimate of the counterfactual outcome, leading to a systematic over- or underestimate of the true treatment effect. The amount of selection bias in a study cannot be directly observed, but in some cases, the bias may be small enough that it would not affect policy decisions about whether the treatment was worthwhile.

When a randomized study is available for comparison, the extent of selection bias has sometimes been assessed by comparing the experimental estimate of the treatment effect to the estimate obtained using nonrandomized comparison groups. Some such comparisons for job training programs have found selection bias in the non-RCT case to be substantial. These analyses, however, have been criticized for their use of poorly matched comparison groups (see Box 6.2). More recent studies of educational interventions using better matched comparison groups indicate that the bias may be much smaller.

Bifulco evaluated an experimental study about the impact of attending magnet schools. Students were randomly assigned to schools by lottery. Bifulco created three nonrandomized comparison groups from different geographic areas. Students comprising these comparison groups were different in several respects from the magnet school treatment group, as shown in Table 6.1. Comparison students in the first two were generally less affluent than the magnet schools' treatment group, while comparison students in the third comparison group were more affluent.

Table 6.1   Magnet School Analysis Comparison Groups

Comparison Group	Geographic Area	Significant Differences From Treatment Group
Comparison Group 1	Same school districts as treatment	Fewer white students More free-lunch-eligible students Lower Grade 6 reading scores
Comparison Group 2	School districts in New Haven metropolitan area	More free-lunch-eligible students
Comparison Group 3	All nontreatment school districts in Hartford area	More white students Higher Grade 6 reading scores

(Continued)

(Continued)

In the RCT, the primary outcome were Grade 8 reading scores measured 2 years after the magnet school lottery. The experimental estimated effect of magnet school attendance on the treated was 0.269 reading score standard deviations greater than the pretreatment scores. The forest plot in Figure 6.1 compares the 95% confidence interval for the experimental effect size to the nonexperimental effects estimated using the three comparison groups. Three statistical adjustment methods (which will be discussed later in this chapter) are summarized for each group below:

Method 1: Ordinary least squares (OLS) using student characteristics without pretreatment reading and math scores

Method 2: OLS using student characteristics including pretreatment reading and math scores

Method 3: PS weighting using student characteristics including pretreatment scores

Figure 6.2 shows the nonexperimental effects and confidence intervals estimated with the three comparison groups and three methods. Methods 2 and 3 closely mirror the experimental effect size estimate of attending a magnet school for the first two comparison groups. Failing to adjust for pretreatment scores, Method 1 led to overestimates of the magnet school effect in these two groups. The estimates were uniformly smaller using the third comparison group, suggesting that the available student characteristics did not fully adjust for geographic misalignment. This magnet school example shows that selection bias can be trivial in nonexperimental designs with carefully chosen covariates and comparison groups.

Figure 6.2   Nonexperimental Estimates of Magnet School Effects on Eighth-Grade Reading Scores

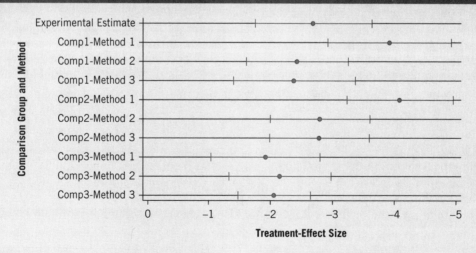

Note: Standard errors based on the midpoint of the range of potential group variance covariances.

matches in the comparison group is sufficient for estimating ATT. For estimating ATE, it is also required that the combinations of characteristics in the comparison group are observed in the treatment group.[10]

Improving Overlap

If results are unsatisfactory for any of the models, Rosenbaum and Rubin recommend modifying the initial PS model by adding interaction or nonlinear terms to model the relationship between continuous covariates and treatment status.[11] In considering these alternate models, statistical significance should not be used as a guide for covariate inclusion because it is confounded by sample size. Similarly, the c-statistic (which indicates the degree to which the PS model discriminates between subjects who are treated and those who are untreated) should not be used to assess balance as it provides no information as to whether the PS model has been correctly specified.

After the iterative process of optimizing covariate balance, one might wonder just how well do PSs perform in approximating the counterfactual when compared to estimates derived from RCTs. Box 6.8 presents work on this question.[12,13]

Regression and Regression on the Propensity Score to Estimate Treatment Effects

After PS matching or weighting, the PS-adjusted comparison group along with the treatment group can be used to estimate treatment effects in the outcome model. We begin our discussion of estimating treatment effects with a simple regression model. Later in this chapter, we will discuss situations in which the information available (such as the structure of the data or the study design) can be exploited by more complex modelling to yield treatment effects. The remainder of this chapter utilizes linear regression techniques extensively. Box 6.9 presents a brief refresher on multiple regression. Readers familiar with regression may skip Box 6.10.

Regression

The key to unconfounded regression adjustment methods is to ensure that the average outcomes of the intervention and comparison groups reflect the corresponding true counterfactual means after adjusting for potential confounders. On the assumption of sufficient covariate overlap between the comparison and intervention groups, estimation of the mean outcome for the comparison group and the mean outcome for the treatment group is straightforward using linear regression,[14] which can work well provided we have good approximations to the conditional mean functions.[15] The technical details of how one might use regression to control for confounders and estimate treatment effects is given in Box 6.10.

Box 6.9
How to Interpret Regression

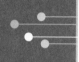

Linear regression is a method for modelling the relationship between a response variable (sometimes called dependent variables) and a set of one or more explanatory variables (sometimes called regressors, independent variables, or predictors). For each observation, the value of the response and the explanatory variables is observed. The classical linear regression model has fundamental underlying assumptions, and from that starting point, regression theory has been developed to relax those assumptions. Rather than list the assumptions, something one could find in an introductory econometrics or statistics textbook, we highlight a few important aspects of linear regression that will help the reader understand the material in this chapter.

First, linear regression assumes that the relationship between the response variable and the explanatory variables is linear. Symbolically, we can write the relationship as

$$y_i = \beta_0 + \beta_1 x_{i1} + \cdots + \beta_K x_{iK} + \varepsilon_i, \quad i = 1, \cdots, n \tag{6.2}$$

where y_i is the response variable for the i-th observation, $x_{i1}, \ldots, x_{iK}$ are a set of K predictors observed on the i-th observation, $\beta_0, \ldots, \beta_K$ are unknown parameters to be estimated, and ε_i is an unobserved error term. Although linearity may seem restrictive, some nonlinearities can be accommodated; in some cases, it is possible to transform regressors to ensure linearity. At other times, it may be necessary to use nonlinear regression, a topic that we will not address in this regression refresher.

Second, most linear regression analyses, and all of those in this chapter, give us information about what happens *on average* to the response variable for different levels of the explanatory variables. Mathematically we have,

$$E[y|x_1, \ldots, x_K] = \beta_0 + \beta_1 x_1 + \cdots + \beta_K x_K \tag{6.3}$$

that is, for fixed values of $x_1, \ldots, x_K$, the average value of y is a linear combination of $x_1, \ldots, x_K$ and to compute this average, all that is needed are estimates of the unknown parameters $\beta_0, \ldots, \beta_K$. *Regression* in *linear regression* just refers to the method for estimating $\beta_0, \ldots, \beta_K$. Once they are estimated, the average of the dependent variable given set values of the explanatory variables can be ascertained.

Sometimes in linear regression analyses, we are interested in a specific parameter estimate, say β_k. We put a "hat" on β_k to distinguish it as the regression estimate of β_k. Why would one be interested in β_k? Careful examination of Equation 6.2 elucidates one important reason: β_k estimates the partial effect of x_k on the response variable y ceteris paribus. In other words, β_k estimates how much y will increase or decrease when x_k increases by one unit, while holding all the values of the other explanatory variables fixed. Of course, increasing x_k by 1 does not make sense if x_k is not continuous, such as the case when x_k is a dummy variable for the treatment group. The interpretation of β_k is slightly different in this case: Suppose $x_k = 1$ for observations in the treatment group and 0 for observations in the comparison group. Then the estimate β_k is the average difference in y observed for those in the treatment group compared to the comparison group ceteris paribus (controlling for the other explanatory variables).

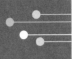

Box 6.10
Using Regression to Estimate the Average Treatment Effect and Average Treatment Effect on the Treated

Considering a single covariate, x, we have:

$$\mu_1(x) = \alpha_1 + x\beta_1 \tag{6.4}$$

$$\mu_0(x) = \alpha_0 + x\beta_0 \tag{6.5}$$

where μ_0 and μ_1 are the regression models for the intervention and comparison groups, respectively, conditioned on x. The ATE, a measure based on the entire population, can then be estimated by averaging the covariate x. Thus,

$$\hat{\tau}_{ATE,reg} = \hat{\mu}_1 - \hat{\mu}_0 = (\hat{\alpha}_1 - \hat{\alpha}_0) + x^*(\hat{\beta}_1 - \hat{\beta}_0) \tag{6.6}$$

where x^* is the average of the covariate, $\hat{\alpha}_1$ and $\hat{\beta}_1$ are the estimated parameters from Equation 6.4, and $\hat{\alpha}_0$ and $\hat{\beta}_0$ are the estimated parameters from Equation 6.5. Although we have illustrated the regression adjustment method using a single covariate, it is easily extended to cases with a vector of covariates.

An equivalent regression specification that pools all the intervention and comparison data can be used to obtain the ATE. Illustrating this specification with a single covariate, x, we have

$$Y_i = \alpha + \beta_1 W_i + \beta_2 X_i + \beta_3 W_i \left[X_i - x^* \right] + \varepsilon_i \tag{6.7}$$

Here, the ATE is estimated by $\hat{\beta}_1$, the regression estimated coefficient on assignment (W_i). To estimate the more restricted ATT effect, we simply center the covariate x about the average of the covariates x^* in the *treated* subsample.

Regression on the Propensity Score

If a PS has been established using matching methods, the PS can be used as a regression covariate. Results from this approach are referred to as "adjusted means" or "adjusted odds ratios," depending on whether a linear or logistic model is estimated. The regression specification is given in Box 6.11.

One might wonder why regression on the PS would be used when we could use regression on the covariates. Both methods assume that all potential confounders are observable and control for them, either directly as in regression or indirectly through the PS. However, the confounders controlled for in the regression model are those that confound the outcome of the treatment, and

Box 6.11
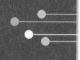

Regression on the Propensity Score

In this method, the outcome variable is regressed on a variable indicating treatment status, W_i, and on the estimated PS, $e(X_i)$,

$$Y_i = \alpha + \beta_1 W_i + \beta_2 e(X_i) + \varepsilon_i \qquad (6.8)$$

The impact of treatment is the estimated regression coefficient $\hat{\beta}_1$ from the fitted regression model. That is, after controlling for the probability of assignment to the treatment group, $\hat{\beta}_1$ is the effect on the treated compared to the comparators.

the confounders that are controlled for in the PS are those that confound selection into the treatment group. Often, it is easier to select and obtain the variables that might bias selection than the variables that might bias the outcome. Furthermore, we recall from our discussion of the PS that it has been shown that controlling for the probability of treatment, the PS, is enough to eliminate bias due to observable covariates.

Combining Regression and Propensity Score Weighting

Weighting intervention and comparison groups by their respective inverse probability weights produces mean differences with the smallest asymptotic variance possible.[16,17] Given this, why should we combine multivariate regression adjustment with PS weighting? Recall that if assignment is unconfounded conditional on covariates, then assignment also is unconfounded conditional on the PSs,[18] and we can base regression adjustment *solely* on estimates of the PS rather than on the entire set of covariates in a second regression. However, it is known theoretically that combining regression adjustment and PS estimation can lead to "doubly robust" estimates of the ATE—on the assumption that *either* the conditional mean *or* PS models are correctly specified.[19] Box 6.12 discusses some of the technical details of combining regression and PS weighting. Further details on use of the PS in unconfounded design can be found in Appendix B.

Box 6.12

Estimation Details for Combining Regression and Propensity Score Weighting

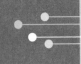

In the case of linear regression with covariates, one should estimate two models, one for the treated sample using $1/PS_i$ as weights and a second for estimating the parameters for the comparison group using $1/(1 - PS_i)$ as weights. Having obtained the estimates, the expression for the ATE is the same as the difference in average predicted values of the intervention and comparison groups.

If outcomes are binary or take values in the unit interval, one should use the logistic function. One other useful case is when outcomes are greater or equal to zero, in which case exponential mean functions should be used, and the primary function should be the log-likelihood for the Poisson distribution.

SUMMARY

This chapter surveyed the machinery of modeling observational data in health care program evaluation. It began with comparison group construction, using PSs to create a comparison group with baseline characteristics similar to those of the treatment group. In some cases, once a comparison group is available, simple regression techniques can adequately model the data and yield treatment effects. In other cases, other statistical approaches are required.

DISCUSSION QUESTIONS

1. Explain selection bias and how it could affect evaluation results.

2. How do PSs methods address selection? Under what conditions are they a complete solution?

3. What might you consider to assess whether a PS method was ameliorating the quality of the comparison?

4. What does "doubly robust" mean in this chapter?

NOTES

1. See Imbens and Rubin (2015, Chapter 12) for an extensive discussion of such situations. Imbens, G. W., and D. B. Rubin. *Causal Inference in Statistics, Social, and Biomedical Sciences* (Cambridge University Press, 2015).

2. Imbens, G. W. "Nonparametric Estimation of Average Treatment Effects Under Exogeneity: A Review." *Review of Economics and Statistics*, 86 no. 1 (2004): 4–29.

3. Unconfoundedness cannot be tested, only assessed. Imbens and Rubin (2015, Chapter 12) offer three methods: Estimate the effect of treatment on unaffected outcome, estimate the effect of pseudo-treatment on outcome, and assess the sensitivity of treatment estimates to choice of pretreatment variables.

4. LaLonde, R. J. "Evaluating the Econometric Evaluations of Training Programs with Experimental Data." *The American Economic Review* 76 no. 4 (1986): 604–20.

5. Rosenbaum, P. R., and D. B. Rubin. "The Central Role of the Propensity Score in Observational Studies for Causal Effects." *Biometrika*, 70 no. 1 (1983): 41–55.

6. Pearl, J. "Comment: Graphical Models, Causality and Intervention." *Statistical Science*, (1993): 266–69.

7. Imbens, 2004.

8. Heinrich, C., A. Maffioli, and G. Vazquez. *A Primer for Applying Propensity-score Matching: Inter-American Development Bank* (Washington, DC: IADB, 2010).

9. Simulation evidence by Busso, Dinardo, and McCrary shows that the weighting used in Equation 6.5 does not produce estimators with the best finite-sample properties, primarily because the weights on Y_i are not guaranteed to sum to unity. A weighted least squares formulation tends to work better. Thus, to obtain μ_1, regress Y_i using the treated observations on 1.0 with weights $1/\hat{e}(X_i)$, producing a fully nonparametric regression. Perform the same regression model using control observations with weights $1/[1 - \hat{e}(X_i)]$ to obtain μ_0. The evaluator can use a pooled regression of Y_i on 1 and W_i using weights $[W_i/\hat{e}_i + (1 - W_i)/[1 - \hat{e}_i]]$. The coefficient on W_i is the estimate of τate. If the weights are chosen as $[W_i + (1 - W_i)/e_i[(1 - \hat{e}_i)]]$ in the regression, the W_i coefficient is a consistent estimator of ATT. Busso, M., J. DiNardo, and J. McCrary, "New Evidence on the Finite Sample Properties of Propensity Score Reweighting and Matching Estimators," *The Review of Economics and Statistics* 96 no. 5 (December 2014): 885–97.

10. Bryson A., R. Dorsett, and S. Purdon. *The Use of Propensity Score Matching in the Evaluation of Labour Market Policies*, Working Paper No. 4 (Department for Work and Pensions, 2002).

11. Rosenbaum P. R., and D. B. Rubin, "Reducing Bias in Observational Studies Using Subclassification on the Propensity Score." *Journal of the American Statistical Association* 79 (1984): 516–24.

12. Bifulco, R. "Can Nonexperimental Estimates Replicate Estimates Based on Random Assignment in Evaluations of School Choice? A Within-Study Comparison." *Journal of Policy Analysis and Management*, 31 no. 3 (2012): 729–51.

13. Ibid.

14. Depending on the nature of the outcome, *Y*, we might want to use other functional forms. For example, if *Y* is a count variable, we can use an exponential functional form and a quasi-maximum likelihood method. Several possibilities are discussed in Wooldridge (2010, Chapter 21).

15. One way to address an overlap problem is to estimate the ATE for a restricted subpopulation determined by values of X_i. Using local estimation methods, such as kernel regression or local linear regression, provides more flexibility and will tend to make any overlap problems apparent. There should be none of these, however, because the evaluator should already have addressed any concerns with overlap before applying any regression adjustment. Heckman, J. J., H. Ichimura, and P. E. Todd. "Matching as an Econometric Evaluation Estimator: Evidence from Evaluating a Job Training Programme." *The Review of Economic Studies*, 64 no. 4 (1997):

605–54; Heckman, J., H. Ichimura, J. Smith, and P. Todd. *Characterizing Selection Bias Using Experimental Data* (No. w6699) (Cambridge, MA: National Bureau of Economic Research, 1998).

16. Hirano, K., G. W. Imbens, and G. Ridder. *Efficient Estimation of Average Treatment Effects using the Estimated Propensity Score.* Research Paper Number C02-13. (Los Angeles, CA: USC Center for Law, Economics and Organization, University of Southern California Law School, 2003).

17. Li, Q., J. S. Racine, and J. M. Wooldridge. "Estimating Average Treatment Effects with Continuous and Discrete Covariates: The Case of Swan–Ganz Catheterization." *The American Economic Review* 98, no. 2 (2008): 357–62.

18. Imbens, 2004.

19. Imbens, G. M., and J. M. Wooldridge. *Recent Developments in the Econometrics of Program Evaluation* (No. w14251) (Cambridge, MA: National Bureau of Economic Research, 2008).

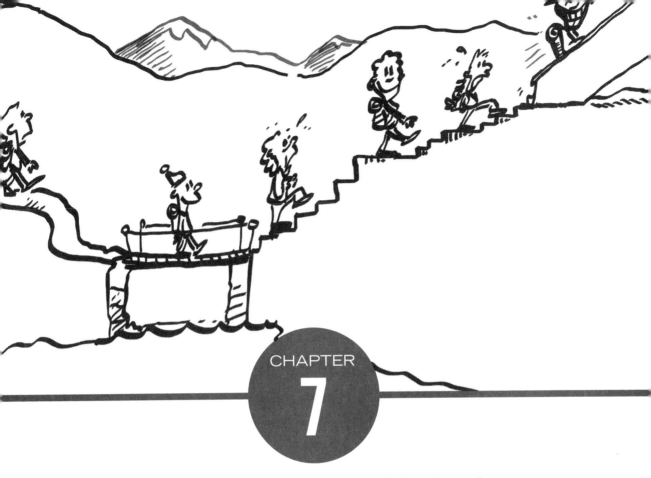

Quasi-experimental Methods

Regression Modeling and Analysis

Jeff Wooldridge

Guido Imbens

Nikki Freeman

Rachael Zuckerman

Steven Sheingold

John Orav

If we have managed to create a comparison group, assess covariate balance, and feel comfortable that we have met the standards for an unconfounded design, there are several modeling options available. In this section, we address interrupted time series (ITS) designs, comparative interrupted time series (CITS) designs, and difference-in-difference (DID) models. In a following section, we address models appropriate for situations where we cannot meet the requirements of unconfoundedness.

Interrupted Time Series Designs

ITS models have become increasingly popular as quasi-experimental designs used to evaluate policies and programs. Under appropriate conditions, these designs can be used to imply causality, and indeed, they have been shown to produce similar results to randomized experiments.[1] One reason for the growing popularity and use of these methods is the availability of longitudinal data. The term *longitudinal data* describes data collected on the same units for the same variables at intervals over time. It is particularly useful for when data are available for the preintervention period and the postintervention period, and when the intervention takes place at a specific, identifiable point in time. The time relationship between the data points can be used to estimate treatment effects. In this section, we consider three study designs when longitudinal data are available, and the statistical techniques that can be used to implement these designs:

1. Interrupted time series

2. Comparative interrupted time series

3. Difference-in-difference

For the first of these designs, the counterfactual is established based on the intervention group's preintervention trend. In the second two designs, a comparison group's trend postimplementation is used as the counterfactual.

Basic Interrupted Time Series

The term *interrupted time series* refers to the situation in which multiple observations for the treatment group are available both before and after the intervention. That is, the intervention is the potential interruption in the trend. In this basic ITS design, there is no comparison group of individuals or units that were not exposed to the intervention or program. The design is based on repeated measurements before and after the implementation of an intervention. That is, it makes full use of the longitudinal data by enabling the comparison of pre- and postintervention trends. The trends from the preintervention period establish a baseline that is used to project what would be expected in the absence of intervention. Intervention effects are demonstrated when the observations gathered after the intervention deviate from the expectations derived from the baseline projections.

Requirements for Using Interrupted Time Series

Making inferences using an ITS approach requires data for a time period before and after when intervention is implemented. That is, we assume that the intervention happens at a distinct point in time. As such, the intervention is the interruption—there is a clear distinction between pre- and postperiods. This does not mean the implementation must occur quickly, as in flipping an on/off switch, but the implementation period must be well known so that it can be modelled separately if needed.[2]

The timing of outcomes is also important in determining the appropriateness of ITS. The expected change in the measured outcomes should occur within a relatively short time period after the intervention is implemented. For example, ITS may be appropriate for examining the impact of a stress reduction program on measured blood pressure, but not for the potential impact on medical events such as strokes—an impact that would likely occur only after a much longer time period. Finally, regardless of which outcome is chosen, it must be defined and measured consistently across the entire pre- and postperiods chosen.

There is no strict answer to the question of how many time points are needed in the pre- and postperiods. The power of the study depends on the variability and distribution of the data, strength of the effect, and confounding influences such as seasonality.[3]

Assumptions for Drawing Inferences

The ITS design is often considered a powerful method for evaluating the effects of an intervention and the next best alternative to the randomized experiment. However, such credentials for drawing inferences about causality can only be realized under a strict set of conditions. In basic ITS, there is no comparison group, so the counterfactual is established as the continuation of the preintervention trend for the treated group. The intervention impact is estimated as the difference between the actual postintervention trend and the preintervention trend extended. Thus, the most important of these assumptions is there are no other external events occurring, which would affect the postintervention trend. Likewise, it must be assumed there are no changes occurring naturally in the sampled units that would cause a change in the postintervention time period absent from the intervention.

A good example of these issues and their effect on evaluation conclusions comes from the Partnership for Patients (PfP) program implemented in 2011 by The Center for Medicare and Medicaid Innovation (CMMI). The campaign was launched with the ambitious goals of reducing preventable hospital-acquired conditions (HACs) by 40% and 30-day hospital readmissions by 20%. To reduce harm at this level of magnitude, the campaign implemented a strategy to align all health care stakeholders, including federal and other public and private health care payers, providers, and patients, to focus on this issue concurrently. By influencing everyone to move in the same direction at the same time, the program strove to overcome the inherently limited reach of any single initiative operating in a complex environment. The program was national in scope, due to its level of implementation. For example, over 70% of general acute care hospitals in the United States, representing over 80% of admissions, worked with PfP-funded Hospital Engagement Networks (HENs) during 2012–2013. This meant that constructing a valid comparison group was impossible and that ITS was an option for evaluating the program.

At the same time, Medicare was implementing several other policies and programs to affect similar hospital outcomes. Despite finding large reduction in some of the key outcomes, the evaluation could not attribute them to the PfP.

> Since hospital payment policies and other U.S. Department of Health & Human Services (HHS) programs that played an important role as part of the PfP campaign were in place and making changes over time, it is not possible at this time for the evaluation to identify the portion of these harm reductions and savings attributable to the PfP campaign's direct work with hospitals versus alignment of forces for harm reduction versus other harm reduction work that would have continued with or without PfP.[4]

In other words, it was easy to identify other external factors that would likely influence the outcomes. Therefore, while it was clear that quality as measured by several indicators was improving, CMMI could not use the evaluation results to clearly demonstrate that PfP was an effective program. In a following section, we discuss one method of avoiding such situations: using comparative ITS designs.

There are also other issues to consider in using time series data. Particularly when using relatively small time increments (weekly, monthly, or quarterly data), it is necessary to detect whether there are cyclical or seasonal influences that normally affect outcomes in a way that could bias the difference between pre- and postperiods. Likewise, the outcome in any period may be most closely related to the previous period, meaning autocorrelation may be a problem. Once visualization and diagnostics determine these issues exist, appropriate adjustments can be made to the data before applying the regression techniques described in the next section.

Estimation Methods for Interrupted Time Series

The most popular current statistical method for analyzing ITS data is called *segmented regression*.[5] Segmented regression focuses on two parameters: the level (intercept) and the trend (slope). For the observations before the intervention, one will have a level (intercept), trend (slope), and maybe even cyclicity. After the intervention, the data may exhibit changes in any one of these features. The change may be permanent or transient, and immediate or delayed. The fundamental idea behind segmented regression is to estimate a linear regression model for the data points from before the intervention and estimate a linear regression model

Figure 7.1   Graphical Analysis of Interrupted Time Series Models

Analysis: Graphical

a. An interrupted time series model with good results:
   Immediate, but no long-term, benefit

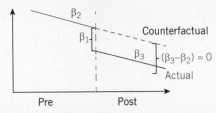

b. An interrupted time series model with ideal results:
   Both immediate and long-term benefits

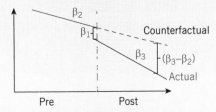

c. An interrupted time series model with good results:
   Long-term, but no immediate, benefit

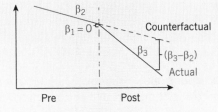

for the data points from after the intervention. The level and trend before and after the intervention are then compared. Box 7.1 provides the estimation details.

As an example, let's assume a program is implemented with an intention to reduce hospital-related adverse events for patients. Figures 7.1a to 7.1c demonstrate three situations that might occur if the program meets its objectives. In Figure 7.1a, there is an immediate reduction in the target rate of adverse events, but the trend continues on the same trajectory as before the intervention period (change in intercept but not the slope for the post). In Figure 7.1b, there is both an immediate- and a longer-term effect, while Figure 7.1c represents a situation in which there is only a longer-term change in the trend.

Box 7.1
Segmented Regression

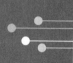

With only the treatment group under consideration (no comparison group), we can estimate the treatment effect with the following regression:

$$Y_t = \alpha + \beta_1 T_t + \beta_2 X_t + \beta_3 X_t T_t + \varepsilon_t \tag{7.1}$$

where

- Y_t is the outcome variable measured at time t,
- T_t is the time since the start of the study, and
- X_t is an indicator variable for the intervention.

Interpretation of Equation 7.1 is straightforward. The parameter α is the starting level of the outcome variable, β_1 is the outcome variable trend before the intervention begins, β_2 captures the change in the level of the outcome variable immediately after the intervention takes place, and β_3 is the difference between the preintervention and postintervention trends. A statistically significant estimate of β_2 indicates an immediate treatment effect; a statistically significant estimate of β_3 indicates a treatment effect over time.

Comparative Interrupted Time Series

In the basic ITS described above, there is no comparison group so the counterfactual is based on the assumption that the preintervention trend would have continued for the treated group in the absence of the intervention. Drawing inferences about causality relies on the strong assumption that there are no factors other than the intervention that would have affected the trend. In many cases, this assumption is not reasonable. Thus, the best way to strengthen ITS is by adding a comparison group that would be exposed to all the same factors other than the intervention. These analyses are called comparative interrupted time series (CITS).[6] CITS compares trends in the outcomes measure between the treatment and comparison groups. Indeed, exactly the same segmented regression models can estimate by adding separate intercept and slope terms for the two groups.

CITS controls for the differences in the time trend between the two groups by comparing how much the treatment group deviates from its preintervention trend and how much the comparison group deviates from its preintervention trend. If the change in the trend for the treatment group is bigger than that of the comparison group, then the intervention has an effect. In Box 7.2, we detail the regression specification for CITS analysis. Figures 7.2 and 7.3 provide a graphical illustration. Figure 7.3a represents a preferred situation in which the preintervention trends for the treatment and comparison groups are parallel, that is, although they may be at different levels, the slopes are the same. The difference between the pre- and postintercepts and slopes between intervention and comparison groups are then easily compared. In Figure 7.3b, the preintervention trends differ between the two groups. In this case, comparing the differences of slopes and intercepts between the pre- and postperiods is still acceptable, but acceptability of the results likely requires greater explanation of the factors that may have been affecting the two groups during the preintervention period.

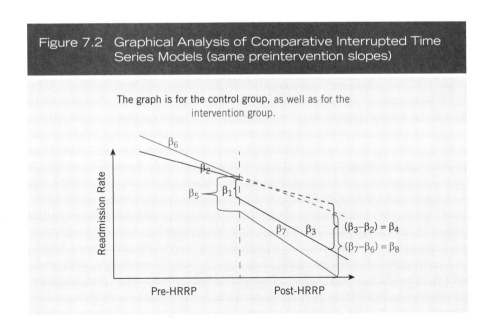

Figure 7.2 Graphical Analysis of Comparative Interrupted Time Series Models (same preintervention slopes)

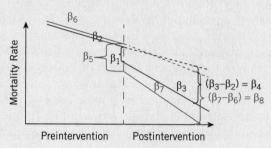

a. *Ideally:* We would like the mortality to start at the same
point, with the same preintervention slopes.

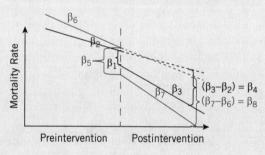

b. *Practically:* We are satisfied with comparing the immediate
changes ($\beta_5-\beta_1$) and the long-term changes ($\beta_8-\beta_4$).

Figure 7.4 provides an example of the latter situation from a recent study
of the effects of Medicare's Hospital Readmission Reduction Program (HRRP).[7]
The HRRP was intended to reduce unnecessary hospital readmissions. The study
examined whether the program had been effective. For the same reasons as
described above related to PfP, a basic ITS did not seem appropriate. Therefore, a
CITS design was used.

The HRRP also represents a case in which more than one "interruption" point
is prudent and thus, segmented regression is applied to three time periods. The
HRRP was authorized by the Affordable Care Act (ACA) in March 2010 for implementation in fiscal year 2013. As in most public programs, the parameters of the
program must be announced well in advance of implementation. In this case, it
was almost immediately clear that penalties in the fiscal year 2013 would be based
on readmissions in 3 prior years, meaning hospitals were effectively already in the
program and had incentives to respond immediately. Thus, the passage of ACA
(March 2010) and the HRRP implementation date (October 2012) were used as

the interruption points. Because the HRRP only applied to specified target conditions, the trends for nontarget conditions could be used as a comparison.

The pre-ACA trends were slightly negative for both sets of conditions—more so for the target conditions. Once the program was legislated, the trend for the targeted conditions deviated from its trend by a significantly greater amount than did the nontarget conditions. Interestingly, both trends became flat once the penalties went into effect in October 2012. The evidence was considered strong enough to conclude that HRRP did provide sufficient incentives for hospitals, at least initially, to reduce readmissions within the targeted conditions. Although the effect took place prior to actual implementation, this result was consistent with the roll-out of program information and reaction of hospitals to past payment policy changes.

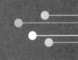

Box 7.2
The Comparative Interrupted Time Series Model

The comparative interrupted time series regression model can be specified as

$$Y_t = \alpha + \beta_1 T_t + \beta_2 X_t + \beta_3 X_t T_t + \beta_4 Z + \beta_5 Z T_t + \beta_6 Z X_t + \beta_7 Z X_t T_t + \varepsilon_t \qquad (7.2)$$

where

- Y_t is the outcome variable measured at time t,

- T_t is the time since the start of the study,

- X_t is an indicator variable for the intervention, and

- Z is an indicator for the treatment group.

Equation 7.2 can be interpreted as follows. The coefficients α and β_1 are the level and trend, respectively, for the comparison group before the intervention; β_4 is the difference in the level, and β_5 is the difference in the trend between the treatment and controls before the intervention. β_6 is the difference between the treatment and control groups' level immediately following the intervention. Finally, β_7 is the difference between the treatment and control groups' trend after the intervention.

Difference-in-Difference Designs

DiD might be considered as a specific type of CITS. It takes advantage of the natural experiments that occur when policies, practices, or interventions are introduced, which affect certain groups, but not others. In DiD, the estimated

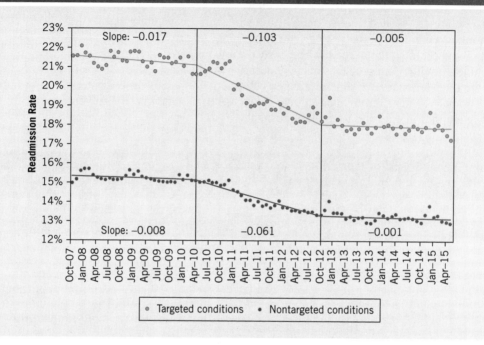

Figure 7.4 Graphical Analysis of Comparative Interrupted Time Series Model for Readmissions

counterfactual is the comparison group's change in its baseline mean. That is, under a DiD estimation strategy, it is assumed that the treatment group would have had the same trend (average gain or average loss) as the comparison group, if not for the intervention. For DiD, the intervention takes place at a specific point in time, as it did in the ITS and CITS models, but instead of multiple time points for both the treatment group and the comparison group, data were available for two time periods: the preintervention period and the postintervention period. While ITS and CITS compare pre- and postintervention trends, DiD compares means for the two periods.

While there are many variations on the basic design, the simplest design is when outcomes are observed for two groups for two time periods. One group is exposed to a treatment in the second period, but not in the first period. The comparison group is not exposed to the intervention during either period. This simple DiD design is shown in Table 7.1.

When the same units within a group are observed in each time period, the average gain in the comparison group is subtracted from the average gain in the treatment group. This removes biases in second-period comparisons between the treatment and control group that could be due to permanent differences between the groups, as well as biases from time attributable trends common to

Table 7.1   A Simple DiD Design

	Time Period	
	Preintervention	Postintervention
Treatment Group	Not exposed	Exposed
Comparison Group	Not exposed	Not exposed

both groups. Compared to some of the other methods in which we have tried to minimize bias, the DiD design controls for the common time trend between the treatment and comparison groups. An example of this approach is provided in Box 7.3.

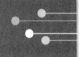

Box 7.3
The Impact of Medicare Part D on Prescription Drug Use by the Elderly

The Medicare Prescription Drug, Improvement, and Modernization Act, established on January 1, 2006, is a federal entitlement benefit for prescription drugs for Medicare beneficiaries (Medicare Part D) implemented through tax breaks and subsidies. Medicare Part D is a voluntary plan that provided new drug coverage for Medicare beneficiaries without prior coverage or that could replace the drug coverage they had under Medicare health maintenance organizations, Medigap, or Medicaid. Those with credible drug coverage through alternative sources could keep the drug coverage they had, while those without any credible coverage could choose not to enroll or be subject to late enrollment penalties. The 2006 enrollment period ended May 15, 2006. As of June 2006, approximately 90% of Medicare's 43 million beneficiaries had credible drug coverage.

Using a 50% sample (every other week) of prescriptions filled by one of the nation's largest retail pharmacy chains during the period September 2004–December 2006, Lichtenberg and Sun (2007) used a DiD design to compare prescription drug claims for elderly (affected by the Part D legislation) and nonelderly (not affected by the legislation) patients to estimate the impact of Part D legislation on drug utilization and drug costs.[8] Their analysis suggests that Medicare Part D reduced user drug cost among the elderly by 18.4% and increased their prescription drug use by about 12.8%. Medicare Part D reduced the total amount paid by patients by about 5.6%, while it increased the amount paid by third parties by 22.3%. They conclude that although Medicare Part D had a negligible impact on the overall price of prescription drugs (expenditure per day of therapy), it is likely an economically efficient program in that increased compliance with drug therapy is associated with reductions in other Medicare Parts A and B medical spending.

The DiD model gets its name from how its estimation can be conceptualized. Estimation can be thought of as two steps. First, the difference in the outcome variable before the treatment and after the treatment takes place is computed for the comparison group. Because the comparison group does not receive the treatment, any difference between the two time periods is attributable to natural changes over time. The difference in the outcome variable before and after the treatment takes place is also computed for the treatment group; any changes observed could be due to the underlying time trend or because of the treatment. To isolate the treatment effect, the difference over time for the comparison group is subtracted from the difference over time for the treatment group. This subtracts out the time trend, leaving just the effect of the treatment. Estimating the treatment effect using a DiD model can be done using regression or taking differences as we described. Box 7.4 details this.

The evaluator will usually want to add covariates, Xi, to the DiD analysis to strengthen unconfoundedness and to check whether the ATE estimates change and improve their precision. If treatment Wi is independent of Xi, then adding the covariates helps reduce the error variance without inducing multicollinearity. Yet another reason covariates are added is to account for compositional changes within the groups.

If the covariates have a stable distribution over time so that the types of subjects do not change in their characteristics, then methods other than basic regression adjustments are available. More generally, if the unexplained difference in

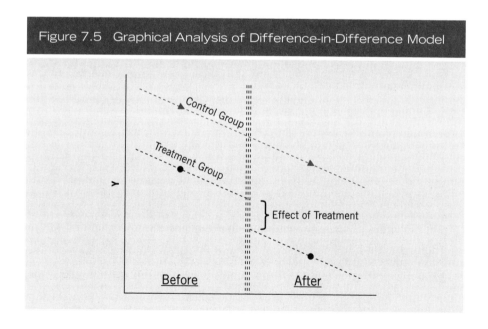

Figure 7.5 Graphical Analysis of Difference-in-Difference Model

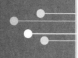

Box 7.4
The Difference-In-Difference Model

The DiD model assumes that both treatment and comparison groups share a common outcome trend from the base period. This assumption is manifested in the lack of an interactive baseline effect between time periods and group assignment. Supposing that the treatment affects all individuals the same, so that the outcome for the treatment group equals the sum of the outcome for the comparison group plus the ATE, τ, we have the following specification:

$$Y_i = \alpha + \beta T_i + \gamma G_i + \tau W_i + \mu_i \tag{7.3}$$

where $W_i = T_i G_i$.

In Equation 7.3, T_i is an indicator for the postperiod, and G_i is an indicator for the group that receives the treatment. In this model, the ATE is the coefficient of W_i, the term that interacts treatment with the postperiod.

The intuition for why the ATE is the coefficient, τ, is given in the following conditional expectations. Assuming no correlation of the error term, μ_i, with the group by time interaction term, W_i, we have

$$E\left[Y_i \mid G_i = 1, T_i = 1\right] - E\left[Y_i \mid G_i = 1, T_i = 0\right] = \beta + \tau \tag{7.4}$$

$$E\left[Y_i \mid G_i = 0, T_i = 1\right] - E\left[Y_i \mid G_i = 0, T_i = 0\right] = \beta \tag{7.5}$$

Equation 7.4 is the average gain (or loss) for those in the treatment group between the postperiod and the preperiod. It is the sum of the time trend, β, and the gain (or loss) attributed to treatment, τ. Similarly, Equation 7.5 is the average gain (or loss) between the postperiod and preperiod, except it is computed for the comparison group. Because the comparison group did not receive the treatment, any gains (or losses) observed for the comparison group are attributed to the time trend, β. Now, the second Equation 7.5 can be subtracted from the first (7.4) to remove biases associated with a common time trend unrelated to the intervention, β, and isolate the average treatment effect (ATE).

The regression interaction estimator, $\hat{\tau}$, can be described either as (1) the change in prepost period means for the intervention minus comparison group, or (2) the difference in study-comparison group means in the postperiod minus the difference in the base period. Ordinary least squares (OLS) regression is very convenient for conducting inference; the standard heteroscedasticity-robust standard error for the ATE is valid, which means that confidence intervals and tests of significance can be conducted.

groups is constant across time, then subtracting the estimated ATE from the base period from the ATE estimate from the postperiod should remove sample group differences and consistently estimate the overall ATE. Heckman, Ichimura, and Todd suggest estimating the two ATE estimates by using full regression adjustment in *each* of the two periods.[9] Abadie proposes propensity score (PS) and regression adjustment combined with PS weighting to obtain the two estimates.[10] (See Imbens and Wooldridge for further discussion.[11]) There is no reason one cannot, in each period, use blocking on the PS or matching to obtain ATE estimates in the pre- and postperiods.

It is important to note that, without further information, the assumptions underlying the DiD approach we have discussed cannot be tested. If allowance is made for the possibility of an unknown time trend and unknown preintervention group difference, there are four parameters to estimate, but there may be data on just the four (mean) cells. A more general DiD design is introduced in the next section that allows for unequal study comparison trends.

Unequal Base Period Trends. In some applications, the common trend assumption (also commonly referred to as the parallel trends assumption) may be too strong (in the previous model, it is the assumption that the time trend, β, is common to both the treatment and comparison groups). Consider the case of a state introducing a new health system for its public employees. The decision to do so may be due not only to the *average* health costs of its workers, but also to *trends* in the state's health costs. If the health trends in state B differ from those in comparison state A, then the DiD estimator of public insurance reform may simply reflect differences in underlying trends in health care costs. We can obtain a more convincing estimate of the policy effect by refining the comparison group. In the current example, suppose data can be collected on individuals who are and are not government employees from each state. There are now four groups: (1) state employees in State A, (2) nonstate employees in State A, (3) state employees in comparison State B, and (4) nonstate employees in comparison State B (see Table 7.2).

Table 7.2 Unequal Base Period Trends

		Time Period	
		Preintervention	Postintervention
State A	State Employees	Not exposed	Exposed
	Nonstate Employees	Not exposed	Not exposed
State B	State Employees	Not exposed	Not exposed
	Nonstate Employees	Not exposed	Not exposed

To estimate the new health system for public employees, we utilize the triple difference model (DiDD). Similar to the DiD estimator, the DiDD estimator attempts to difference out underlying trends (this time due to both state-specific trends and time trends) to obtain the treatment effect. Box 7.5 details DiDD regression specification.

Box 7.5
Triple Difference Model

The DiDD estimator can be obtained from a regression that pools all the data:

$$Y_i = \alpha + \gamma_1 A_i + \gamma_2 E_i + \gamma_3 A_i E_i + \beta_1 T_i + \beta_2 T_i A_i + \beta_3 T_i E_i + \tau_{didd} W_i + U_i \qquad (7.6)$$

where $W_i = T_i A_i E_i$.

Here, T_i, A_i, and E_i are dummy variables for the pre-/postintervention time period, being a resident of State B, and being a state employee, E, respectively. The DiDD treatment effect estimate, $\hat{\tau}_{didd}$, is the estimated coefficient associated with the triple interaction term.

As with the DiD estimator, we can understand the DiDD estimate by considering the expected value of Y_i conditional on whether the individual is from State A or State B, a government employee or not, and whether the observed outcome is from the preintervention period or the postintervention period. We consider the conditional expectations of interest in Table 7.3; we also introduce suppressed notation for the conditional expectations of the form $Y_{A,E,1}$, where the first subscript indicates the state (A or B), the second subscript indicates employment (E for state employee, N otherwise), and the third subscript indicates the time period (0 for the preperiod and 1 for the postperiod).

Table 7.3   Triple Difference Model

		Time Period	
		Preintervention	**Postintervention**
State _A_	**State Employees**	$E[Y_i \mid A_i = 1, E_i = 1, T_i = 0]$ $= Y_{A,E,0} = \alpha + \gamma_1 + \gamma_2 + \gamma_3$	$E[Y_i \mid A_i = 1, E_i = 1, T_i = 1]$ $= Y_{A,E,1} = \alpha + \gamma_1 + \gamma_2 + \gamma_3 + \beta_1 + \beta_2 + \beta_3 + \tau_{didd}$
	Nonstate Employees	$E[Y_i \mid A_i = 1, E_i = 0, T_i = 0]$ $= Y_{A,N,0} = \alpha + \gamma_1$	$E[Y_i \mid A_i = 1, E_i = 0, T_i = 1]$ $= Y_{A,N,1} = \alpha + \gamma_1 + \beta_1 + \beta_2$

(Continued)

(Continued)

		Time Period	
		Preintervention	Postintervention
State *B*	State Employees	$E[Y_i \mid A_i = 0, E_i = 1, T_i = 0]$ $= Y_{B,E,0} = \alpha + \gamma_2$	$E[Y_i \mid A_i = 0, E_i = 1, T_i = 1]$ $= Y_{B,E,1} = \alpha + \gamma_2 + \beta_1 + \beta_3$
	Nonstate Employees	$E[Y_i \mid A_i = 0, E_i = 0, T_i = 0]$ $= Y_{B,N,0} = \alpha$	$E[Y_i \mid A_i = 0, E_i = 0, T_i = 1]$ $= Y_{B,N,1} = \alpha + \beta_1$

Estimation begins with two DiD specifications,

$$\tau_{did,E} = \left(Y_{A,E,1} - Y_{A,E,0}\right) - \left(Y_{B,E,1} - Y_{B,E,0}\right) = \beta_2 + \tau_{didd} \tag{7.7}$$

$$\tau_{did,N} = \left(Y_{A,N,1} - Y_{A,N,0}\right) - \left(Y_{B,N,1} - Y_{B,N,0}\right) = \beta_2 \tag{7.8}$$

The first DiD estimate (7.7) is the estimate only for state employees in the two states. The second DiD estimate (7.8) is the DiD estimate for the unaffected nonstate employee group that factors out state differences in underlying health cost trends. If $\tau_{did,N}$ is statistically different from 0, the conclusion follows that States A and B did indeed have different trends in health costs in the absence of intervention. To account for this, we use the DiDD estimator,

$$\tau_{didd} = \tau_{did,E} - \tau_{did,N} \tag{7.9}$$

It is also useful to rearrange Equation 7.10 so that the DiDD estimator debits changes between public and nonpublic employees in the control state from corresponding changes in the intervention state, that is,

$$\tau_{didd} = \left[\left(Y_{A,E,1} - Y_{A,E,0}\right)\right] - \left[\left(Y_{A,N,1} - Y_{A,N,0}\right)\right] - \left[\left(Y_{B,E,1} - Y_{B,E,0}\right) - \left(Y_{B,N,1} - Y_{B,N,0}\right)\right] \tag{7.10}$$

If one thinks the trends in health care costs for government and nongovernment employees is the same in the absence of intervention, the second term in brackets should not be statistically different from 0. In essence, it can act as a test that can be used to validate the DiD study only using State A.

As in the case of two groups and two time periods, the assumptions underlying the DiDD estimator are not testable unless one makes assumptions about the means and variances in the different groups in the absence of treatment. Generally, one needs to estimate the unrestricted eight means from the different group and time pairs.

In both the DiD and the DiDD regressions, covariates, Xi, can be introduced to check if the estimates of the treatment effect change and to improve precision by reducing the equation's error variance (hopefully without inducing multicollinearity). In some cases, covariates are added to account for compositional changes in the sample over time if, for example, the kinds of people who become state employees change after the new health plan is introduced.

Confounded Designs

So far, we have assumed that bias due to nonrandom assignment to the treatment group can be controlled by observable covariates. Sometimes, this is not a reasonable assumption. We now present two strategies—instrument variables and regression discontinuity—for treatment effect estimation in a confounded design.

Instrument Variables to Estimate Treatment Effects[12]

The instrumental variable (IV) estimation method is a technique used to control for bias in an otherwise uncontrolled comparison study. When the estimated treatment effect of an intervention is correlated with the error term, a variable can sometimes be created based on additional characteristics of the participants. The IV should not be directly related to the outcome but to treatment status. If these conditions are met, the IV can be incorporated into the regression analysis to reduce this bias. An instrumental variable can be one of two types:

1) A binary instrument—for example, the presence or absence of a single characteristic in a program participant related to treatment status but thought nevertheless to be only indirectly correlated with the outcome of treatment for an individual.

2) A "multivalue" instrument—for example, a medical study in the early 1990s—found correlation between the intervention outcome and the distance of a participant's home from a particular type of hospital. Distance is the IV, because it is not directly related to treatment outcomes, and multivalued, because it is a continuous variable that can take on any number of values.

In 1994, Mark McClellan, Barbara McNeil, and Joseph Newhouse[13] conducted an observational study of the effects on mortality rates of different levels of aggressiveness in acute myocardial infarction (AMI) treatment for the elderly. Intensity was measured by use of catheterization or revascularization procedures. They found that the distance of a participant's home from a particular type of hospital indirectly influenced the outcome of treatment despite having no relation to the participant's health status. They found that this distance influenced the rigor of a participant's treatment, effectively influencing their assignment to a treatment group and indirectly affecting the outcome. Their research design used "analysis of incremental treatment effects using differential distances as instrumental variables to account for unobserved case-mix variation (selection bias) in observational Medicare claims data." Given the retrospective nature of an observational study, the researchers were unable to remove selection bias in their sample; the inclusion of this distance as an instrumental variable therefore allowed them to compare outcomes for patients who were identical in all ways, except for their values of this distance.

They first compared unadjusted outcomes between the treatment groups and used "fully interacted analysis of variance (ANOVA) methods to adjust" for differences in observable characteristics of the groups (sex, race, age, geography [urban/rural]), and health status (presence or absence of comorbid diseases). Then they did the same but included the instrumental variable; comparing the estimates of both methods thus allowed them to "isolate the effect of treatment variation in the observational data that is independent of unobserved patient characteristics."

To test the validity of their assumption that proximity to a certain type of hospital would affect the treatment status, they first tested whether different hospitals have differing propensities to use certain, more intensive treatments for AMI. They did so by estimating "the average effect of hospital capability on procedure use," also using ANOVA. This then allowed them to isolate the selection bias resulting from being first admitted for AMI to a hospital of a particular type—noncatheterization, catheterization, and revascularization hospitals—due to the degree of proximity. They found "selection bias in hospital choice" and thus were able to incorporate their instrumental variable into regression estimates and finally isolate "the incremental effects of more intensive treatments on mortality without selection bias."

After demonstrating the independence of health status and differential distance to a particular type of hospital, differential distance could function as an instrumental variable to effectively randomly distribute health status among hospital types. In comparing these groups, differing only in likelihood of receiving a more intensive treatment, the researchers ultimately found that "the impact on mortality at one to four years after AMI of the incremental use of invasive procedures in Medicare patients was at most five percentage points."

Regression Discontinuity to Estimate Treatment Effects

We now turn to regression discontinuity (RD). It exploits the precise rules that govern whether an experimental unit is treated or not. The design often arises in cases of administrative decisions where clear transparent rules (rather than discretion by administrators) are used for treatment allocation. In contrast to the situations we have seen so far, in an RD design, the factor(s) that determine assignment are completely known. Two types of RD designs exist: sharp and fuzzy. The premise of both designs is that a predictor called the forcing variable, X_i, meets a two-fold criterion. First, assignment to treatment is determined completely or partly by the forcing variable being on either side of a common threshold. If you were to plot the forcing variable and the probability of treatment, you would observe a discontinuity in the probability of treatment at the cutoff value. The second assumption about the forcing variable is that the relationship between the forcing variable and the treatment outcome is smooth. If a discontinuity in the outcome is observed at the cutoff, it is interpreted as evidence for a causal effect of treatment.

Sharp Regression Discontinuity Design

In a sharp RD design, treatment status is completely determined by the forcing variable. Unlike propensity score matching and weighting, you cannot match the treated and the untreated on a full set of covariates; by design, the forcing variable will not be balanced. Consequently, the treatment effect is estimated by observing and comparing the outcomes of units with forcing variable values very close to the cut off. Box 7.6 provides the technical details, and Box 7.7 presents a sharp RD design.

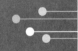

Box 7.6
Sharp Regression Discontinuity Design

In the sharp regression discontinuity (SRD) design, the assignment W_i is a deterministic function of one of the covariates, the forcing (or treatment-determining) variable X_i

$$W_i = 1[X_i \geq c] \qquad (7.11)$$

where $1[\cdot]$ is the indicator function (equal to 1 if $X_i \geq c$ and 0 otherwise) and c is the cutoff. All units with a covariate value of at least c are in the treatment group, and participation is mandatory for these individuals. All units with a covariate value less than c are in the control group; members of this group are not eligible for the treatment. In the SRD design, we focus on estimation of

$$\tau_{SRD} = E[Y_i(1) - Y_i(0)|X_i = c] = E\left[Y_i(1)|X_i = c\right] - E\left[Y_i(0)|X_i = c\right] \qquad (7.12)$$

where $Y_i(1)$ is the outcome for individual i in the case of being in the treatment group, and $Y_i(0)$ is for individual i in the case of being in the comparison group. By design, there are no units with $X_i = c$ for whom $Y_i(0)$ can be observed. Thus, to estimate $E[Y_i(w)|X_i = c]$, one uses units with covariate values arbitrarily close to c. The statistical problem becomes one of estimating a regression function nonparametrically at a boundary point. Once the two conditional expectations are estimated, the effect size can be estimated.

Fuzzy Regression Discontinuity Design

In a fuzzy RD design, the probability of receiving the treatment need not change from 0 to 1 at the threshold. Instead, the design only requires a discontinuity in the probability of assignment to the treatment at the threshold. In practice, the discontinuity needs to be sufficiently large to be seen easily in simple graphical analyses. These discontinuities can arise if incentives to participate in a program change discontinuously at a threshold, without the incentives being powerful enough to move all units from nonparticipation to participation. Box 7.7 formalizes this mathematically.[14]

Box 7.7
Fuzzy Regression Discontinuity Design

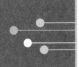

Fuzzy regression discontinuity (FRD) design looks at the ratio of the jump in the regression of the outcome on the covariate to the jump in the regression of the treatment indicator on the covariate. Formally, the function of interest is

$$\tau_{\text{FRD}} = \frac{\lim_{x \downarrow c} E\left[Y_i \big| X_i = x \right] - \lim_{x \uparrow c} E\left[Y_i \big| X_i = x \right]}{\lim_{x \downarrow c} E\left[W_i \big| X_i = x \right] - \lim_{x \uparrow c} E\left[W_i \big| X_i = x \right]} \tag{7.13}$$

Hahn, Todd, and van der Klaauw (2001) provide an estimation technique for the FRD design when the effect of the treatment varies by unit. They define compliers as those whose participation is affected by the cutoff point. A complier is someone with a value of the forcing variable $X_i = x$ close to c, who would participate if c were chosen to be just below x, but not if c were chosen to be just above x. The estimand τ_{FRD} is estimated as the average effect of the treatment, but only for units with $X_i = c$ (by regression discontinuity) and compliers (people affected by the threshold). The analysis generally does not have much external validity, because it is only valid for the subpopulation who are compliers at the threshold and for the subpopulation with $X_i = c$. Nevertheless, the FRD analysis may do well in terms of internal validity because, in contrast to the SRD case, an unconfoundedness-based analysis is possible in the FRD setting since some treated observations will have $X_i \leq c$, and some comparison observations will have $X_i \geq c$.

Estimation and inference for RD designs is unlike other analyses we have seen thus far, because estimation is done in the vicinity of the cutoff value. Mathematically, this is regression at a boundary point. Naturally two questions arise: (1) How does one do regression at a boundary? (2) How does one pick the vicinity of the cutoff value on which to do analysis? In Box 7.8, we discuss possible answers to these questions. Those who are not methodologically interested are encouraged to skip Box 7.9.[15,16,17,18,19,20,21]

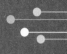
Graphical Methods

Graphical analyses are typically an integral part of any RD analysis. RD designs suggest that the effect of the treatment of interest can be measured by the magnitude of the discontinuity in the conditional expectation of the outcome on the forcing variable at the cutoff. Inspecting the estimated conditional expectation is a simple yet powerful way to visualize the identification strategy.[22]

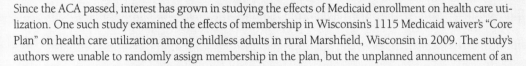

(Continued)

early cutoff date for enrollment in the plan resulted in the formation of a quasi-experimental comparison group, lending the program's evaluation perfectly to an RD design. As enrollment in the Core Plan began to outpace the state's allocated funding, the governor announced—without prior public notification—that the enrollment window would close early: in 4 days at noon. Applications submitted after that date and time were put on a waitlist; no one from the waitlist was ever enrolled.

Using records from the Marshfield clinic matched with Medicaid eligibility and enrollment data, the researchers were able to compare utilization by Core Plan beneficiaries to that of waitlisted eligible beneficiaries. They specifically looked at outpatient days, preventative care days, mental health or substance abuse days, ER days, and inpatient days per beneficiary over the 2 years following the cutoff date. They implemented an SRD design, with the date of application functioning as the treatment assignment variable and the sudden enrollment deadline as the cutoff date.

Underlying the model were the critical assumptions that characterize an RD design: applicants prior to and following the early deadline were similar to one another except for the date of application, which they assumed to have varied randomly. The assumptions are reasonable given the scenario. The data showed a spike in enrollment between the early deadline announcement and the deadline itself, suggesting "heaping bias" in which eligible beneficiaries rushed to enroll in the Core Plan for fear of missing the deadline. To remedy this, the researchers excluded from their study Core Plan enrollees whose application date fell between the governor's announcement and the cutoff. Furthermore, acknowledging the tradeoff between accuracy and precision in selecting the bandwidth (in what vicinity of the "cutoff" should the analysis take place), the study's authors decided to "estimate a variety of bandwidths and present graphical depictions of all estimates and their 95% confidence intervals."

The regression output varied by bandwidth but generally showed statistically significant increases in utilization by Core enrollees over waitlisted eligible beneficiaries. Table 7.4 summarizes the regression results at a bandwidth of 14 days (i.e., excluding enrollees whose application date fell within 1 week of the cutoff date on either side):

Table 7.4 Table Summary of Regression Discontinuity Results

	Any Outpatient	Preventive	Behavioral Health	Emergency	Inpatient
Baseline values for core enrollees	2.783	0.275	0.297	0.056	0.034
Coefficient	1.076	0.256	−0.064	0.060	0.042
P-value	0.026	0.000	0.655	0.086	0.081

The main plot in an SRD setting is a histogram. The histogram should be constructed with the threshold c on the edge of one of the bins with some bins to the left and some to the right of the threshold. For each bin, the number of observations and the average outcome is calculated. The question is, Around the threshold c, is there any evidence of a jump in the conditional mean of the outcome? If the basic plot shows no evidence of a discontinuity, there is little chance that more sophisticated analyses will lead to credible estimates with statistically and substantially significant magnitudes.

One should also inspect the graph to see whether there are any other jumps in the conditional expectation of Y_i given X_i that are comparable in size to, or larger than, the discontinuity at the cutoff value. If so, and if one cannot explain such jumps, this calls into question the interpretation of the jump at the threshold as the causal effect of the treatment. To optimize the visual clarity, it is recommended to calculate averages that are not smoothed across the cutoff point c. It is also recommended not to artificially smooth on either side of the threshold in a way that implies that the only discontinuity in the estimated regression function is at c.

Figure 7.6 is a sample of the graphical output generated by the RD analysis of the Wisconsin 1115 Medicaid Waiver's Core Plan that we discussed in Box 7.9. Presented in pairs, the graphs on the left show the actual RD produced by the model, plotting the assignment variable against the output variable. Plots on the right display the coefficient of the assignment variable and its 95% confidence interval plotted against bandwidth where bandwidth is the vicinity of the cutoff point on which the analysis takes place. Although only a subset of those produced by the Core Plan study were discussed in Box 7.9, the graphs on the left side of pairings clearly show a break in model output at the cutoff date (where $x = c$), allowing a fairly straightforward interpretation of the results.

In panels A and B, illustrating utilization of outpatient and preventative care services respectively, a wide gap in care utilization is observed at the cutoff. Utilization is greater for those where x is negative—those whose application date was earlier than the deadline and thus were Core Plan beneficiaries. The right-hand side graphs for panels A and B indicate a consistent, positive relationship between Core Plan enrollment and health care utilization because the coefficient is fairly consistent and positive regardless of bandwidth. As a point of comparison, the left-hand side graph in panel C shows a smaller gap between the regression segments, thereby calling into question the significance of any difference between utilization on either side of the cutoff. The panel C right-hand side graph shows that the sign of the coefficient is depending on the bandwidth and indicates the lack of a clear relationship between treatment status and output. Consistent with the regression analysis, the researchers concluded that enrollment in the 1115 Waiver plan resulted in greater utilization of outpatient and preventative health care services, but it had no significant impact on beneficiaries' utilization of mental health or substance abuse services.

Validity and Regression Discontinuity

There are two important validity concerns in RD designs.

1) Other changes at the same threshold value of the covariate—for example, the same age limit may affect the eligibility for multiple programs. If all the programs whose eligibility changes at the same cutoff value affect the outcome of interest, an RD analysis may mistakenly attribute the combined effect to the treatment of interest.

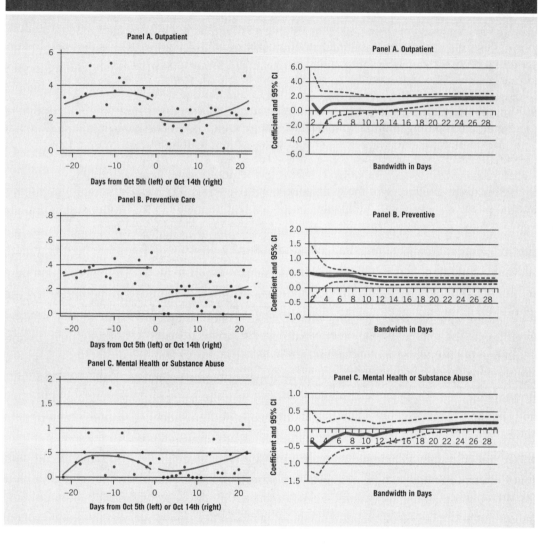

2) Manipulation by the individuals of the covariate value that underlies the assignment mechanism—for example, when eligibility criteria are known to potential participants and are based on variables that are affected by individual choices. If thresholds are known to students, they may take a qualifying exam multiple times in an attempt to raise their score above the threshold.

These concerns can sometimes be assuaged by further investigation. Nonetheless, the researcher should take care to address them if they are suspected to be at play.

Additional Considerations: Dealing With Nonindependent Data

Nonindependent data exist when knowing something about one observation helps predict the outcome for a different observation. Traditional regression methods assume that each observation is independent; when this assumption is violated, special methods are required to account for the dependencies. In this section, we discuss three types of nonindependent, or correlated, data:

1) Multilevel data where individual observations belong to larger clusters that might affect their outcomes

2) Geographic data where the distance between observations might affect their outcomes

3) Longitudinal data with repeated measurements of an outcome over time

Multilevel Data

Multilevel data occur when individual observations belong to a larger cluster, such as patients within a physician practice or members of a family. Multilevel data are generally described from the smallest to the largest units. Throughout this section, we will use hospital readmissions to describe multilevel models where patients are nested within hospitals. Thus, patients are Level 1 units, while hospitals are Level 2 units. The outcome of interest is a patient's readmission within 30 days of discharge. It is likely that whether a patient from a particular hospital is readmitted provides information about the likelihood of another patient from the same hospital having a 30-day readmission. Hence, Level 1 units are not statistically independent because knowing something about one unit (patient) in a cluster (hospital) provides information about other units in the same cluster. Although data with two levels are the simplest to model, some evaluations may involve more than two levels of clustering. For example, students (Level 1) could be nested in classrooms (Level 2), which are nested in schools (Level 3), which are nested in school districts (Level 4).

When using statistical methods to evaluate multilevel data, the goal, as with other regression models, is to accurately model the data to determine, when possible, the causal relationship between the intervention and the outcome. However, if group membership is likely to affect the outcome of interest, then it must be accounted for in the impact analysis. Furthermore, the nonindependent observations of multilevel data always violate the assumption of unconfoundedness between observations.

Models of multilevel data must address two shortfalls of the linear regression models we have encountered so far. First, because of their group membership, members are associated with each other and do not provide as much information as they would if they were not in hierarchical clusters (like the situation discussed in Chapter 5). Having less information is equivalent to having a smaller sample size; this is called the effective sample size and is always smaller than the observed sample size. The smaller effective sample size decreases the precision of estimates, but it does not change (bias) the estimates.

Second, because outcomes may be associated with characteristics at both the member and cluster level, the assumption of unconfoundedness between observations in the traditional linear model is violated. This is particularly important for member level covariates, which are often described as having a total effect comprised of Level 1 and Level 2 effects. In the language of statistics, these are called *within* and *between cluster effects*, respectively. In the example of hospital readmissions, there is no question that both a patient's health status and the hospital to which they are admitted are associated with the likelihood of readmission, and additionally, the hospital may moderate the effect of health status. If only Level 1 effects (the patient's health status) are included in a model, while the Level 2 effects (hospital that the patient was admitted to) are not, then the total effect will be attributed to the Level 1 covariates. However, if both Level 1 and Level 2 effects are included, the total effect can be decomposed into the within (patients from the same hospital) and between (hospitals) effects. In many cases, we are only interested in the within-cluster association. That is, given the hospital a patient is admitted to, how does health status affect a patient's likelihood of being readmitted? To accurately assess this within effect, both Level 1 and Level 2 covariates must be included in the model.

Below, we discuss three methods for modeling group structures with multilevel data:

1. Marginal models

2. Conditional models (commonly called random effect models)

3. Fixed effects models

Each of these types of models can appropriately account for multilevel data. Thus, the decision of which model to use depends primarily on the question of interest.

Marginal Models

Marginal models use generalized estimating equations (GEE) to model the correlation between observations. They are useful for evaluating either the total or within-cluster effect on an outcome as well as prediction.

In the simple linear model, we assume that observations are independent. Mathematically, this independence means that the covariance of the residuals of the regression model between observations is equal to 0. In contrast, marginal models allow the residuals of observations within a cluster to be correlated, or not equal to 0. Typically, the correlation is assumed to be the same across all clusters, meaning that all groups have the same influence on their group members. The clusters are assumed to be independent of each other.

Marginal models require that the covariance structure be specified for estimation to take place. A few of the most common structures for multilevel data include independent, unstructured, and exchangeable.[23] An independent covariance structure, as the name implies, models units within groups as uncorrelated. This structure estimates the total effect of covariates. In contrast, unstructured and exchangeable covariance structures allow for within-group correlations and estimate within-cluster effects. An exchangeable structure assumes that all pairs of observations within a group have the same correlation, while an unstructured correlation structure estimates a separate correlation coefficient for each pair. To appropriately adjust standard errors for clustered data, GEE models should use a robust standard error estimate. Most statistical programs include the Huber–White sandwich estimator for this purpose.

Marginal models can be estimated with both individual- (such as health status) and cluster-level (such as hospital size) covariates. One important disadvantage is the assumption that correlations are the same across clusters, or in other words, that group membership has the same affect for all groups. To illustrate when this assumption may not be correct, consider two hospitals: hospital A has instituted an intervention to reduce readmissions, and hospital B has not. If the intervention were effective, being admitted to hospital A would have a stronger effect on a patient's likelihood of being readmitted than being admitted to hospital B. However, this cannot be captured in a marginal model because it assumes that this effect is the same across hospitals. In some cases, adding a cluster-level effect (such as whether the hospital has implemented an intervention) may address this issue.

Conditional Models

Conditional models, also referred to as random effects, mixed, or hierarchical models, explicitly include cluster-level random effects in the regression model. These models decompose estimates into individual and cluster components. This can be done for the intercept term, resulting in a group-specific intercept, or for covariates, resulting in a group-specific slope. We show this mathematically in Box 7.10. Readers not interested in methodology are encouraged to skip Box 7.10.

By producing estimates for group specific intercepts and slopes, conditional models can estimate how much the average readmission rate differs across hospitals after controlling for health status. Conditional models can also easily account for more than two levels by allowing cluster-specific effects for both Level 2 and Level 3 clusters. One significant disadvantage of conditional models is their treatment of small groups. In conditional models, the deviation of cluster-specific effects from the overall mean is dependent on group size. Effects for small clusters

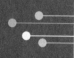

Box 7.10

Model Specification for Conditional Models

To estimate the association between health status and readmission rates with a simple linear model, we have

$$Y_{hi} = \beta X_{hi} + C \tag{7.14}$$

for patient i in hospital h, where Y_{hi} is whether or not patient i was readmitted, βX_{hi} is patient i's health status, and C is the intercept. We can expand this model to include a hospital specific intercept, a hospital random effect, by writing

$$Y_{hi} = \beta X_{gi} + \left(C + c_h\right) \tag{7.15}$$

where c_h is the hospital specific intercept. We assume that the hospital specific intercepts (c_h) are normally distributed around the mean intercept (C). For, example, if the average readmission rate across all patients in all hospitals were 18%, we would assume that individual hospitals' mean readmission rates would be normally distributed around 18%. In the same way, we could decompose β, the effect of health status, into an overall and hospital specific effect. This would mean that being sicker is associated with a different change in the probability of readmission in hospital A as compared to hospital B.

are nearly equal to the mean, even if the observed values are far from the mean. Thus, these models are not particularly good for predicting values for small clusters (see Appendix B for more discussion of the problem with small clusters). This becomes even more of a problem if there is a relationship between cluster size and the outcome of interest. For example, if smaller hospitals on average have high readmission rates, these models will predict readmission rates that are disproportionately near the mean and too low for small hospitals.[24]

Fixed Effects

The final method for modeling multilevel data is group fixed effects. This method includes a categorical variable for each group. In the readmissions example, this would be a variable indicating which hospital admitted the patient. As compared to marginal or conditional models, fixed effects models do not require a specification that is very different from the simple linear model.

The biggest disadvantage of fixed effects models is that they cannot include group level covariates. In the readmissions example, this would include measures like hospital size or profit status. Mathematically, any group level covariate is collinear with the group variable, and thus it would be dropped during model estimation. This is mainly a problem when the policy variable(s) of interest vary only at the group level; although, not needing to collect information on group-specific covariates can be an advantage. Finally, group-level covariates can be interacted with the treatment variable to model treatment heterogeneity.

Geographic Data

Location data such as address, ZIP code, or county may provide additional information that should be included in a modeling strategy. Here we assume that observations that are closer together are more alike than observations far apart; this is referred to as spatial correlation. Multiple techniques for addressing spatial correlation in statistical models exist. The appropriate model to use depends on the type of geographic information included and the evaluation questions at hand. In this section, we will discuss only two methods for modeling spatial data (for further reading on geographic data, spatial correlation, and spatial modeling, see Cresse's text[25]):

1. Treating the geographic information like a group and using multilevel modeling strategies
2. Using distance to identify correlation between observations

Multilevel Modeling With Geographic Data

Geographic information can be used to determine groups for the multilevel strategies described in the prior section. Data containing individuals (Level 1) within a ZIP code (Level 2) or hospitals (Level 1) within a county (Level 2) can be evaluated this way. However, this strategy generally assumes that the Level 2 groups are independent. If, for example, counties next to each other are likely to have similar outcomes, this should be specified in the model. An approach for including this information is described next.

Distance-Based Approach to Modeling Geographic Data

In some cases, it is likely that the correlation between observations does not depend on group membership, but rather on proximity to other observations. Specific modeling techniques have been developed to evaluate this type of spatial dependence. Here, we discuss the use of marginal models to incorporate spatial correlation with only one level of data.

We use the example of a health marketing campaign in some counties to promote insurance take-up rates. In this case, we have insurance rates at the county level and whether or not the county participated in the marketing campaign. It is unlikely that any effect of the campaign would be entirely restricted to the county in which it was implemented; spillover effects might be observed in surrounding counties, affecting their insurance rates.

To use a marginal model to account for the correlation between insurance rates of nearby counties, we first need to know which counties are next to each other. We then construct a measure of the minimum distance between two counties. This might be measured by the number of other counties between the two. Based on this distance measure, we can specify a correlation structure for a marginal model for insurance rate by county. Two covariance structures that can be used to model the distance between two observations are Toeplitz and autoregressive. The Toeplitz specification estimates a single correlation parameter for each distance. All counties adjacent to each other are assumed to have the same correlation, counties with only one other county in between them are assumed to have a different correlation, etc. The model then estimates a correlation parameter for each distance. In contrast, for an autoregressive structure, only one parameter is estimated, and the correlation is assumed to decay as distance increases to a specified distance. Thus, if the correlation between two adjacent counties is ρ, then the correlation between counties with one county in between them is ρ^2. If all further counties are assumed to be independent with a correlation of 0, then we have an autoregressive (1) structure. If counties with two other counties are assumed to have a correlation of ρ^3, but further counties are assumed to be independent, the structure would instead be autoregressive (2).

The health insurance and counties example is based on area-level data, and the distance between observations is determined by adjacency. If, instead of area-level data you have point data, such as addresses, it is possible to use a correlation structure based on the measured distance between observations. For more detail on modeling spatial point data, see Waller and Gotway.[26]

SUMMARY

At other times, more complex statistical models are necessary either because of the program's design (e.g., a regression discontinuity and administrative cutoffs) or because of the nature of the data (hierarchical, geographic, longitudinal).

Treatment effects are not the only end-goal in an evaluation. With many demonstrations leaving the model of health care being implemented up to the participants (practices, accountable care organizations, etc.), describing the variation in models and outcomes has become increasingly important to put evaluation findings in context. In the next two chapters, we address the sources of treatment effect heterogeneity and how to analyze them.

DISCUSSION QUESTION

1. Describe the necessary conditions for a CITS approach.

2. Find an example of an instrumental variables approach in the literature and discuss how one might assess the strength of the application of IV methods.

3. Discuss how different quasi-experimental methods may be used together. For example, how might propensity scores and DiD designs be utilized together?

NOTES

1. St. Clair, T., T. D. Cook, and K. Hallberg, "Examining the Internal Validity and Statistical Precision of the Comparative Interrupted Time Series Design by Comparison With a Randomized Experiment," *American Journal of Evaluation* 35 no. 3 (2014).

2. Ibid.

3. Ibid.

4. *Mathematica Policy Research, Project Evaluation Activity in Support of Partnership for Patients: Task 2 Evaluation Progress Report*, February 2014; Pronovost, P., and A. K. Jha, "Did Hospital Engagement Networks Actually Improve Care?" *New England Journal of Medicine* 371 (2014): 691–93

5. Wagner, A. K., S. B. Soumerai, F. Zhang, and D. Ross-Degnan, "Segmented Regression Analysis of Interrupted Time Series Studies in Medication Use Research" *Journal of Clinical Pharmacy and Therapeutics* 27 (2002): 299–309. doi: 10.1046/j.1365-2710.2002.00430.x

6. Somers M., P. Zhu, R. Jacob, and H. Bloom. *The validity and precision of the comparative interrupted time series design and the difference-in-difference design in educational evaluation.* MDRC working paper in research methodology (New York, NY: MDRC, 2013).

7. Zuckerman, Rachael, Steven Sheingold, John Orav, Joel Ruhter, and Arnold Epstein. "Readmissions, Observation, and the Hospital Readmissions Reduction Program," *New England Journal of Medicine* 374 (April 21, 2016): 1543–51.

8. Lichtenberg, F. R., and Sun, S. X., "The Impact of Medicare Part D on Prescription Drug Use by the Elderly," *Health Aff (Millwood)* 26 no. 6 (November–December 2007): 1735–44.

9. Heckman, J. J., H. Ichimura, and P. E. Todd. "Matching as an Econometric Evaluation Estimator: Evidence from Evaluating a Job Training Programme," *The Review of Economic Studies* 64 no. 4 (1997): 605–54.

10. Abadie, A. "Semiparametric Difference-in-Differences Estimators," *The Review of Economic Studies* 72 no. 1 (2005): 1–19.

11. Imbens, G. M., and J. M. Wooldridge. *Recent Developments in the Econometrics of Program Evaluation* (No. w14251). (Cambridge, MA: National Bureau of Economic Research, 2008).

12. This section is based on the article "Does more intensive treatment of acute myocardial infarction in the elderly reduce mortality? Analysis using instrumental variables" by Mark McClellan, Barbara J. McNeil, and Joseph P. Newhouse, *JAMA* 272 no. 11 (1994): 859–66.

13. Ibid.

14. Hahn, J., P. Todd, and W. Van der Klaauw, "Identification and Estimation of Treatment Effects with a Regression-Discontinuity Design," *Econometrica* 69 no. 1 (2001):

201–9. Retrieved from http://www.jstor.org/stable/2692190.

15. Fan, J., and I. Gijbels. (1996). *Local Polynomial Modelling and its Applications: Monographs on Statistics and Applied Probability* (Boca Raton, FL: CRC Press, 1996).

16. Porter, M., "The Economic Performance of Regions," *Regional Studies* 37 no. 6 (2003): 545–46.

17. Seifert, B., and T. Gasser, "Data Adaptive Ridging in Local Polynomial Regression," *Journal of Computational and Graphical Statistics* 9 (2000): 338–60.

18. Ichimura, H., and P. E. Todd. (2007). "Implementing Nonparametric and Semiparametric Estimators," *Handbook of Econometrics* 6 (2007): 5369–468.

19. Lee, David S., and T. Lemieux, "Regression Discontinuity Designs," *Journal of Economic Literature* 48 (June 2010): 281–355. Accessed September 23, 2014, from https://www.princeton.edu/~davidlee/wp/RDDEconomics.pdf.

20. Imbens, G., and K. Kalyanaraman. "Optimal Bandwidth Choice for the Regression Discontinuity Estimator." *The Review of Economic Studies*, rdr043 (2011).

21. Code i4en Matlab and Stata for calculating the optimal bandwidth is available on their website.

22. Burns, Marguerite E., Laura Dague, Thomas DeLeire, Mary Dorsch, Donna Friedsam, Lindsey Jeanne Leininger, Gaston Palmucci, John Schmelzer, and Kristen Voskuil. "The Effects of Expanding Public Insurance to Rural Low-Income Childless Adults," *Health Services Research* 49, no. S2 (2014): 2173–87.

23. For a more detailed discussion of correlation structures, see Chapter 6 in Rabe-Hesketh S. and A. Skrondal, *Multilevel and Longitudinal Modeling Using Stata* (Stata Press, College Station, TX, 2012).

24. The problems and potential solutions with predicted values for small groups is discussed in O'Brien, S. M., E. R., DeLong, and E. D. Peterson. "Impact of Case Volume on Hospital Performance Assessment," *Archives of Internal Medicine* 168 no. 12 (2008): 1277–84.

25. Cressie, Noel. *Statistics for Spatial Data* (New York, NY: Wiley, 2015).

26. Waller, Lance A., and Carol A. Gotway. *Applied Spatial Statistics for Public Health Data.* Vol. 368. (New York, NY: Wiley, 2004).

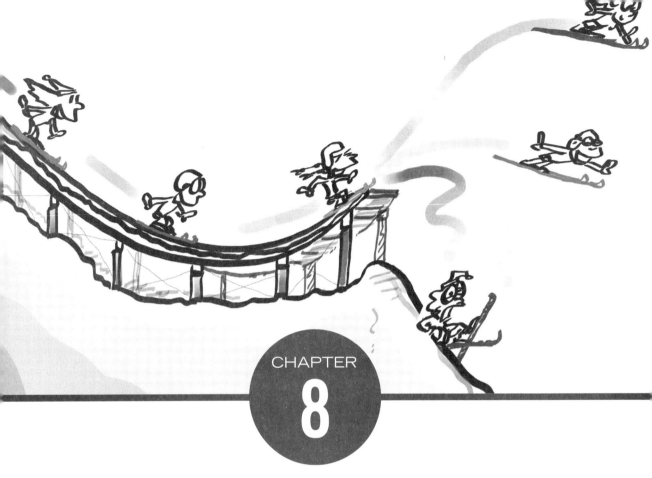

Treatment Effect Variations Among the Treatment Group

Steven Sheingold

Kevin Smith

Lok Wong Samson

Learning Objectives

Evaluation does not need to conclude with a focus solely on the overall average treatment effects (ATE). Indeed, the ATE may not be the experience of most or

(Continued)

(Continued)

even any units in the study. This chapter provides an overview of the source of heterogeneity (variation) in treatment effects (HTE) and what can be learned from understanding when and why the impact of a treatment may differ. HTE may occur because of differences at the environmental level, the organization level, the individual level, or at multiple levels. Analyzing an intervention's contextual factors provides not only a rich description of the intervention, but also a more refined lens through which quantitative findings can be considered. Finally, we discuss some special consideration for assessing contextual factors and heterogeneity in complex interventions.

The previous chapters provide a comprehensive description of methods to estimate program impacts. These methods are generally designed to estimate average treatment effects (ATE). Being able to provide estimates of ATE in the most methodologically rigorous manner possible is critical to summative evaluation. Nonetheless, ATE should not be the end of the line for a full impact analysis that maximizes the information available for program and policy decisions, as well as diffusion of information to support change. The ATE is a convenient overall measure, but it is important to remember that there may be considerable variability, called heterogeneity in statistical terminology, between subjects in their responses to treatment and how the treatments are delivered. Small average effects may reflect a mixture of substantial improvement, little improvement, and declines among the outcomes. To understand heterogeneity of treatment effects (HTE), researchers need to have an appreciation of the likely sources of heterogeneity and of methods that can be used to assess it.

For clinical studies, understanding variation in treatment effects and how the effectiveness of an intervention applies to individual patients is critical. In particular, practitioners need to understand the patient factors associated with variation in effects, that is, which patients might benefit and which patients might be harmed. Ignoring this heterogeneity in responses can lead to situations in which some patients continue to be offered ineffective interventions, while others are denied treatments that could help them. Since many clinical studies are conducted by high-quality institutions and under strict protocols for how care is provided to both treatment and control groups, researchers focus on patient-level characteristics as sources of HTE, as opposed to differences in the quality of the research institutions or how they deliver the treatments.

Social, economic, and health services research (for example, research into effects of changes in the health care delivery system) is more complex with regard to the nature and sources of treatment effect variation. Rather than being delivered under strict protocol by equally capable entities, the treatment/intervention itself often requires the delivering organizations to undertake complex changes in their structure, processes, and possibly organizational culture. Some entities will be more capable and ready than others to undertake these changes, at least initially. Moreover, there may be a variety of potentially viable methods to make these complex changes to implement the intervention. Thus, it is reasonable to expect variation in how the treatment is delivered and in its potential effectiveness across participating organizations. In addition, the effectiveness of the treatment may be influenced by the environment in which it is delivered (such as by local culture, economic, and demographic factors). As discussed in Chapter 2, a planned comprehensive evaluation will identify, and measure to the extent possible, each potential source of variation theorized to influence treatment effectiveness.

Thus, evaluations of complex interventions may need to analyze HTE in terms of factors internal to the delivering organization, external to the organization, and differences in those being served by the program or intervention. The first two are often called context for assessing the intervention and its effects. As with other topics discussed in this book, the relevant literature contains different labels or terminology for these concepts. For example, The Consolidated Framework for Implementation Science offers three possible domains called *inner setting*, *outer setting*, and *individual characteristics*.[1] Other models use treatment contrast, program context, and client characteristics to identify these concepts, with context being associated with external factors.[2]

In this chapter, we refer to these sources of heterogeneity as

1) Factors internal to the organization that may result in variation in how the treatment/intervention is structured and delivered, such as

   a. Differences in cultures, readiness to change, and effectiveness of delivering organization to provide the intervention/treatment

   b. Differences in composition and intensity of methods used in delivery

2) Factors external to the organization (e.g., environmental factors) that affect the delivery or potential effectiveness of the treatment

3) Individual-level factors that may cause the effect to vary among participants receiving the same treatment

The chapter describes each of these factors and then discusses methods that might be applied to evaluate their effect on treatment outcomes. Finally, we discuss statistical methods for analyzing data at these different levels, often called nested data. For example, we may have patient-level data from multiple hospitals, some of which implemented a program expected to reduce hospital readmissions. It may be important to examine variation in effects at both the patient and hospital levels.

Context: Factors Internal to the Organization

Particularly for the large initiatives or legislation-inspired social, health, and economic programs, thinking in recent years on how to conceptualize and examine variation in treatment effects has become more sophisticated.[3] Whether related to evaluating education, training, or health-related programs such as delivery system transformation, there is a growing recognition that the internal and external context in which treatments are delivered can vary greatly from setting to setting, and that this variation may influence effectiveness. For the internal context, several factors have been identified, including those related to the delivering organization and the intervention itself. Often, such programs or initiatives do not specify a specific rigid intervention protocol. That is, they do not require a specific composition or intensity of services in delivering the intervention. Such interventions may be subject to greater heterogeneity in composition and intensity than highly routinized interventions, and hence, they are subject to greater heterogeneity in outcomes. It should be noted, however, that even when there is greater specification concerning the delivery of an intervention, contextual factors may result in differences in delivery. Below we discuss how differences in composition and intensity of methods used in delivery, or the effectiveness of delivery, may be influenced by a number of organizational factors; including structural characteristics, leadership, organizational culture, and focus on quality/value of care.

To introduce how contextual consideration may affect implementation, consider how a patient medication management education program may be implemented across hospitals with varied resource levels. Well-resourced hospitals may implement a pharmacist-led patient education medication management intervention, while hospitals with more limited resources may decide to use nurses to provide patient education on medications. If a protocol for patient medication management is not provided to pharmacists, the content, duration, and frequency of the patient education and frequency of follow-up may vary substantially between individual pharmacists and hospitals and patients. Moreover, there may be substantial differences in the content and quality of education delivered by pharmacists and nurses. A health care system implementing and evaluating this intervention will need to decide how much variation to allow, whether the test should be a rigidly prescribed intervention (as in randomized controlled trial), and whether to allow different hospitals or providers to respond to a general intervention given differences in their resources, policies, and the markets they serve. The important point here is that, even when intervention and treatment protocols are rigidly prescribed, there is often unplanned and unexpected variation in the actual adoption and delivery of any protocol.

Differences in organizational factors that affect staff training, workload, and resource availability may also influence the method and intensity of services delivered, and these differences may impact the intervention or treatment outcomes. For example, clinics that employ nurses in conjunction with training community health workers may provide more frequent home visits for high-risk patients than another clinic that relies only on nurses for patient follow-up.

The business model and strategy pursued by an organization will also help determine its potential effectiveness in delivering services, its profitability, and how it interacts with the external environment. For example, a competitive market environment may lead hospitals to pursue an acquisition/merger strategy. A hospital that decides to buy up physician practices to expand its market share may not yet have developed the internal systems to integrate and deliver services as efficiently and effectively as a vertically integrated health care system; but such a collection of physician practices may be better positioned than an independent hospital to reduce unnecessary readmissions.

An additional important aspect of context is the delivering entity's willingness and ability to adopt an intervention, which in turn affects the intervention's potential effectiveness. Many programs require that organizations make complex changes to deliver the appropriate treatment. Multiple factors may affect an organization's willingness and ability to fully undertake these changes. These factors include an organization's internal culture, structure, leadership, staffing, and human resource policies, and/or whether the organization focuses on internal performance, quality improvement, and client-centered services. Having internal "champions" to support and encourage the adoption of new protocols or technologies is also strongly related to adoption. Experience with change adds a dynamic dimension to these organizational factors. An intervention that seeks to change client outcomes through requiring fundamental organizational change may vary depending on an organization's prior history with implementing change. For example, because teaching hospitals are frequently testing innovations, they may be more comfortable implementing a new practice relative to hospitals in which changes in protocol are less frequent.

Evaluation Approaches and Data Sources to Incorporate Contextual Factors

Understanding the sources of heterogeneous treatment effects is critical to evaluating complex interventions. This is true both from the standpoint of knowing what factors are effective for achieving desired outcomes and which are not, but also for provision of information intended to assist the diffusion of effective intervention into practice. Because of the complex array of organizational characteristics that may in turn result in variation in how the intervention is delivered, there is likely no one analytic solution for explaining the heterogeneous treatment effects, however. On a case-by-case basis, evaluators must decide how to appropriately contextualize the intervention and develop a set of methodological tools for assessing how organizational factors affect the delivery of the intervention and its outcomes. Often, addressing these factors will require mixed methods research—that is, finding the right mix of quantitative and qualitative tools to complement each other for explaining difference in outcomes.

Systematic analysis of the contextual factors in which the intervention takes place is needed for evaluations to address the internal and external threats to validity. Systematic study involves conceptualizing context as a theoretical construct, then operationalizing it as a variable, and including variability of that contextual variable in the evaluation. Researchers and evaluators often find the limited context in which an intervention takes place is a limitation to the generalizability of study findings. Without explicitly including contextual variables in the evaluation at baseline, during implementation and postintervention, the interdependencies between levels of contextual factors and relationship to how the intervention is implemented and how they ultimately impact the outcomes cannot be studied.

Contextual factors often require qualitative methods to elicit information about complex processes that are not housed in databases. The complexity of relationships and interdependencies may require in-depth qualitative methods such as participant observation, archival document analysis or key informant interviews to understand the role of context in the intervention in conjunction with direct measurement through surveys. For example, organizational assessments and surveys seek to understand and quantify differences in roles, attitudes, readiness for change and behaviors among leaders, and management and front line workers within an organization. Below we describe a recent framework for evaluating complex interventions, and then Chapter 9 provides additional detail on the measurement framework for organizing these concerns and introduces several validated tools for measuring organizational context.

Complex, multicomponent, and multilevel interventions, especially those that seek broader systems change, need special attention to be given to contextual factors in evaluation and implementation. Alexander and Hearld identified key issues and challenges from conducting delivery-systems research and provided their recommendations to identifying and analyzing HTE from contextual factors, including time.[4] The following issues and challenges are relevant to most evaluations:

1) Modeling intervention context—intervention is mediated by a complex host of factors that affect the relationship between the intervention and outcomes

2) Readiness and capacity for adopting and implementing the proposed intervention or change, which may be confounded by readiness for/ resistance to change

3) Assessing intervention fidelity and sustainability—variation due to contextual factors that are difficult to assess in the short term

4) Assessing multicomponent interventions

5) Incorporating time as an analytic variable

The Alexander and Hearld recommendations to address these issues can be applied through mixed methods research, incorporating both qualitative and quantitative methods. Qualitative approaches include

- contextualization of the intervention through detailed description and reflection of the role of context,

- assessing capacity and readiness for implementing the intervention and change through surveys or interviews,

- measuring factors that influence implementation of the intervention,

- monitoring implementation and fidelity to the intervention, and

- assessing dynamic, multifaceted aspects of interventions.

Quantitative approaches to addressing these issues include

- incorporating key aspects of multicomponent interventions in longitudinal monitoring and models,

- identifying temporal patterns in data (including time-varying predictors), and

- exploring interactions between the intervention and participant outcomes.

Synthesizing contextual factor findings among an array of programs in an evaluation may benefit from more recently developed methods. For example, qualitative comparative analysis is a method for analyzing qualitative data that uses set theory to help with causal understanding of sufficient factors in an intervention's success. This approach complements quantitative regression-based study designs in understanding causal relationships and is addressed in Chapter 10. Furthermore, meta-analytic techniques can be employed to identify and quantify program heterogeneity. Dubbed "meta-evaluation," this method utilizes both qualitative and quantitative evaluation findings; we discuss meta-evaluation in further detail in Chapter 14.

Context: External Factors That Affect the Delivery or Potential Effectiveness of the Treatment

Factors external to the organization and professions that should be considered for understanding the heterogeneity of treatment effects include local economic characterisics, regional market pressures, local policy or regulatory changes, interests of professional societies, and area resources and culture. For example, a history and culture of engaging in collaborative learning across organizations in a market may facilitate these organizations' effective adoption of new interventions compared to a similar market without this history and learning environment. Secular trends in the environment may also impact the outcomes of interest—such as focus on quality improvement by medical professional societies in their training and re-certification programs—which may directly influence professionals' delivery of services independent of an organization's employee training on quality improvement. The ability to capture and describe this larger environmental context, as well as to target key groups through sampling or stratification, may help to identify sources of heterogeneity of treatment effects that will be important for appropriate generalization of observed effects.

Environmental factors relevant to the individual patients/clients receiving the intervention typically include the characteristics of the neighborhood and community resources where a person lives and works, such as transportation, access to and availability of high-quality services, history and concentration of poverty and unemployment, community support services, availability of fresh produce, and local policies. Several of these environmental factors may influence the effectiveness of an intervention. For example, the availability of housing support for low-income seniors in assisted living communities may affect the impact of an intervention designed to reduce length of nursing home stays, due to the influence of an individual's access to other services. Environmental factors may also influence where individuals seek and obtain services and treatment. For example, physicians serving poor neighborhoods may have weaker specialist referral networks, reducing the effectiveness of a cancer screening program to improve timely cancer diagnosis and treatment outcomes for patients seeking care from those clinics. For many behavioral interventions, social support, religious affiliation, and other social and cultural features of patient/client lives may be important influences of intervention uptake.

It is possible that such external factors could influence HTE in two ways: (1) by influencing the internal contextual factors described above (e.g., market characteristics, laws, regulation may influence organizational culture); and (2) by moderating or mediating the effect of an intervention on outcomes (e.g., the impact of school-based programs may vary among local areas based on the overall educational infrastructure available). The first of these influences would best be examined along with the internal contextual factors. The potential for the external factors to moderate or mediate the treatment effect can generally be quantified and controlled for with standard statistical techniques such as regression—as long as evaluators can identify and measure them.

Individual-Level Factors That May Cause Treatment Effect to Vary

Individual level factors may influence both the professionals delivering the intervention and the clients/patients receiving the treatment or intervention. If the intervention is targeted at the professionals who will deliver the intervention, how they perceive, understand, and respond to the intervention is another individual source of heterogeneity. Their prior training, skills, orientation toward team work, age, beliefs, and languages spoken may also lead to differences in how the intervention is delivered to clients/patients. Individual factors of the persons receiving the treatment, such as disease type and severity and sociodemographic factors—educational level, housing situation, and economic status—may affect the effectiveness of an intervention on impacting outcomes relevant to the individual, especially if the intervention does not directly address those factors. There may also be an interaction of factors between the professional and the client/patient, such as language or culture concordance, which likely impact outcomes that are influenced by the effectiveness of a professional to motivate behavior change in a client/patient.

Individuals delivering the intervention are also influenced by the external and organizational environment through organizational training, staffing, and reimbursement/incentives policies. In addition, external or organizational factors may influence the behavior or types of individuals seeking care or services. For example, high concentrations of poverty may lead to fragmented social and community supports in a neighborhood; people residing in these areas may be more likely to seek emergency medical care, and hospitals serving them may find individual case management programs less effective than approaches to build community support services and linkages to them.

In terms of measurement, it is useful to examine key sources of heterogeneity for HTE analyses:

In clinical studies, four dimensions can affect a patient's response to a particular treatment:[5]

1) The risk of incurring an adverse event without treatment (benefits to patients usually increase with risk)

2) Responsiveness to the treatment (genetic or metabolic factors that produce bigger effects in some patients than others)

3) Vulnerability to adverse side effects (genetic and environmental influences on susceptibility, including drug metabolism and receptor binding)

4) Preferences for different health states (patient preferences for specific outcomes can vary 10-fold for the same disease)

The sources of heterogeneity are likely to be quite different for social programs and community health interventions where individual biology is less important. In these settings, potential sources include the following:

- In health care interventions, HTE may be related to patient adherence, initial health status, disease severity, or duration of disease. A particularly good candidate is often a baseline measure of the primary outcome because effects might be expected to be largest among those with highest baseline risk. For expenditure and utilization outcomes, effects might be strongest for previous high-cost patients or high utilizers.

- Program effects may vary by socioeconomic status or by levels of social support.

- HTE is a situation in which the magnitude of the treatment effect is correlated with the probability of receiving treatment. This correlation may emerge whenever a subject attempts to increase her chances of being selected because she (correctly) believes that the treatment will be more beneficial for her than for others. The same situation can occur when care providers or social service representatives act on behalf of a client.

- In multisite studies, HTE may result from variations in program delivery, uneven implementation, or variations in program fidelity.

Methods for Examining the Individual Level Heterogeneity of Treatment Effects

There are three methods that might be used as part of an evaluation to examine individual level sources of heterogeneity. These are described below.

1. Subgroup Analysis

    The most common method for testing for HTE involves subgroup analysis. In this method, subgroups within the target population are identified (e.g., male vs. female; insured vs. uninsured; diabetes vs. no diabetes; low, medium, and high adherence). Treatment effects are then estimated from a regression model containing indicators for the subgroups, the treatment, and an interaction term formed by the product of the subgroup and treatment indicators. A significant interaction term is evidence of HTE.[6] ATE is a weighted composite of the subgroup effects. More favorable results in one group must be offset by less favorable results in another subgroup.

    Consider, for example, an intervention that assigns nurse coaches to work with patients in an effort to improve patient's self-management skills. The goal of the program is to reduce health care expenditures. An observational study is conducted in which the coaching treatment is compared to a group of patients receiving usual care. The investigators suspect that the program may be more beneficial for patients who have two or more chronic conditions than for those with fewer conditions.

    Ordinary least squares (OLS) regression results for this hypothetical study are shown in Table 8.1. The primary outcome is monthly health care expenditures. Age, gender, Medicare eligibility, and an indicator for two or more chronic conditions are covariates in the regression model. The first column of the table shows the results for a standard analysis. The coefficient for the coaching treatment group indicator, the ATE, shows small, but statistically insignificant monthly savings ($b = \$150$, $SE = 116.9$, $p > 0.05$). Potential heterogeneity is tested in the second column of results, which adds the conditions by treatment group interaction to the model. The interaction term is statistically significant, indicating that heterogeneity is present in the treatment effects. The overall cost savings are greater among patients with two or more chronic conditions than for those with fewer conditions by $255 per month.

Subgroup analyses require that individual characteristics be specified prior to the analyses. These subgroups should be based on strong theoretical reasons for suspecting treatment effect heterogeneity. When a potential source of HTE can be identified in advance on conceptual grounds, there still remains the problem of measuring the hypothesized factor in a manner that lends itself to subgroup classification. If standardized instruments are available to measure the factor (e.g., depression levels or self-efficacy to perform self-management activities), then the instruments can be incorporated into the study protocol, and subgroups can be delineated based on the instrument scores.

While the subgroup method is the most popular approach for testing heterogeneity, it has several potential shortcomings. First, the method tends to invite exploratory fishing expeditions in which multiple subpopulations are tested in an attempt to find something that will yield significant findings.[7,8] Searches should be limited to only a few a priori subgroups with a sound theoretical basis for heterogeneity, a criterion that is increasingly enforced by scholarly journals.[9] A useful set of guidelines developed for reporting subgroup methods in clinical trials also has broad applicability to observational studies.[10] Second, analyses are typically underpowered to detect anything other than large interaction effects. Simulations show that subgroup analyses have only 29% power to detect an effect as large as the overall treatment effect.[11] Moreover, for a range of study characteristics, statistically significant false-positive subgroup effects were found in 7% to 21% of simulations in which there was no overall treatment effect. Third, subgroup effects are often of dubious generalizability since the effects found in a single study may not be representative of the target population. This is especially true for ad hoc tests.[12,13]

2. Propensity Score Approach

Another approach for exploring HTE uses propensity scores. A propensity score (PS) is the probability that a subject is a member of the treatment group conditional on observed covariates. Rather than specifying characteristics to be tested as in subgroup analysis, the PS approach examines whether treatment effects vary by the likelihood that subjects have been selected for treatment. Different effects for different levels of PSs are evidence for HTE.

The basic approach involves the following steps:

1) Estimate propensity scores for probability of treatment for all subjects using a logistic regression model.

2) Divide the entire sample into strata with similar ranges of PS scores. Quintiles are frequently used to define strata.

3) Estimate treatment effect separately within each stratum.

4) In a second stage model, regress the estimated stratum effects on the PS stratum rank.

5) Linear effects in second-stage model are evidence of HTE, indicating that treatment effects systematically increase (or decrease) with the probability of being selected for treatment.

In essence, the PS strata take the role of subgroups in this approach. Detailed procedures are given in Xie et al. (2012)[14] who also describe methods for using continuous PSs and smoothing techniques.

An example of the approach is provided by Brand and Davis (2011)[15] who were interested in the impact of college attendance on

	Model 1 (no interaction effect)	Model 2 (with interaction effect)
	Coefficient (S.E.)	Coefficient (S.E.)
Age	8.4 (5.8)	12.7 (5.1)
Female	−12.6 (82.5)	22.3 (91.8)
Medicare	1305.8** (120.3)	1283.4** (131.7)
Two or more conditions	1424.1** (116.9)	1348.2** (119.4)
Treatment group	−150.2 (80.5)	−88.3 (96.7)
Treatment * Two or more conditions	— —	−254.5* (125.6)
Intercept	−386.7 (306.6)	−433.2 (273.6)

Table 8.1 Regression Estimates of Subgroup Interaction Effects for Hypothetical Coaching Treatment

N = 1000; * p < 0.05; ** p < 0.01

women's fertility. Their initial analysis showed that by the time women were 41 years old, attending college reduced childbearing by 17%. They then estimated a PS model for the probability that the women in their sample attended college, divided the sample into six propensity strata, and examined the trend in attendance effects across strata. The results of the second stage regression indicated that attendance effects were negatively correlated with propensity stratum. This is a heterogeneous effect since the impact of college attendance was smaller for those who were the most likely to attend college.

3. Impact Variation Approach

In randomized trials, HTE can be detected by comparing the outcome variances of the treatment and control groups.[16] If there is no heterogeneity, these variances should be similar. This is tested statistically by computing the F-test for the ratio of the two variances. A significant F value indicates that effects vary across individuals.

It should be noted that this approach is valid only in the case of randomized studies. Furthermore, the difference in group outcome variances is not the same as the variance of individual treatment effects. As noted earlier, that comparison requires knowledge of the correlation between impacts and counterfactual outcomes.

Multilevel Factors

Conceptualizing context at different levels—group, organizational, external, or geographic environment, as well as individuals—will also add richness to understanding context in a multilevel evaluation. Existing data may be available at these different levels that can be utilized in quantitative analysis. However, multimethod approaches to analyzing both quantitative and qualitative data will help with interpreting heterogeneous treatment effects, instead of concluding null effects from the average treatment effect.

The different levels of contextual factors previously described—organizational, environmental, and individual—result in a multilevel environment in which an intervention is implemented and evaluated. For example, how an organization chooses to respond to a national policy (such as a hospital pay-for-performance program) may be based on a constellation of local environmental and organizational factors such as local market competition—the presence of competing (or complementary) initiatives by other key stakeholders or payers that interacts with the strength of the performance incentives. Such external environmental factors also interact with an organization's mission, culture, and financial standing to influence how a national policy changes hospital behavior and how its staff deliver services to patients.

This interplay among national, regional, local, organizational, and individual level factors can all influence who gets treatment, how that treatment is delivered, and the extent to which benefit from the treatment can be estimated. A multilevel approach to evaluation can help describe and document those potential sources of influence and can elucidate the mechanism in which an intervention targeting organizations at one level impacts behavior of professionals at another level, and individual client/patient outcomes at still another.[17]

Importance of Incorporating Contextual Factors Into an Evaluation

Systematic analysis of the contextual factors in which the intervention takes place is needed for evaluations to address the internal and external threats to validity. Systematic study involves conceptualizing context as a theoretical construct, then operationalizing it as a variable, and including the variability of that contextual variable in the evaluation.[18] Researchers and evaluators often find the restrictive context in which an intervention takes place to be a limitation to the generalizability of study findings. In other words, without explicitly including contextual variables in the evaluation at baseline, during implementation, and postintervention, the interdependencies between levels of contextual factors, and their relationship to how the intervention is implemented and how they ultimately impact the outcomes cannot be studied.

Conceptualizing context at different levels—group, organizational, external, or geographic environment, as well as individuals—will also add richness to understanding context in a multilevel evaluation. Existing data may be available at these different levels for use in quantitative analysis. However, mixed methods approaches to analyzing both quantitative and qualitative data may also help with interpreting heterogeneous treatment effects, instead of concluding null effects from the ATE, when in reality, half the patients benefited and half worsened when exposed to treatment.

SUMMARY

Evaluation does not need to conclude with a focus solely on the overall ATE. An assessment of HTE may deepen a policymaker's understanding of what programs work and in which settings. This chapter describes different types of HTE and points to key elements of successful HTE analyses. We have paid special attention to heterogeneity in complex interventions, detailing the need for mixed methods research to meet the challenge of analyzing these interventions, and in the next chapter, we discuss the tools that can be used to evaluate the implementation of an intervention. Carefully designed HTE analyses do not only reveal a more complete picture of an intervention, but they can also provide the empirical basis for expanding, modifying, rescaling, or terminating programs in the future.

DISCUSSION QUESTIONS

1. How does the level of the heterogeneity of treatment effects impact an evaluator's decision to estimate the average treatment effect, the average treatment effect on the treated, or the intent to treat effect?

2. How can evaluators strike a balance between restricting the context of an intervention to make an evaluation valid and maintaining a sufficient level of generalizability of study findings?

3. Discuss the implications of analyzing subgroups to understand heterogeneity. Do subgroups need to be specified a priori so that power can be considered?

NOTES

1. Kathryn M. McDonald, "Considering Context in Quality Improvement Interventions and Implementation: Concepts, Frameworks and Application," *Academic Pediatrics* 13 no. 6 Supplement (November– December 2013): S45–S53.

2. Michael J. Weiss, Howard S. Bloom, and Thomas Brock, "A Conceptual Framework for Studying the Sources of Variation in Program Effects," *MDRC*, June 2013.

3. Ibid.; Jeffrey A. Alexander, and Larry R. Hearld, "Methods and Metrics Challenges for Delivery System Research," *Implementation Science* 7 no. 15 (2012).

4. Alexander and Hearld, 2012.

5. Richard L. Kravitz, Naihua Duan, and Joel Braslow, "Evidence-Based Medicine, Heterogeneity of Treatment Effects, and the Trouble with Averages," *Milbank Quarterly* 82, no. 4 (December 2004): 661–87.

6. Pocock, S. J., M. D. Hughes, and R. J. Lee (1987). "Statistical Problems in the Reporting of Clinical Trials. A Survey of Three Medical Journals." *New England Journal of Medicine* 317 no. 7 (1987): 426–32. doi: 10.1056/NEJM198708133170706

7. Ibid.

8. Assmann, S. F., S. J. Pocock, L. E. Enos, and L. E. Kasten, "Subgroup analysis and other (mis)uses of baseline data in clinical trials," *Lancet* 355 no. 9209 (2000): 1064–69. doi: 10.1016/S0140-6736(00)02039-0

9. Rothwell, P. M. "Treating Individuals 2. Subgroup Analysis in Randomised Controlled Trials: Importance, Indications, and Interpretation." *Lancet* 365 no. 9454 (2005): 176–86. doi: 10.1016/S0140-6736(05)17709-5

10. Wang, Rui, Stephen W. Lagakos, James H. Ware, David J. Hunter, and Jeffrey M. Drazen, "Statistics in Medicine—Reporting of Subgroup Analyses in Clinical Trials," *New England Journal of Medicine* 357 no. 21 (2007): 2189–94.

11. Brookes, S. T., E. Whitely, M. Egger, G. D. Smith, P. A. Mulheran, and T. J. Peters, "Subgroup Analyses in Randomized Trials: Risks of Subgroup-Specific Analyses; Power and Sample Size for the Interaction Test," *Journal of Clinical Epidemiology* 57 no. 3 (2004): 229–36. doi: 10.1016/j.jclinepi.2003.08.009

12. Parker, A. B., and C. D. Naylor "Subgroups, Treatment Effects, and Baseline Risks: Some Lessons from Major Cardiovascular Trials." *American Heart Journal* 139 no. 6 (2000): 952–61. doi: 10.1067/mhj.2000.106610

13. Yusuf, S., J. Wittes, J. Probstfield, and H. A. Tyroler, "Analysis and Interpretation of Treatment Effects in Subgroups of Patients in Randomized Clinical Trials." *JAMA* 266 no.1 (1991): 93–98.

14. Brand, J. E., and Y. Xie, "Who Benefits Most From College? Evidence for Negative Selection in Heterogeneous Economic Returns to Higher Education." *American Sociological Review* 75 no. 2 (2010): 273–302. doi: 10.1177/0003122410363567

15. Brand, J. E., and D. Davis, "The Impact of College Education on Fertility: Evidence for Heterogeneous Effects." *Demography* 48 no. 3 (2011): 863–87. doi: 10.1007/s13524-011-0034-3

16. Bloom, H. S., S. S. Raudenbush, and M. Weiss, "Estimating variation in program impacts theory, practice and applications." Unpublished draft manuscript (New York, NY: Manpower Demonstration Research Corporation, 2011).

17. For example, Burke et al. (2014) show how Hierarchical Linear Modeling can be applied to health plans nested within issuers, rating areas, and states to disentangle the effects of these characteristics on health insurance premiums. Burke, A., A. Misra, and S. Sheingold, "Premium affordability, competition, and choice in the health insurance marketplace" (June 18, 2014). ASPE Research Brief, accessed October 20, 2014, from http://aspe.hhs.gov/health/reports/2014/Premiums/2014MktPlacePremBrf.pdf.

18. Rousseau, D. M., and Y. Fried "Location, Location, Location: Contextualizing Organizational Research." *Journal of Organizational Behavior* 22 (2001): 1–13. doi: 10.1002/job.78

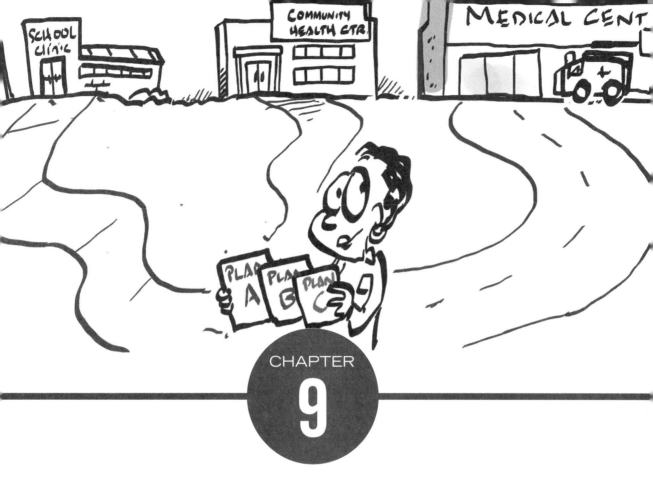

9

The Impact of Organizational Context on Heterogeneity of Outcomes

Lessons for Implementation Science

Thomas Nolan

Leila Kahwati

Heather Kane

Learning Objectives

The implementation process is critical to innovation and often holds lessons, not only for implementation success in that particular case, but for the scalability of that intervention model as well. Understanding when an intervention works or doesn't, or what is required for successful implementation of a particular model, is a critical learning step. This chapter presents commonly used frameworks for implementation research, including the Action on Research Implementation in Health Research Framework and the Consolidated Framework for Implementation Research, followed by a review of tools that can be used to analyze organizational readiness for change. Finally, it presents an introduction to Qualitative Comparative Analysis, a technique used to assess which of the numerous features of an intervention, context, individuals, and organization(s) can be identified sufficient for implementation success.

The previous chapter explored the issue of analyzing heterogeneity in outcomes as part of a comprehensive evaluation. One potential source of heterogeneity is the characteristics of the organizations delivering the intervention, particularly when doing so requires these organizations to undertake complex system changes. Analyzing these factors internal to the organization can involve a variety of quantitative and qualitative approaches. In this chapter, we describe these approaches in greater depth.

The chapter also introduces the topic of implementation science, which is often defined as the scientific study of methods to promote the systematic uptake of research findings and other evidence-based practices into routine practice, and hence, to improve the quality and effectiveness of health services. One difference between the evaluation strategies we have discussed and implementation science is that the former assesses whether an intervention is effective; the latter assesses its adoption when shown effective. Nonetheless, evaluation and implementation science are related in important ways. For one, assessing how effective innovation diffuses into practice often uses traditional evaluation methods. More importantly, implementation science emphasizes methods and measures to establish the appropriate organizational context for adopting innovations; these same methods and measures can be used to establish context for evaluations. In this chapter, we explore the applicable lessons from implementation science, while using recent Centers for Medicare and Medicaid Innovation (CMMI) models as examples.

Context for the Evaluation: Some Examples From Centers for Medicare and Medicaid Innovation

In many demonstrations, the intervention is delivered at the level of a health care organization (for example, primary care practices or hospitals). The impact of the intervention on patient outcomes may then depend on the characteristics of the organization. At the same time, these characteristics can have a direct effect on outcomes, independent of the intervention. Understanding the environment in which the intervention is delivered is therefore crucial to a successful evaluation. For example, in the Multipayer Advanced Primary Care Practice Demonstration (see Chapter 6, Box 6.5 for description) participating medical homes practices are matched to comparison practices on the basis of several observable characteristics. However, it is quite possible that participating medical homes practices are more innovative risk-takers and more responsive to financial and other program incentives than nonparticipants, irrespective of the demonstration. Such characteristics can be expected to explain some of the observed change in outcomes, yet they may be difficult to quantify.

Other demonstrations may deliver the intervention across organizational boundaries. This poses an even greater challenge for the evaluator seeking to establish causal links between the intervention and the performance. Examples include the Accountable Care Organizations and the Community-Based Care Transitions demonstrations. In addition to the characteristics and capabilities of individual organizations, the outcomes of such demonstrations are likely to be affected by the characteristics of the multiorganization coalition.

Several themes emerge after a review of the demonstrations sponsored by CMMI that are germane to design of an evaluation and analysis of the outcomes:[1]

1) Centers for Medicare and Medicaid Services (CMS) is changing which services it pays for or how it pays for them, and is leaving it to the participating organizations to decide how to redesign care.

2) The specified interventions may be technical in nature: specific payment agreements or shared savings contracts. Interventions like these do not change care itself. They are hypothesized to create the environment to promote the improved models of care, which combine new processes and social systems.

3) Many initiatives allow providers to share in any cost savings that result from their efforts to give them a financial incentive to redesign care.

4) Some of the initiatives involve complex design efforts, for example, developing an effective Accountable Care Organization (ACO) or statewide innovations. Others seek to spread evidence-based improvements across multiple sites (such as primary care practices or long-term care facilities).

Certain evaluation challenges related to organizational characteristics arise given these circumstances. The ability of organizations and coalitions to execute such complex system changes will vary substantially. Heterogeneity of outcomes is quite probable, even for participants that choose similar models of care to implement. If not recognized and managed, the variation across organizations may be misattributed to patient mix characteristics or provider skill, or simply remain as unexplained error variance (increasing the likelihood of a Type II error, that is, mistakenly failing to reject the null hypothesis when an effect is present).

Because of the pertinence of demonstrations at and across the organization-level and the complexity of assessing their characteristics, this chapter expands the discussion of organization-level characteristics and heterogeneity from Chapter 8. It provides methods that enable evaluators to recognize variation in organizational capability for improvement, instruments for measuring implementation effectiveness, and tools to take such variation into account in designing an evaluation and interpreting its results.

Evaluation for
Complex Systems Change

In demonstrations of large or complex systems with loosely specified interventions, heterogeneity of treatment effects should be assumed.[2] The class of "theory-based evaluations" is apt to address interventions in which behavior change and new models are utilized to affect the outcomes of interest. One of the evaluation methods in this category has been termed Realist Evaluation by Pawson and Tilley.[3] It assumes that the pattern in outcomes is a function of the intervention mechanism and the context in which the mechanism is applied. Included under context is the capability of the organizations to improve, as measured by the Promoting Action on Research Implementation in Health Services (PARIHS) framework or other organizational assessments. Table 9.1 outlines several of the CMMI demonstration projects using the Realist Evaluation Framework.

The table makes clear why an organization assessment may be an important aspect of the evaluation of CMMI demonstrations (as in non–health system demonstrations as well). In each demonstration, the intervention and outcomes are only indirectly linked. The intervention is often a payment mechanism that incentivizes a participant to improve processes or design new models of care. The capability of each participant to perform this task is a source of heterogeneity. This does not mean the CMMI demonstrations can only succeed for the highest performing health care systems. Formative research could lead to a more well-defined set of interventions that include an understanding of the environment created by the payment mechanism. In addition, effective technical assistance ("facilitation" in the PARIHS framework) may also be used to support organizational capabilities for improvement.

Demonstration and Outcomes	Mechanism	Context
Advanced Payment ACO Model (January 13, 2013) – Medicare expenditures per attributed members – Quality measures	Accountable Care Organizations (ACOs) create incentives for health care providers to work together to treat an individual patient across care settings. The Medicare Shared Savings Program will reward ACOs that lower their growth in health care costs, while meeting performance standards on quality of care. Provider participation in an ACO is purely voluntary, and Medicare beneficiaries retain their current ability to seek treatment from any provider they wish.	– Across care settings including doctor's offices, hospitals, and long-term care facilities. – Improvement capability of individual organizations in the ACO – Characteristics and capabilities of the ACO
Physician Group Practice Demo (First report to Congress 2006) – Medicare expenditures per attributed members – Quality measures	Goals: (1) testing the use of incentives for health care groups; (2) encouraging coordination of health care furnished under Medicare Parts A and B; (3) encouraging investment in care management infrastructure and processes for efficient service delivery; and (4) rewarding physicians for improving health care processes and outcomes. Programs include chronic disease management programs, high-risk/high-cost care management, transitional care management, end-of-life/palliative care programs, and initiatives designed to standardize and improve the quality of care.	Demonstration participants represent large physician-driven organizations with diverse organizational structures including free-standing multispecialty group practices, faculty group practices, integrated delivery systems, and a physician network made up of small and individual one-physician practices.
Bundled Payments for Care Improvement 2 (Accessed June 29, 2013) – Medicare expenditures per episode – Quality measures	Research has shown that bundled payments can align incentives for providers—hospitals, postacute care providers, doctors, and other practitioners—to partner closely across all specialties and settings that a patient may encounter to improve the patient's experience of care during a hospital stay in an acute care hospital, and during postdischarge recovery.	In Model 2, the episode of care will include the inpatient stay in the acute care hospital and all related services during the episode. The episode will end either 30, 60, or 90 days after hospital discharge. Participants can select up to 48 different clinical condition episodes.

Frameworks for Implementation Research

Using standard methods and tools to assess organizational characteristics may increase the evaluator's understanding of the link between organizational characteristics, performance, and demonstration success. PARIHS is a framework for guiding implementation of evidence-based practice.[5,6] Since it was first developed, it has been revised and widely cited and used.[7] The PARIHS framework is built on the hypothesis that successfully implementing evidence-based practice is a function of three components—evidence, context, and facilitation:

1. Evidence is characterized by findings from prior research, clinical experience, patient experience, and local data.
2. Context is characterized by culture, leadership, and evaluation.
3. Facilitation is characterized by purpose, role, skills, and attributes.

The three elements and the multiple sub-elements of the PARIHS framework have shown up in various formats in other research. For example, Gustafson, et al. developed 18 criteria and used them to predict the success or failure of improvement projects in health care organizations.[8] Their criteria addressed involvement of the organizations' leadership, staff involvement, clinical leadership, the nature of the change itself, evidence for the change, and investment in the change process. Another framework with the same fundamental purpose is the Consolidated Framework for Implementation Research (CFIR) (see Box 9.1).[9]

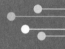

Box 9.1
Consolidated Framework for Implementation Research

The Consolidated Framework for Implementation Research (CFIR) is a commonly used framework in assessing the implementation of health service delivery interventions. To the extent that this framework is applied across studies, it can allow for common features and processes to be defined and understood not only within one particular study, but across a number of studies, thereby improving our understanding of the implementation process.

CFIR has five major domains (the intervention, inner setting, outer setting, the individuals involved, and the process by which implementation is accomplished). This basic structure is also partially echoed by the Promoting Action on Research Implementation in Health Services framework, which describes the three key domains of evidence, context, and facilitation.

1. The intervention is being implemented into a particular organization. Without adaptation, interventions usually come to a setting as a poor fit, resisted by individuals who will be affected by the intervention, and requiring an active process to engage individuals to accomplish implementation. Interventions are conceptualized as having core components (the essential and indispensable elements of the intervention itself) and an adaptable periphery (adaptable elements, structures, and systems related to the intervention and organization into which it is being implemented).

2. The inner setting includes features of structural, political, and cultural contexts through which the implementation process will proceed.

3. The outer setting includes the economic, political, and social context within which an organization resides.

4. The individuals involved with the intervention and/or implementation process have agency; they make choices and can wield power and influence on others with predictable or unpredictable consequences for implementation. Individuals are carriers of cultural, organizational, professional, and individual mindsets, norms, interests, and affiliations.

5. The implementation process, to be successful, usually requires an active change process aimed to achieve individual and organizational level use of the intervention, as designed.

These processes—which may be formally planned or spontaneous, conscious or subconscious, linear or nonlinear—are all aimed, ideally, in the same general direction: effective implementation. More detailed subdomains and descriptions are available at www.biomedcentral.com/content/supplementary/1748-5908-4-50-S3.pdf.

Organizational Assessment Tools

A common framework that can be used to describe components of the intervention, the setting into which it will be implemented, the individuals involved, and the implementation process provides a useful backdrop for tools that assess organizational readiness for change. In the CFIR framework, for example, most of these tools would be considered to assess the inner context. Assessment of organizational capability can be used to check for balance between the intervention and comparison sites, or as a qualitative or quantitative covariate in analyzing the results. Several possibilities for doing this type of assessment are presented later in this section.

A recent literature review broadly categorizes the different organizational characteristics that may affect readiness for change into four areas: structural characteristics, leadership, organizational culture, and focus on quality or value of care.[10] Each of these areas can be further deconstructed into more specific organizational characteristics:

1) *Structural characteristics*: size, ownership, financial performance, membership in a provider network, and institutional resources

2) *Leadership*: alignment of goals, creating an effective training and learning environment, and level of leadership engagement in the change process

3) *Organizational culture*: shared values, emphasis on learning and development, clear articulation and alignment of organizational goals, participation in external collaboratives, and employee incentive programs

4) *Focus on quality/value of care*: use of reporting systems and feedback loops, empanelment (whether or not patients are assigned to a single provider), quality-improvement strategies, measuring of clinical performance and patient satisfaction, patient-centered interactions, care coordination, and evidence-based care[11]

Each of the survey instruments shown in Table 9.2 investigates many but not all of these characteristics. This list, which is far from exhaustive, offers useful options for organizational assessment for health care delivery change.

Table 9.2 Organizational Readiness Characteristic Domains, by Survey Instrument[12]

Survey Instrument	Structure	Leadership	Culture	Focus on Value
1. Organizational Learning Capacity Scale (OLCS)	✓	✓	✓	✓
2. Patient-Centered Medical Home Assessment (PCMH-A)	✓	✓		✓
3. Organizational Readiness for Change (ORCA)	✓	✓	✓	✓
4. AHRQ[13] Change Process Capability Questionnaire (CPCQ)		✓	✓	✓
5. TeamSTEPPS Teamwork Perceptions Questionnaire	✓	✓	✓	

1. *Organizational Learning Capacity Scale (OLCS):* This instrument contains 13 questions assessing the individual-level experience, 6 questions on team- or group-level experience, 24 questions on individual perceptions of the organization, and 15 questions regarding organization performance or characteristics. All survey questions except 3 solicit scalar responses to prompts on the topic area (e.g., never, rarely, sometimes, often, always).[14]

2. *Patient-Centered Medical Home Assessment (PCMH-A):* Designed to evaluate an organization's progress toward PCMH accreditation or a PCMH's "current level of 'medical homeness,'" this instrument contains 33 items spanning the 8 topical areas: engaged leadership, quality improvement strategies, patient empanelment, continuous and team-based healing relationships, evidence-based care, patient-centered interactions, enhanced access to care, and care

coordination. Respondents are asked to assign a point value to each prompt on a 12-point scale, indicating the level of care they believe their organization (or site within an organization) exhibits. Each section's score is an average score of the questions within that section; the overall score is an average of the eight section averages.[15]

3. *Organizational Readiness for Change Assessment (ORCA)*: As its name suggests, this instrument examines respondent perceptions of organizational readiness for adopting and implementing changes, using a 5-point scalar response instrument (e.g., "strongly disagree" to "strongly agree"). This tool can be adapted to evaluate gaps in readiness to implement different organizational changes. An example of this tool (in an evaluation of readiness for process changes at Veterans Health Administration sites) can be found in DesRoches, Jaszczak, and Situ's *Environmental Scan*.[16]

4. *AHRQ's Change Process Capability Questionnaire (CPCQ)*: AHRQ provides a 32-question survey instrument to evaluate degree of interest and dedication to implementing change, and different strategies that may have been used in an organization's transition. AHRQ fielded this Internet-based survey to over 40 quality improvement coordinators or directors and achieved a 100% response rate. This instrument may be useful as is in a given program or demonstration evaluation, or it may serve as a reference point for future survey samples.[17]

5. *TeamSTEPPS Teamwork Perceptions Questionnaire (T-TPQ)*: This 35-question instrument assesses the degree to which respondents agree or disagree with various prompts, spanning such topics as team structure, leadership, situation monitoring, mutual support, and communication. The RTI evaluation of the Health Care Innovation Awards (HCIA) for CMMI incorporated this tool into its own survey instrument to evaluate implementation effectiveness in the ongoing HCIA demonstrations. (More information on the HCIA evaluation can be found in Chapter 13.)[18]

These tools, among others, have been used over time by CMS to evaluate capacity for and progress toward change in numerous demonstrations. Box 9.2 provides a snapshot of the different organizational characteristics currently being evaluated for four CMMI demonstrations.[19]

None of the organizational assessment models described above make the claim to be predictive of positive results. Most mention that as more aspects of the model present at a high level in the organization, the more "likely" the project will be to accomplish its desired results. The implication is that the framework elements are best thought of as necessary but not sufficient for a successful demonstration.

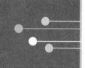

Box 9.2

Organizational Characteristics Currently Being Evaluated By CMMI

Organizational Characteristics	CMMI Demonstration			
	MAPCP[1] Provider Survey	CPC[2] Provider Survey	CPC Practice Survey	FQHC-APCP[3] Staff Survey
Enhanced access to care	✓			
Team-based relationships	✓	✓	✓	
Patient-centered care	✓			
Care coordination	✓	✓	✓	✓
Data exchange	✓			
Use of HIT	✓	✓	✓	
Focus on quality improvement	✓	✓	✓	✓
Staff burnout		✓	✓	✓
Teamwork		✓	✓	
Career/job satisfaction		✓	✓	✓
Leadership		✓	✓	✓
Work responsibilities				✓
Structural characteristics	✓			
Provider characteristics	✓	✓	✓	✓

Acronyms: (1) MAPCP, Multipayer Advanced Primary Care Practice Demonstration; (2) CPC, Comprehensive Primary Care Initiative; (3) FQHC-APCP, Federally Qualified Health Center Advanced Primary Care Practice Demonstration.

Analyzing Implementation Characteristics

Once organizational and implementation characteristics have been assessed, how does one analyze the information? Qualitative comparative analysis (QCA) has been applied to evaluation data to relate explanatory factors to outcomes. Box 9.3 describes this method.[20,21,22,23]

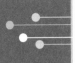

Box 9.3
Qualitative Comparative Analysis

Qualitative comparative analysis (QCA) is a case-oriented method originating from the comparative social sciences that applies formal logic and set theory, a branch of mathematics, to identify noncorrelational relationships using qualitative data or quantitative data or both derived from the cases included in the analysis. Case-oriented methods and variable-oriented methods have a role in research that advances understanding of effective health care intervention. Quantitative variable-oriented methods excel for hypothesis testing and making population generalizations; qualitative approaches are useful for developing hypotheses and comprehensively exploring a few cases. As a complement to these approaches, case-oriented methods seek to examine or interpret theory through an in-depth examination within and across cases (e.g., patients, hospitals, communities) that share some degree of similarity. Consistent with a case-oriented approach, QCA was originally developed for use with a small to medium number of cases (N = 10 to 50) to explore causal complexity. More recently, analysts have used QCA for large samples.

QCA is a configural comparative method in that it focuses on the relationship between combinations of explanatory factors and outcomes, as opposed to the independent effect of any single factor. The goal of QCA analysis is to determine which combination of features are necessary, sufficient, or both to produce an outcome. Relationships of necessity and sufficiency are types of relationships found among causally complex phenomena and are mathematically represented as superset and subset relationships within empiric data. Figure 9.1 shows how these relationships can be visualized.

In "crisp set" QCA, key patient or design variables are calibrated dichotomously (e.g., Condition A present/Condition A absent, Condition B high/Condition B low), and researchers assign each case as either "fully in" the condition set (represented as a set membership value of "1") or "fully out" (represented as a set membership value of "0"). Whether a case is "in" or "out" is determined using an external standard or referent threshold that has substantive meaning. "Fuzzy set" QCA allows for qualitative and quantitative differences in set membership by assigning set membership values between 0 and 1. Similarly, each case is assigned a set membership value for the outcome set. The calibration and scoring process yields a data matrix of condition set membership values for each case, which is converted into a "truth table," the key analytic device used in analysis. Specialized software (e.g., "R QCA library") is used to analyze the truth table in terms of subset, and superset relationships between combinations of features and the outcome. These set relationships are interpreted in the context of statements of necessity (superset relationships) and sufficiency (subset relationships).

QCA complements qualitative and quantitative methods. Conventional qualitative methods often examine processes and themes for a small number of cases and entail deductive and inductive analyses of nonnumeric data. Traditional multivariate regression seeks to estimate the independent contribution of a specific variable to an outcome holding all other variables constant at their respective average values. QCA maintains each case's own configuration of variables, allowing each configuration of

(Continued)

(Continued)

conditions to be evaluated as a whole toward the outcome. QCA recognizes more than one solution (or pathway) to an outcome and allows researchers to unravel different types of relationships that may not be evident using probabilistic methods and common combinations of features across more cases that may not be evident using traditional qualitative approaches. But because QCA is not a probabilistic method, no statistical tests of causal inference are used; however, measures of consistency and coverage are calculated to assess the degree to which the derived solution formulas fit the empirical data.

Figure 9.1 QCA Example: Visualizing Qualitative Characteristics With Set Logic

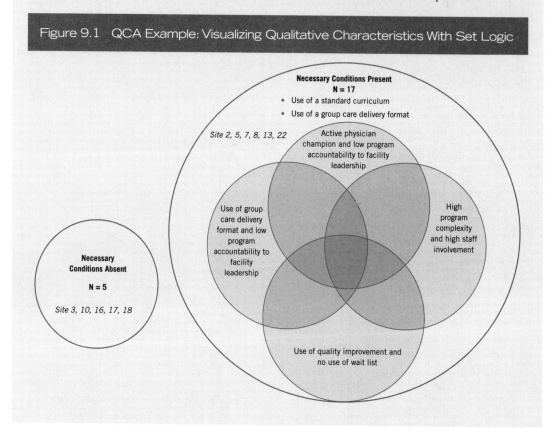

SUMMARY

This chapter recognizes that comprehensive evaluation may produce findings to help answer the questions of what works, for whom, and in which contexts. Program demonstrations often consist of financial or other policy mechanisms aimed at igniting the improvement capability of the participating organizations, to redesign care systems with the intent of reducing cost while maintaining or improving quality. The chapter suggests realist evaluation methods as relevant to the evaluation of these types of demonstrations. Such methods aim to identify the combinations of mechanism and contexts that interact to produce the desired patterns of outcomes. One aspect of context is the improvement capability of the participating organization. Without the ability to redesign complex systems, the policy mechanism will be unlikely to produce the intended results. Several organizational assessment tools are introduced for use in helping describe the context of the evaluation. Finally, QCA is presented as a technique that can complement other quantitative analyses to understand impacts through the characteristics of interventions, organizations, and implementation processes.

DISCUSSION QUESTION

1. In addition to the organizational assessment tools described in this chapter, how can interviews with organizations' leadership staff improve an evaluation?

2. Describe one situation to which you might apply QCA and discuss what might be learned.

3. How might you consider combining organizational assessment with difference-in-difference modeling?

NOTES

1. Centers for Medicare and Medicaid Services. "Innovation Models" (website). Available at http://innovation.cms.gov/initiatives/index.html.

2. Davidoff, F., "Heterogeneity Is Not Always Noise," *JAMA* 302 no. 23 (2009): 2580–86.

3. Pawson, Ray, and Nick Tilley. *Realistic Evaluation.* (Thousand Oaks, CA: Sage, 1997).

4. Centers for Medicare and Medicaid Services. Innovation Center (website). Available at http://innovation.cms.gov/.

5. Helfrich, Christian D., Laura J. Damschroder, Hildi J. Hagedorn, Ginger S. Daggett, Anju Saha, Mona Ritchie, Teresa Damush, Marylou Guihan, Philip M. Ullric, and Cheryl B. Stetl, "A Critical Synthesis of Literature on the Promoting Action on Research Implementation in Health Services (PARIHS) Framework" *Implementation Science* 5 (2010): 82. Available at http://www.biomedcentral.com/content/pdf/1748-5908-5-82.pdf.

6. Kitson, A., G. Harvey, and B. McCormack. "Enabling the Implementation of Evidence Based Practice: A Conceptual Framework," *Quality in Health Care* 7 no. 3 (1998): 149–58.

7. Rycrojt-Malone, J., "The PARIHS Framework—A Framework for Guiding the Implementation of Evidence-based Practice," *Journal of Nursing Care Quality* 19 no. 4 (2004): 297–304.

8. Gustafson, D. H., David H. Gustafson, François Sainfort, Mary Eichler, Laura Adams, Maureen Bisognano, and Harold Steudel, "Developing

and Testing a Model to Predict Outcomes of Organizational Change," *Health Services Research* 38 no. 2 (2003): 751–76.

9. Damschroder L. J., D. C. Aron, R. E. Keith, S. R. Kirsh, J. A. Alexander, and J. C. Lowery, "Fostering Implementation of Health Services Research Findings into Practice: A Consolidated Framework for Advancing Implementation Science," *Implementation Science* 4 no. 1 (2009): 50.

10. DesRoches, C., A. Jaszczak, and A. Situ, "Measuring Characteristics of High Performing Health Care Organizations: An Environmental Scan," *Mathematica Policy Research, Inc.* (April 2014): 9–10.

11. Ibid.

12. Ibid, pp. 6–21.

13. Agency for Healthcare Research and Quality.

14. See "Dimensions of the Learning Organization Questionnaire." Available at http://www.partnersforlearning.com/questions.php.

15. PCHM-A MacColl Center for Health Care Innovation, Group Health Cooperative (May 2013).

16. DesRoches et al., 2014, pp. 67–73.

17. "Change Process Capability Questionnaire (CPCQ), Module 6 Appendix," Agency for Healthcare Research and Quality, Rockville, MD (May 2013). Available at http://www.ahrq.gov/professionals/prevention-chronic-care/improve/system/pfhandbook/mod6appendix.html

18. "TeamSTEPPS Teamwork Perceptions Questionnaire (T-TPQ) Manual," American Institutes for Research (June 2010).

19. DesRoches et al., 2014.

20. Ragin, Charles C. "Qualitative Comparative Analysis Using Fuzzy Sets (fsQCA)," pp. 87–121 in Benoit Rihoux and Charles Ragin (eds.), *Configurational Comparative Analysis* (Thousand Oaks, CA: Sage, 2008).

21. von Eye, A., G. Anne Bogat, and J. E. Rhodes. "Variable-oriented and Person-oriented Perspectives of Analysis: The Example of Alcohol Consumption in Adolescence." *Journal of Adolescence* 29 no. 6 (2006): 981–1004. doi:http://dx.doi.org/10.1016/j.adolescence.2006.06.007.

22. Schneider, C. Q., and C. Wagemann. *Set-theoretic Methods for the Social Sciences: A Guide to Qualitative Comparative Analysis* (Cambridge, UK: Cambridge University Press, 2012).

23. Ibid.

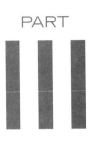

Making Evaluation More Relevant to Policy

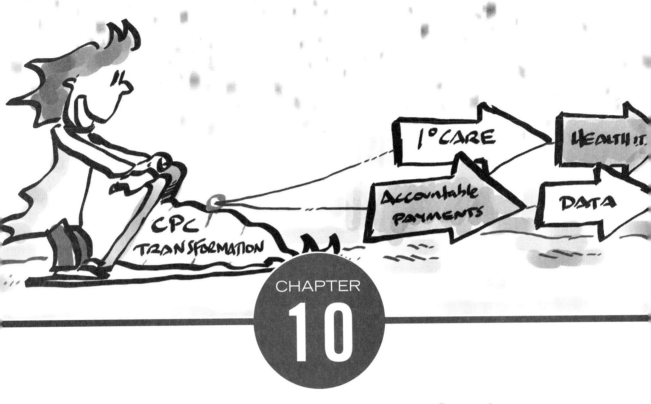

Evaluation Model Case Study

The Learning System at the Center for
Medicare and Medicaid Innovation

Rocco Perla

Bruce Finke

Learning Objectives

Previous chapters lay out the background and a series of tools for evaluating innovative health care system demonstrations. This chapter describes the learning

(Continued)

(Continued)

system at the Centers for Medicare and Medicaid Innovation as a case study of a generalizable model. Traditional approaches to evaluate change ask, "Did the change work?" in a properly controlled setting. A learning system, in contrast, is designed in part to address the question, "How can we make the change work?" as it unfolds in real time. The answer involves adaptive course corrections driven by learning from the results of the rapid-cycle evaluation approach and sharing those results with participants quickly to shape future outcomes that ideally translate into program success as defined at the summative level.

Over the past several years, pioneers in health care delivery around the world have begun considering how to harness systems engineering, improvement science, rapid-cycle evaluation (RCE), and management theory to accelerate testing and learning and improve execution in health care.[1] This multidisciplinary approach is quickly becoming the standard for large-scale change initiatives in health care and informs the learning system approach used at Centers for Medicare and Medicaid Innovation (CMMI). CMMI defines a learning system as a systematic improvement framework used to manage change across a mix of health systems, gain an understanding of the context in which change occurs, and increase the likelihood of successful tests of change in payment policy and care delivery.

An effective learning system will

- Provide a clear focus on achievable and measurable aims and goals

- Guide early identification of critical success factors or "drivers" to achieve the desired results

- Identify changes that both program participants and policymakers can test and implement to achieve program aims

- Encourage rapid testing and refinement of strategies in the field, with locally derived (practice level) data playing a key role in driving sequential cycles of improvement

- Use expert faculty and provide ideas (technical content) to support active testing of changes

- Build a collaborative and transparent learning space within which participants can share results of their tests, information about challenges and opportunities, and tools and resources

This chapter identifies seven major areas of activity (or seven steps) in development of a systematic approach to managing change across multiple systems in

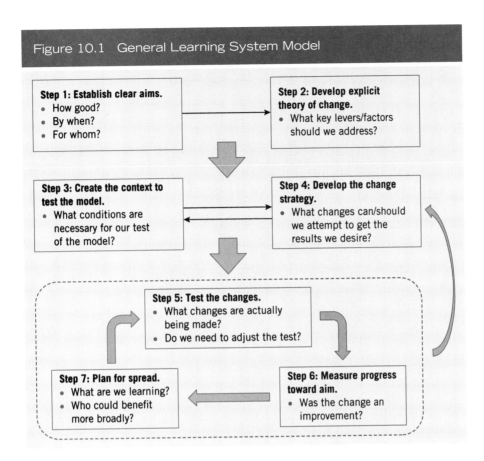

Figure 10.1   General Learning System Model

Step 1: Establish clear aims.
- How good?
- By when?
- For whom?

Step 2: Develop explicit theory of change.
- What key levers/factors should we address?

Step 3: Create the context to test the model.
- What conditions are necessary for our test of the model?

Step 4: Develop the change strategy.
- What changes can/should we attempt to get the results we desire?

Step 5: Test the changes.
- What changes are actually being made?
- Do we need to adjust the test?

Step 7: Plan for spread.
- What are we learning?
- Who could benefit more broadly?

Step 6: Measure progress toward aim.
- Was the change an improvement?

complex payment and delivery settings. Each step in the model is demonstrated with examples drawn from two CMMI models: the Pioneer Accountable Care Organization (ACO) program and/or the Comprehensive Primary Care (CPC) initiative.

The seven steps outlined here are not new; they are the application of lessons learned from previous work in the areas of improvement science,[2] systems theory,[3] and research in large-scale change.[4] These steps are presented in a linear fashion to demonstrate their logical relationship with each other; in reality, the process is often nonlinear, with activities cooccurring in multiple ways (see Figure 10.1).

Step 1: Establish Clear Aims

Answers the question: How good, by when, for whom?

As a steward of public funds, the Centers for Medicare and Medicaid Services (CMS) has adopted the three-part aim of better care, smarter spending, and healthier people through improvement.[5] These high-level aims provide the orientation for the agency's efforts to improve health care. The work of CMMI is to test and evaluate payment and delivery models through which these goals might be reached, and to do that requires translating the three-part aim into specific and quantifiable targets. Every model tested must provide an answer to these three questions: What constitutes better care in this specific model? What health outcomes can be expected to improve, and by how much? How much cost savings can we predict from this change over what period of time?

The path to high-level outcomes goes through a range of intermediate aims and objectives. If the high-level and intermediate aims are not clearly in place, teams lose the opportunity for a shared focus and the early phase of work tends to be uncoordinated. The ideal aim is often described as specific and quantifiable, answering how much improvement is expected and by when. But that level of specificity is not always necessary for an aim to provide the focus a model test requires. For example, the Pioneer ACOs are working to provide greater coordination of care for patients across care settings, thereby allowing these provider groups to move more rapidly from a shared savings payment model to a population-based payment model. This program-level view was translated into the following aim statement early in the program:

> *100% of the original ACOs will generate sufficient cost savings and quality improvements to qualify for population-based payments in Year 3 of the program.*

A good aim statement will generally answer the question: "How good by when?" Sometimes in the early stages of a large and complex initiative, the team gets a better understanding of what is possible over time, and the aim (and sub-aims) gets clearer. With a clear aim established, teams can get to work thinking about the levers they need to push to achieve the objectives. To the extent goals are limited to high-level generalities—such as "improve access to care" or "reduce the total cost of care"—the opportunity is lost to deepen understanding of the situation and to learn how to move forward in an effective manner, especially during the early stages of work. Clear aims set the stage for Step 2, which defines an explicit theory of change and identifies the central drivers or critical factors needed to achieve the aim.

Step 2: Develop an Explicit Theory of Change

Answers the question: What are the key "drivers" (factors or levers) needed to achieve the aim?

Implicit in every effort to improve something is a theory of change driving the work, that is, a hypothesis about the actions that must be taken to achieve the results desired. These theories, stated or unstated, inevitably guide and shape the work. Within that theory of change is a set of assumptions, an understanding of what will be required to make the particular change happen. Articulating these assumptions increases the likelihood of success and is a necessary precursor to learning. When the theory of change is explicit, the evaluator can test it against reality, as tests in the field generate data. Were the actions the evaluator thought were required to produce the results successful? If so, confidence in the hypothesis is increased. If not, then theory and practices need to be adjusted accordingly. Either situation contributes to learning and can guide next steps.

Of the many ways to depict a theory of change, a model CMMI has found particularly useful for working toward a specific aim is called a "driver diagram."[6] A driver diagram depicts the relationship between the aim, the primary drivers that contribute directly to achieving the aim, and the secondary drivers necessary to achieve the primary drivers. The process of clearly defining an aim and its drivers helps a team develop a shared view of the theory of change in a system and reduces the risk of having team members working at cross purposes. A driver diagram comes to represent the team members' current and developing theories of "cause and effect" in the system—their thinking about what changes will likely cause the desired effects. It sets the stage for defining the "how" elements of a project—the specific changes or interventions that will lead to the desired outcome. It is an action-oriented logic model.

Figure 10.2 depicts the early "generalized" driver diagram for Pioneer ACOs. The aim is to the left, and the drivers believed to have the greatest direct impact on the aim are positioned to the right. Secondary drivers are activities or changes that logically follow from, and support, the primary drivers. For example, the first *primary driver* listed is "continuous care improvement driven by data," which is linked to the following *secondary drivers*:

- Peer-based learning

- Strong data systems

- Appropriate staff and resources

- Capacity to test at point of care

- Population based measurement

The assumption being tested by the Pioneer ACOs is that continuous improvement will occur more rapidly, and be sustained, when these five aspects of data and measurement are realized. During testing, some of these secondary drivers may prove more valuable than others, which will be shared with the collective group and may also lead to modifications of the theory of action. In reality, once testing begins, new drivers are likely to be identified that need to be incorporated into the model. The driver diagram in Figure 10.2 that also separates the drivers linked to the ACOs themselves from those CMS/CMMI can impact to achieve the aim. Individual Pioneer ACOs will have modified

Figure 10.2 Driver Diagram for Pioneer ACOs

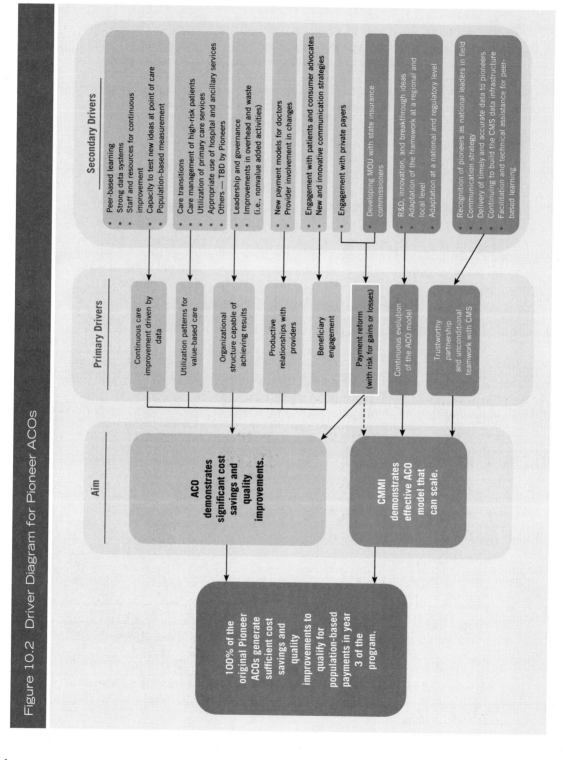

versions of this generalized driver diagram that reflect adaptation to the specific environment and conditions of their work.

Creating a driver diagram is valuable in the initial planning of a performance improvement initiative and should be seen as a tool that is updated regularly as the team refines the theories of action. It also helps in defining which aspects of

Figure 10.3 CPC Driver Diagram With Four Primary Drivers

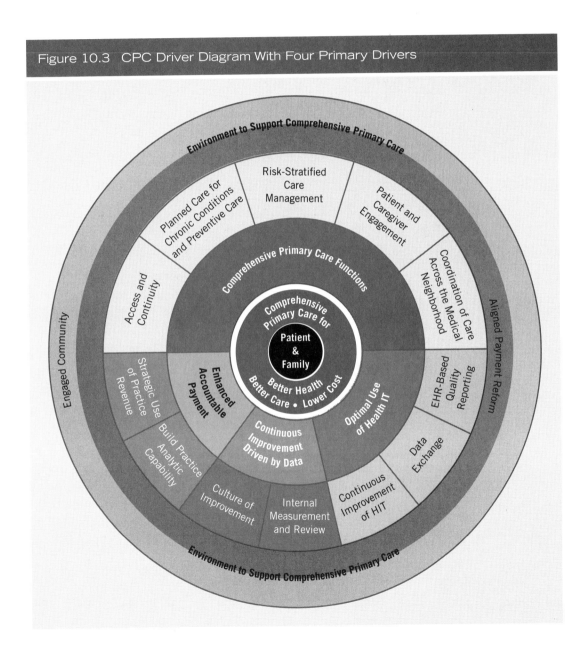

the system should be measured and monitored, to see if the changes/interventions are effective, and to determine whether the underlying "causal" theories are valid. When the diagrams are used as regular references for the improvement work, they can assist teams in staying focused and on course. In addition to aiding leadership and implementation decisions, driver diagrams are helpful in strategically guiding curriculum decisions—identifying where content or assistance is necessary to support actions that lead toward the aim.

The CPC driver diagram in Figure 10.3, in a slightly different form than the Pioneer ACO driver diagram in Figure 10.2, again demonstrates how a well-constructed driver diagram can guide implementation and also communicate the underlying theory of action and critical features of the model.

Step 3: Create the Context Necessary for a Test of the Model

Answers the question: **What conditions are necessary for the chosen test of the model?**

Most large-scale health care innovation and improvement initiatives take place in the context of a defined system, for example, an integrated health system or the federally funded community health centers. While this is true of some of the CMMI initiatives (e.g., the Federally Qualified Community Health Center Advanced Primary Care Practice demonstration), many CMMI initiatives require development of a new or modified system that provides the context for the changes in how care is delivered and paid for. In large-scale initiatives, an important early step is establishing the contextual requirements for success. Each of the models CMMI is testing has required consideration of new partnerships within and between public and private entities, cooperation among payers and providers, and new payment arrangements or regulatory waivers, as well as creation of new markets and data access avenues.

Establishing the environment in which to test payment and delivery system changes requires both understanding the current operational context and a clear aim and theory of change. The aim and driver diagram anchor this process, and expert faculty, interviews with subject matter experts, and reviews of both published literature and unpublished experience of similar initiatives combine to help define the environment necessary to support a model test. In-person and virtual meetings with potential participants (e.g., accelerated development of learning sessions for the Pioneer ACO program) prior to the formal start of an initiative create awareness and prepare the field for the specific model test.

In the CPC initiative, for example, the test of payment and delivery system reform required (1) establishment of markets in which other health care payers aligned with CMS in the broad outlines of comprehensive primary care and (2) the payment reform and other changes to support it. Within those markets or regions, eligible practices had to be recruited and organized into a community of practice and provided with the support necessary to make the changes required.

Understanding how this process takes form is a critical dimension of the learning system, and it is not done unilaterally. Creating or modifying the context for change requires the support and feedback of commercial payers, practices, medical societies, multiple stakeholders, and other organizations in the regions capable of supporting primary care transformation. This collaborative focus is perhaps the most significant consideration in creating the conditions for health care reform. For the CPC initiative, CMMI defined a new role, that of regional lead, reflecting the heavy requirements of developing and maintaining the multipayer and multistakeholder environment, in which the practices transform the delivery of care. Further, the CPC initiative developed learning communities in each of the seven regions, to support practices as they actively test their way into the new method of delivering care.

Step 4: Develop the Change Strategy

Answers the question: What changes can/should be attempted to get the results desired (i.e., achieve the aim)?

Identification of the aims and drivers sets up the framework for testing specific changes. What changes must be made to a system to develop "effective peer-based learning," "strong data systems," or "capacity to test at point of care"? This is where individual model tests begin to take shape. The set of changes a specific test site selects is often referred to, following accepted practice, as its "change concepts and tactics," or collectively as its "change package."

Table 10.1 is an example from the CPC Initiative of how the program identifies specific changes that can be expected to achieve better care and health outcomes at lower cost and organizes them according to the primary and secondary drivers. In the case of CPC, a core set of changes were identified through inquiry into the published and unpublished literature on primary care transformation as most likely to achieve the CPC aim. At the practice level, there will be further testing using iterative and rapid improvement cycles (Plan-Do-Study-Act or PDSA cycles), to learn how best to actually make these changes.[7] The excerpted portion of the CPC change package in Table 10.1 (for one of the secondary drivers, "Planned Care for Chronic Conditions and Preventive Care") provides a roadmap of changes believed to be required to achieve the CPC aim; the roadmap also serves as a tool for analyzing and understanding what actually happens as the model operates in the real world.

The Pioneer ACO program illustrates an alternative approach to development of a change strategy. The ACO model begins with a clear aim and well-developed theory of action, but no defined set of changes. This model asks that

Table 10.1 Linkage Between Secondary Driver, Change Concepts, and Change Tactics (Example: One secondary driver from the Comprehensive Primary Care Initiative)

Secondary Driver	Change Concept	Change Tactics
Planned Care for Chronic Conditions and Preventive Care	A: Use a personalized plan of care for each patient. B: Manage medications to maximize therapeutic benefit and patient safety at lowest cost.	Provide all patients annually with an opportunity for development of an individualized health plan, including health risk appraisal, gender, age, and condition-specific preventive care services, chronic condition management, and advance care planning.
		Integrate patient goals and priorities into plan of care.
		Use the Medicare *Annual Wellness Visit with Personalized Prevention Plan Services* (AWV with PPPS) for Medicare patients.
		Provide medication reconciliation at each relevant encounter.
		Conduct a periodic, structured, and medication review.
	C: Proactively manage chronic and preventive care for enrolled patients.	Use age, gender, and condition-specific protocols and proactive, planned care appointments for chronic conditions and preventive care services.
		Use panel support tools (registry functionality) to identify services due.
		Use reminders and outreach (e.g., phone calls, emails, postcards, community health workers where available) to alert and educate patients to services due.
	D: Use team-based care to meet patient needs efficiently.	Define roles and distribute tasks among care team members, consistent with the skills, abilities, and credentials of team members to better meet patient needs.
	Use decision support and protocols to manage workflow in the team to meet patient needs.	Manage workflow to address chronic and preventive care, for example through pre-visit planning or huddles.
	Integrate behavioral health services into primary care.	Integrate interdisciplinary team members, e.g., nutrition, behavioral health, pharmacy, physical therapy into primary care.

the pioneers identify and characterize the changes necessary to achieve the program aim. In the true spirit of pioneering, they are asked to create the roadmap as part of the work. Table 10.2 depicts one example of the relationship between secondary drivers and changes being tested in one Pioneer ACO following this process. The pioneers are also working in subgroups based on expertise, interest, or a pressing practical concern to explore new ideas in a loosely structured way—a way that has already led to new insights and solutions that can be shared broadly within and across the program. Table 10.3 provides a sampling of the different activities used to guide this process—including action groups and innovation pods where the focus is on rapid local testing, innovation, and problem solving.

In developing the change strategy, the degree of confidence that a change will lead to the desired aim is critical. If the degree of confidence is high that changes will achieve the desired result (based on research and a body of evidence), the changes will be more sharply defined at the outset, and CMMI will be more open to larger and more sophisticated tests. If there is less confidence in the drivers and associated changes, CMMI may consider exploratory changes to the system and structure smaller tests to guide learning. In the latter case, CMMI realizes that part of the challenge is not only testing changes, but actively developing them. This testing process is guided by ongoing assessment of various data sources (qualitative and quantitative), and involves close interaction between teams responsible for implementing and evaluating the intervention.

Table 10.2 Example of Specific Changes Associated With Secondary Drivers (Example from Michigan Pioneer)	
Secondary Driver	**Changes Being Tested**
Strong data systems	Developing "Episodes of Care" capability in EPIC, a commonly adopted medical software
Care management of high-risk patients	Hired 16 care navigators and embedded them into established care teams
Appropriate use of hospital and ancillary services	Working to identify conditions related to primary care sensitive emergency department use and frequent flier visit
Engagement with patients and consumer advocates	Established a patient engagement team led by patient representative and patient advocate

Table 10.3 Examples of Group-Based Learning Activities Used to Develop New Ideas and Test Changes

Activity	Description	Examples From Pioneer Accountable Care Organization (ACO) Work	Output (example)
Action Groups	A subset of program participants that have a strong interest or expertise in a specific topic that agree to work with each other to address a need or concern over the course of several months or years.	Pharmacy care coordination; population health management; postacute care; beneficiary engagement	Summary report of the findings that are shared with the entire program; collection of presentation materials and case studies
Innovation Pods	A subset of program participants that have an interest in a specific problem and agree to work on an innovation related to that problem with assistance from Centers for Medicare and Medicaid Innovation (CMMI) staff and expert faculty. Innovation pods are usually time limited (e.g., 90-day innovation cycle).	Development of alternative quality sampling methodology for 22 ACO quality measures	White paper (recommendation of cluster sampling)
Face-to-Face Meetings	One- or two-day face-to-face gatherings for program participants to learn from each other and from outside experts, and for program participants to strengthen relationships with each other and with Centers for Medicare and Medicaid Services (CMS)	Mid-year pioneer meeting, where pioneers shared accomplishments, successful tests of change and best practices, new knowledge, challenges, and lessons learned	Collection of presentation materials and case studies
Web-Based Platform for Collaboration	Program participants have access to the CMS Innovation Center Partner Collaboration Site, which is used for knowledge sharing, collaboration, and reporting.	Pioneers use the forum function of the site to communicate and collaborate with each other. Additionally, CMS and pioneers share materials and documents through the site.	Conversation threads; access to outputs of other activities

Step 5: Test the Changes

Answers the question: What changes are actually being made and to what degree?

Anyone engaged in improvement and system redesign in health care (possibly more than in any other area) quickly realizes there is an important difference

Table 10.4 Testing Progress Grid (numbers in table represent the number of program sites in each category)

Key Changes	No Test	Planned Test	Pilot Tested	Implemented	Spread	Sustained
Change 1	20	0	0	0	0	0
Change 2	11	5	3	1	0	0
Change 3	6	8	6	0	0	0
Change 4	13	7	0	0	0	0
Change 5	10	9	1	0	0	0
Change 6	4	3	3	8	2	0
Change 7	Test discontinued—determined to be impractical by group					

between a proposed test and what actually gets tested in the field. In complex systems, we always encounter previously unrecognized challenges that require modification of the test. While fidelity to a test or a model is emphasized in classical evaluation research, fidelity to an aim is prioritized in improvement science; a pure test of a change is of little value if it fails to achieve or contribute to the desired aim. Changed conditions in the field that do not lead to an appropriate change in the specification of what is being tested run a major risk of attributing the results of the actual test to the original test specification. Missing the important differences can lead, not only to confusion of the specific test results, but also to unwitting distortion of the theory of action.[8]

One way to guard against this attribution risk is to develop tracking tools to understand what is actually being tested. Table 10.4 is an idealized version of such a tool that can be adapted to specific programs or models. The set of changes that characterizes each program, whether developed initially as in CPC or over the course of the program as in Pioneer ACO, would be used to populate this tool.

Looking at Table 10.4, it is clear that the 20 participant sites in this example are not at the same point in their testing and learning process. Assuming that all sites were actively testing the six changes could lead to misleading conclusions, especially with regard to linking program results or outcome measures to these tests. What a grid like this instantly shows is that Change 1 has not been attempted by any site, Change 6 has gotten the greatest traction overall, and Change 7 has been discontinued by the group due to implementation difficulties. As a next step, it might be helpful to understand how the eight groups that have reached implementation of Change 6 might be able to help other participants do the same. Since most changes (80%) in Table 10.4 are either not being tested or are in planning, this could reflect either a young program just getting started or a mature program that is not actively testing. The information to populate this table may be collected as part of the monitoring functions, through the survey and data collection activities of the CMMI Research and Rapid Cycle Evaluation Group, or through direct collection as part of the learning system. [9,10] It is also necessary to understand the relationship between participant engagement and the whole range of outcomes. Historically, this type of information has rarely been captured in real time, despite its ability to provide the most important information for shared learning and improvement.

Step 6: Measure Progress Toward Aim

Answers the question: Was the change an improvement?

Measurement within the context of a learning system asks the question: "Are the changes being made leading toward the aim?" In large regional or national programs, it is important to blend, and subsequently study, the relationship between the more formative measures at the practice level and the more summative evaluations performed by evaluators and actuaries.

Learning systems typically use three types of measures that are common in quality improvement work: measures of outcome, process, and unintended consequences. Measurement occurs at the level of the individual organization or participant (reflecting progress of that participant toward the relevant aim) and at the level of the program. To the degree that the measure set is linked to the driver diagram, it provides better understanding of which changes are actually occurring.

The ideal set of measures provides a clear and unambiguous view of the changes occurring, progress toward the aim, and unintended consequences. Clearly, there is no ideal set of measures. The challenge of measurement within the learning system is to measure "just enough" to provide what is needed to guide the next test, and to the degree possible, use measures already being collected as part of the monitoring and evaluation process, thereby reducing the data burden on providers. [11,12]

The CPC program has integrated these three types of measurement into the operational requirements of the program. The CPC practices must complete a complex set of changes, called milestones, derived from the CPC change package. Practices document completion of these milestones, giving the program a set of process measures that indicate progress of the practice toward providing comprehensive primary care. The evaluation of CPC includes administration of a modified CAHPS-CG survey. The data from this survey, from office-based surveys, and from the use of Patient and Family Advisory Councils, provides the practices with balancing measures, allowing them to see unintended consequences on the patient experience of care relative to the changes the practices are making. Finally, CMS and the other payers provide quarterly claims-based data reflecting quality and utilization to the practices, and the practices report to CPC on a set of clinical quality measures, derived from their electronic health records. These measures provide information on both outcomes and unintended consequences. The result is a large, comprehensive, and useful set of measures, linked to the theory of action and fully integrated into the work of the initiative.

Step 7: Plan for Spread

Answers the questions: What is being learned, and who could benefit more broadly?

A central consideration of improvement and redesign efforts is to ensure that new knowledge is disseminated as broadly as possible. This is a complex process, because what works in one setting, of course, may not work in the same way in different settings where the context and conditions may vary greatly.[13] Using techniques such as stratification and rational subgrouping[14] allows the partitioning of variation in a way that reduces within-group variation and maximizes learning between groups. For example, if a set of primary care practices or providers is achieving breakthrough results in a particular area, the evaluator needs to differentiate these practices from other practices, learn about what they did, and consider the contexts and conditions associated with their success. Without this learning, the risk increases that spread attempts will be ill-informed and fail.

Two dimensions are important in spreading knowledge: (1) the spread of successful or promising changes *within* the model test and (2) the spread of successful or promising changes beyond model test participants. The first, spread within the model, is a major consideration in the design of the learning system for all the models tested at CMMI. This requires development of an infrastructure and processes that allow participants to learn with, and from, each other how to achieve their aims. Research suggests five key areas for consideration in fostering the spread of improvements and innovations within and among participating organizations:[15]

- Strong and visible leadership
- Examples of success (in using the new way)
- Development of a spread plan (communication plan, measurement plan, work plan, etc.)
- Consideration of the social system
- Measurement and feedback loops to monitor and guide the spread effort

In the CPC initiative, practices in each of the regions are organized into learning communities, with multiple opportunities to share ideas, tools, and data with each other within the region and across regions. In the Pioneer ACO program, the pioneers work together in action groups on specific challenges, and within affinity groups of like organizations, to share results and resources. Knowledge management—broadly defined as identifying, cataloguing, and enabling the adoption of tools, resources, and strategies that prove useful in local conditions—plays a large part in the spread along the first dimension.

The models in testing at CMMI are subject to rigorous evaluation and actuarial certification, and the decision to spread beyond the initial test phase (second dimension) belongs outside the team managing the test and is truly where policy and practice interface. Important features of a learning system can lay the groundwork for successful spread beyond the model, when supported by policy in the broader statutory context in which the model tests occur. First and foremost is periodic reassessment of the aim, drivers, and changes to ensure the theory of change depicted in the driver diagram accurately matches the reality of change in different settings. For example, the local conditions, payer mix, patient population, technical competencies, and social environments in a small independent provider-based ACO will differ from those of an ACO made up of large academic medical centers. The change package should be revised to reflect the data emerging from the field about what changes were actually implemented and how they were implemented in these different settings. Knowledge management plays an important role here too, in understanding what resources will be needed to effectively spread beyond the test. New knowledge gained in the Pioneer ACO and CPC models, for example, is already finding its way into the broader health care marketplace.

Any discussion of spread, either within or from the model, should take into account factors that are known to influence the rate of adoption and diffusion.[16] These include

- Relative advantage: How improved an innovation is over the previous or existing practice or product

- Compatibility: The degree to which an innovation can be understood by current practitioners

- Complexity: The perceived ease of use of the new approach

- Trialability: How easy it is to test the idea or innovation in local settings

- Observability: The degree to which an innovation is visible to others that may be willing to try it themselves

Failure to address any of these considerations will impair the spread of new knowledge and effective practices both within and beyond the model test.

SUMMARY

The large-scale tests of payment reform and delivery design represented by the models being tested at CMS provide a unique opportunity and set of challenges. Testing changes in care is going on simultaneously with testing changes in the context for that care, and these tests occur in a complex environment of heterogeneous and diverse health care systems.[17]

These opportunities and challenges have stimulated development of a new framework for operational learning, a learning system. An effective learning system increases the likelihood of success in the model being tested; it also offers the opportunity to better understand what is required for that success in a range of different settings. Learning systems, particularly the type of general model outlined here, exist for one simple reason: they enable rapid testing and learning, so program and policy efforts can be adjusted to achieve their intended results. The model presented here provides a general framework for execution in developing these types of large and complex learning systems in a way that provides a line of sight from aims through testing of changes to results.

More health systems engaging in the rapid testing, implementation, and spread of promising changes using systematic models of execution, provides the best way to make significant strides in improving the American health care system—with all stakeholders working together to deliver better care and achieve better health outcomes at lower cost. The value of a systematic framework that serves to coordinate, manage, and guide complex projects with numerous partners across a range of settings goes well beyond health care reform and specific legislation. It has the potential to serve as a general framework for change management in other government programs, enabling the testing of new ideas in a goal-driven manner, with a focus on sustainable results and continuous improvement.

DISCUSSION QUESTIONS

1. Change strategies may be sharply defined and supported by existing evidence, or they may be more exploratory and still in need of development. How does evaluation differ in these two scenarios?

2. What are some limitations that can slow or prevent real-time collection, evaluation, and reporting of data? What, if anything, can be done to avoid these limitations?

3. How does a learning system approach square with a more traditional evaluation approach?

NOTES

1. Berwick D. M., "The Science of Improvement." *Journal of the American Medical Association*, 299(10) (2008): 1182–84; Langley G. L., et al., *The Improvement Guide: A Practical Approach to Enhancing Organizational Performance* (San Francisco, CA: Jossey-Bass Publishers, 2009); McCannon, C. J., and R. J. Perla, "Learning Networks for Sustainable, Large-Scale Improvement," *Joint Commission Journal on Quality and Patient Safety* 35 no. 5 (2009): 286–91; Lanham, H. J., et al., "How Complexity Science Can Inform Scale-Up and Spread in Healthcare: Understanding the Role of Self-Organization in Variation across Local Contexts," *Social Science and Medicine* 93 (September 2013): 194–202; Norton, W. E., et al., "A Stakeholder-Driven Agenda for Advancing the Science and Practice of Scale-Up and Spread In Healthcare *Implementation Science* 7 (2012): 118; Provost, L. P., and S. K. Murray, *The Healthcare Data Guide: Learning From Data for Improvement* (San Francisco, CA: Jossey-Bass, 2011); Hussey P., et al., "From Pilots To Practice: Speeding the Movement of Successful Pilots to Effective Practice," Discussion Paper (Washington, DC: *Institute of Medicine*, 2013), available at http://www .iom.edu/pilotstopractice; Shrank W., "The Center For Medicare and Medicaid Innovation's Blueprint for Rapid-Cycle Evaluation of New Care and Payment Models," *Health Affairs* (2013), doi: 10.1377/hlthaff.2013.0216.

2. Langley G. L., et al., *The Improvement Guide: A Practical Approach to Enhancing Organizational Performance* (San Francisco, CA: Jossey-Bass Publishers, 2009).

3. Ackoff, R. L. Create the Corporate Future. (New York, NY: Wiley, 1981).

4. Norton, W. E., et al., "A Stakeholder-Driven Agenda for Advancing the Science and Practice of Scale-Up and Spread in Healthcare," *Implementation Science* 7 (2012): 118.

5. Burwell S. M. "Setting Value-based Payment Goals—HHS Efforts to Improve U.S. Health Care." *New England Journal of Medicine* 372 (2015): 897–99.

6. Provost L., and B. Bennett, "What's Your Theory? Driver Diagram Serves as Tool for Building and Testing Theories for Improvement," *Quality Progress* (July 2015): 36–43.

7. Langley, G. L., et al., *The Improvement Guide: A Practical Approach to Enhancing Organizational Performance* (San Francisco, CA: Jossey-Bass Publishers, 2009).

8. Pawson, R., and N. Tilley, *Realistic Evaluation* (Thousand Oaks, CA: Sage, 2007); Rossi, P. H., "The Iron Law of Evaluation and Other Metallic Rules," *Research in Social Problems and Public Policy*, 4 (1987): 3–20.

9. Shrank W., "The Center For Medicare and Medicaid Innovation's Blueprint for Rapid-Cycle Evaluation of New Care and Payment Models," *Health Affairs* (2013). doi: 10.1377/hlthaff.2013.0216.

10. Provost, L. P., and S. K.Murray, *The Healthcare Data Guide: Learning From Data for Improvement* (San Francisco, CA: Jossey-Bass, 2011).

11. The use of graphs showing performance over time, such as run charts and Shewhart (control) charts, has become common in guiding healthcare improvement efforts. See Provost and Murray; Perla, R. J., L. P. Provost, and S. K. Murray, "The Run Chart: A Simple Analytical Tool for Learning from Variation In Healthcare Processes," *BMJ Quality and Safety* 20 (2011): 46–51; Brock, J., et al., "Association Between Quality Improvement for Care Transitions in Communities and Rehospitalizations Among Medicare Beneficiaries," *JAMA* 309 no. 4 (2013): 381–91.

12. Such charts are particularly important in clinical effectiveness research, where the stability of systems under study has largely been ignored. Brook, R. H., "Health Systems, Heuristics, and Comparative Effectiveness Research," *Journal of General Internal Medicine* (2012). DOI: 10.1007/s11606-012-2242-y.

13. Rossi, P. H., "The Iron Law of Evaluation and Other Metallic Rules" *Research in Social Problems and Public Policy* 4 (1987): 3–20; Pawson and Tilley; Dixon-Woods, M., et al., "Explaining Michigan: Developing an Ex Post Theory of a Quality Improvement Program," *Milbank Quarterly* 89 no. 2 (2011): 167–205; Parry, G. J., et al., Recommendations for Evaluations of Health Care Improvement Initiatives. *Academic Pediatrics* 13 (6 Suppl) (November–December 2013): S23–S30.

14. Shewhart, W., *Economic Control of Quality of Manufactured Product* (New York: D. Van Nostrand Company, 1931).

15. Langley G. L., et al., *The Improvement Guide: A Practical Approach to Enhancing Organizational Performance* (San Francisco, CA: Jossey-Bass Publishers, 2009).

16. Everett M. Rogers, *Diffusion of Innovations* (4th ed.). (New York: Free Press, 1995).

17. Davidoff, F., "Heterogeneity Is Not Always Noise: Lessons from Improvement." *JAMA* 302 no. 23 (2009): 2589–90.

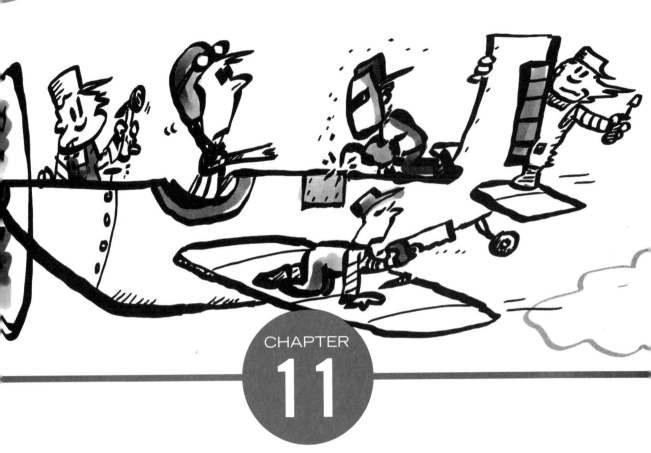

Program Monitoring

Aligning Decision Making With Evaluation

Will Shrank

Sebastian Schneeweiss

K. Malcolm Maclure

Learning Objectives

The increasing amount of electronic health care data available in near real-time in the U.S. health care system provides new opportunities for rapid-cycle evaluation

(Continued)

(Continued)

(RCE) of health care delivery and payment programs, with important implications for decision-making processes.

In this chapter, we draw on case studies and experience of active drug safety monitoring to (1) clarify how RCE can help substantially in the decisions policymakers need to make, (2) develop a framework for synchronizing the timing of decision-making activities with stages of RCE, (3) provide guidelines on evidence thresholds in relation to incremental decision making, and (4) meld these into a proposed process for aligning increments of evidence with incremental decisions in ongoing monitoring and decision making: decisions about, for example, program scale-up, modification, or termination. Rational decision making about program adoption depends on the program effect size in relation to cost of implementation, chance of sustainability, likelihood of broad adoption, and so on.

RCE's early evidence through repeatedly updated effect estimates allows for identification of trends in adjusted effect size, which may stabilize over time, and increasingly precise extrapolation as the evaluation continues. Adapting not only a program in midstream, but also the evaluation strategy in response to interim findings can increase the likelihood that true improvements can be identified and promoted as promptly as possible.

M omentum is increasing to transform the way health care is delivered and paid for in the United States—to reward higher quality and more efficient care, rather than simply paying more for more care. This has greatly disturbed the health care marketplace—as providers, hospitals, health systems, and payers strive to innovate and develop strategies to improve both the cost-efficiency and quality of care delivery.

Time is of the essence here. In a health care environment of constant change, rapid testing of new policies and delivery system approaches is essential for stakeholders to succeed in a competitive marketplace and to deliver on a vision of higher-quality, lower-cost care.

The evaluation norm has been for research studies to wait until enough data have been collected to draw definitive conclusions about program success or failure. This approach may lead to more definitive conclusions at the end of an evaluation, but it fails to allow for the likelihood that learning, and consequent mid-course corrections, can *importantly improve the chances, and the timeliness, of programmatic success.* (See Figure 11.1.)

RCE, as summarized in Chapter 2, is a method that provides interim information on a program's progress. Ideally, it uses the same definitions of process

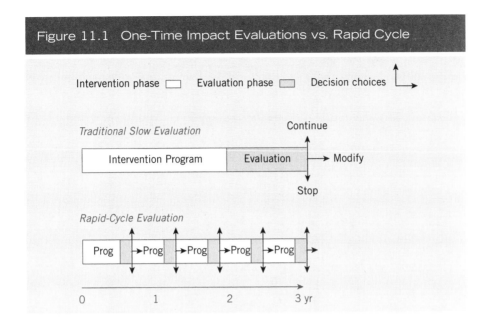

Figure 11.1 One-Time Impact Evaluations vs. Rapid Cycle

Intervention phase ▢ Evaluation phase ▨ Decision choices ⌐→

Traditional Slow Evaluation

Continue

Intervention Program | Evaluation ——→ Modify

Stop

Rapid-Cycle Evaluation

Prog →Prog →Prog →Prog →Prog →

0   1   2   3 yr

and outcome measures as used in the final analysis, but it provides preliminary estimates of them at frequent intervals (e.g., quarterly). RCE is an important addition to program evaluation tools in the quest to support evidence-based decision making, which may greatly increase the chances that programs will achieve their intended goals.

Many key data elements necessary for evaluation are now available electronically in near real-time to support RCE.[1,2] As managing and analyzing such large databases becomes progressively easier, RCE learning is becoming more and more feasible. This type of evaluation is not without its risks, however. Drawing interim conclusions more rapidly and frequently will raise concerns about making inappropriate policy decisions because of undue haste.[3] *Overall* rigor must not be sacrificed for speed. Valid and reliable data that are sensitive to change when it occurs are as important in RCE as they are in comprehensive evaluation.

If RCE reveals a suggestive trend in outcomes that points toward need for a program change, it gives decision makers opportunities to start processes of consensus building while data continue to accrue. Furthermore, if subsequent data updates confirm the trend, the decision makers are ahead of the game—poised to implement without delay the conclusions of the consensus-building process (see Figure 11.2). But if subsequent data updates negate the initial trend, the consensus process can be put on hold and decisions deferred until complete evidence of the program's impact is obtained. The cost of starting an unnecessary consensus process (because the initial trend turns out to be a false positive) must be carefully weighed against the cost of delay in actually implementing a program

Figure 11.2 Evaluation of Decision Makers' Roles and Evaluators' Roles

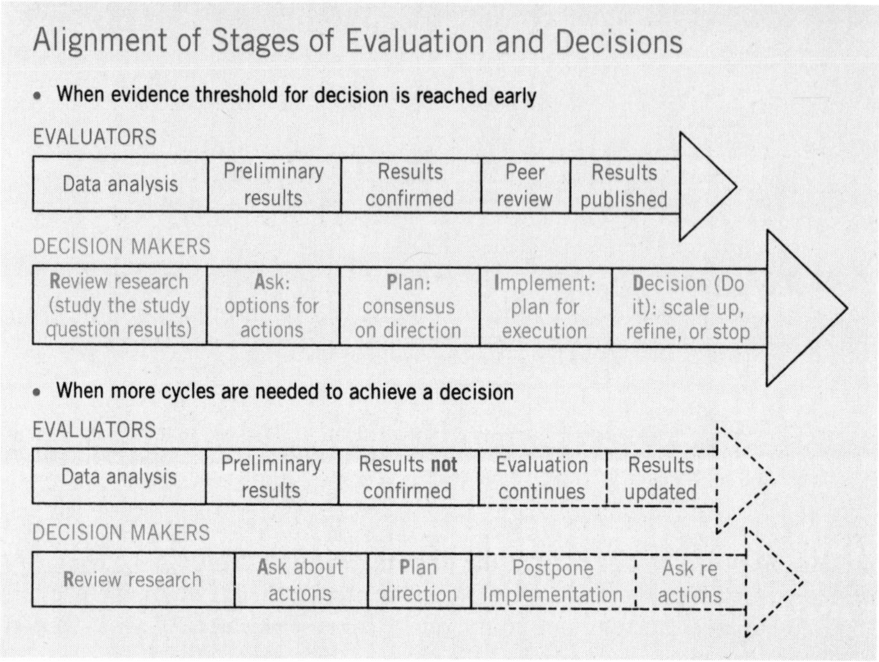

Alignment of Stages of Evaluation and Decisions

- When evidence threshold for decision is reached early

EVALUATORS

Data analysis	Preliminary results	Results confirmed	Peer review	Results published

DECISION MAKERS

Review research (study the study question results)	Ask: options for actions	Plan: consensus on direction	Implement: plan for execution	Decision (Do it): scale up, refine, or stop

- When more cycles are needed to achieve a decision

EVALUATORS

Data analysis	Preliminary results	Results **not** confirmed	Evaluation continues	Results updated

DECISION MAKERS

Review research	Ask about actions	Plan direction	Postpone Implementation	Ask re actions

change when definitive evidence has finally been produced. The complex process of organizational decision making—which requires stakeholder consensus to have a chance of succeeding—requires time, champions, and often intense bargaining. Instead of starting this process at the very end of an evaluation, RCE expedites the process and makes it more inclusive, without sacrificing the ability to make changes as evidence increases over time.

Getting the most out of RCE demands two essentials: (1) understanding the nature of decisions over time, and (2) aligning the timing of related consensus-building processes with the timing of evidence updates. This chapter draws lessons from both the methods of quality improvement using Plan-Do-Study-Act (PDSA) cycles and also the literature on knowledge translation and exchange between researchers and decision makers.[4] The following discussion assumes the evaluation is midway through the first cycle: initial planning is complete, and the doing and the studying are underway. Here the focus is on how to align decisions as the evaluation moves from studying, to acting, to a second cycle of planning and doing. The discussion focuses on an implementation planning stage for scaling up before the final decision is made on whether to do it. This can be summarized in a cyclic 5-step process, called R.A.P.I.D. (see Box 11.1).

Having aligned the *stages* of decision makers' roles with the evaluators' roles (as shown in Figure 11.2), important questions arise about the optimal methods at each stage for linking decision makers' thinking with evaluators' thinking and evidence. This chapter presents a framework and examples to facilitate that linkage.

Nature of Decisions

A key aspect of RCE is that it permits the decision-making process and evaluation process to overlap, so decision makers can improve the alignment of evaluation to the decisions they must make, and evaluators can improve the alignment of decisions to the best evidence available at the time.

The framework for aligning decision making with RCE begins at the heart of the decision-making process: Is the program being tested worthwhile? Typically policymakers face a fourfold decision about direction when provided with

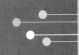

Box 11.1
The Five Steps of R. A. P. I. D.

Review the Research: During the data analysis, a decision maker can pose questions about the analyses to the evaluator. The evaluator will select and/or modify their analytic methods to answer the decision maker's question.

Ask About Actions: As the decision maker reviews the emerging findings from the evaluation and translates them into possible actions, the evaluator may provide guidance by directly linking the findings to the proposed actions.

Plan Direction: The decision maker now faces the daunting options of scaling up a promising program, abandoning a program that people have invested a lot of hope and energy in, or steering a middle course, making refinements and continuing to evaluate it.

Initiate Implementation: Once the decision maker has made a decision about scaling up, coordinating the logistics of implementation not only takes time, but also has an impact on how people think about the problem and the evaluation findings. This provides a golden opportunity—particularly if another cycle of RCE results comes in that casts doubt on the decision maker's implementation plan—for the evaluator and decision maker to postpone implementation if necessary.

Decide to Do It: A point of no return occurs during implementation, and it is not always obvious when that will be.

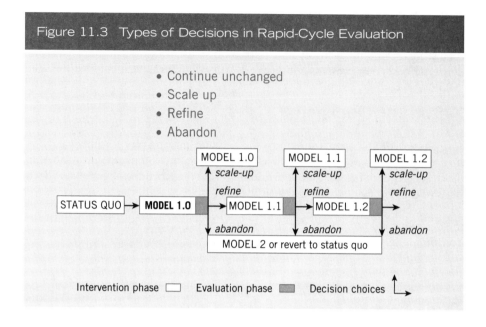

Figure 11.3 Types of Decisions in Rapid-Cycle Evaluation

- Continue unchanged
- Scale up
- Refine
- Abandon

Intervention phase ☐ Evaluation phase ▨ Decision choices

evidence about a program: (1) scaling up a successful program; (2) continuing a partially successful program with modifications, while continuing to monitor its effectiveness; (3) terminating an unsuccessful program; or (4) postpone the directional decision and continue evaluating the intervention. The following sections review factors that can help in choosing which of these paths is best in a given case.

Figure 11.3 shows the three main alternative directions to take when RCE evidence from a program evaluation is presented:

1) Scale up

2) Refine

3) Abandon

We discuss each in turn below.

Scaling Up

RCE can enable earlier discovery and spread of complex health care improvement programs. The RCE of programs is analogous, but not identical, to periodic monitoring of randomized control trials done so a program can be stopped early, when either a statistically significant improvement in outcomes has been achieved earlier than predicted (superiority), or it is unlikely that any difference between therapies will be shown (futility), or even that the outcome looks deleterious. Because so much theory and methodology has been developed over decades for governing the early stopping of clinical trials, it is tempting to assume that the same principles and methods can be transplanted to RCE of complex programs. Unlike a drug with a fixed structure whose efficacy can be assessed in a blinded study, however, a health system program is expected to undergo structural change over time in any case. In addition, its implementation involves people and systems whose attitudes toward change will be influenced by interim results as well as by the Hawthorne effect (performing better when participants are aware of being evaluated).[5] Frequent feedback of interim findings can support change management through cycles of improvement. Moreover, the patient population is not fixed, and both "indicated" and "off-label" use of a program can evolve.

The strong implication is that, unlike drug trials, RCE of complex programs *should not have rigid stopping rules* triggered by reaching threshold p-values or statistical tests. Certainly many lessons can be drawn from the literature on the early stopping of preapproval clinical trials, but such trials are designed to answer a purely scientific question (Is X any better than Y in a controlled setting?) that is loaded with the following ethical challenge (among others): Do the early results of the trial make it unethical to continue giving Y? The legislation for drug approval requires only a binary decision on whether or not there is an effect observed—such an effect may be of any size, which explains the dominance of statistical testing and p-values. Moreover, the drug marketing question (Is X sufficiently better than Y that the company should scale up production, set a high price, and spend a billion dollars on marketing X?) is entirely separated from the scientific question addressed by the trial. Similarly, the adoption and expansion of complex health care improvement programs should not be driven by showing minimal impact, just because that impact is statistically significant at a relevant p-value. Adoption/expansion should, instead, be primarily driven by the size of an effect on key outcome parameters in a sufficiently large trial, which can then be interpreted in the context of other considerations for decision making (implementation cost, chance of sustainability, likelihood of broad adoption by all parts of the system, etc.). In other words, the decision makers' question is not primarily "Is the program working?" but "Is it working well enough to be worth the upheaval of change?" Effect size and continuous improvement are key characteristics for rational program choice.

A good example of an emerging RCE program is the Food and Drug Administration (FDA) Mini-Sentinel (MS) program. The MS program is focused not on whether a drug is effective, but on identifying drug safety issues in an already marketed medication, using a distributed system of 18 longitudinal health care databases with an analysis system that allows pooling adjusted effect estimates. For newly marketed medications, preprogramed analysis modules with extensive confounder adjustment procedures can be re-run every time one of the 18 databases is refreshed. The decisions the FDA is faced with (Figure 11.4) are

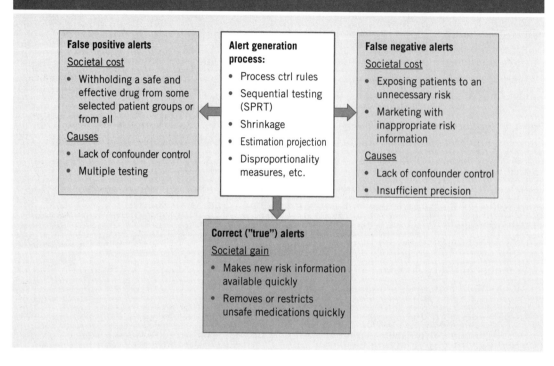

Figure 11.4 FDA's Mini-Sentinel Program and the Consequences of False Decision Making

False positive alerts

Societal cost

- Withholding a safe and effective drug from some selected patient groups or from all

Causes

- Lack of confounder control
- Multiple testing

Alert generation process:

- Process ctrl rules
- Sequential testing (SPRT)
- Shrinkage
- Estimation projection
- Disproportionality measures, etc.

False negative alerts

Societal cost

- Exposing patients to an unnecessary risk
- Marketing with inappropriate risk information

Causes

- Lack of confounder control
- Insufficient precision

Correct ("true") alerts

Societal gain

- Makes new risk information available quickly
- Removes or restricts unsafe medications quickly

different in their specifics from those of program policy decision makers, but both pay a high price for false positive and false negative decisions.

Table 11.1 summarizes differences and similarities between RCE of prescription drug safety by FDA's Mini-Sentinel and RCE of the Centers for Medicare and Medicaid Innovation's complex health system programs.

The decision to scale up a particular health care program could be massively costly if it is made prematurely on the basis of misleading data. It is also risky, because scaling up prematurely will involve spread to clinicians who, being less enthusiastic about the change, might exhibit the opposite of the traditional Hawthorne effect—by purposefully or inadvertently sabotaging the implementation and impact of an intervention. The potential for sabotage or nonrepresentativeness of a pilot demonstration means that RCE should continue after the decision has been made to scale up—to identify unintended consequences, areas for further implementation improvement, and confirmation of generalizability. Further, ongoing RCE may refute or validate skeptics' concerns—either reinforcing the evidence that a program is effective or avoiding the waste associated with scaling up an ineffective program.

Table 11.1   Rapid-Cycle Evaluation of Drug Safety vs. Rapid-Cycle Evaluation of the Effectiveness of Delivery System Innovations

	Mini Sentinel	CMMI Rapid-Cycle Evaluation
Intervention unit	Individual patients	Care delivery systems
Complexity of intervention	Simple: drug of interest vs. comparator	Complex, multifactorial interventions
Outcomes	Infrequent, unanticipated	More frequent, expected
Main data sources	Multiple data sources of similar structure	Single (Centers for Medicare and Medicaid Services) data source?
Data lag time	Frequent asynchronous data refreshes	Near real-time claims data updates
Data availability	Medium lag time (7–12 months)	Short lag time (3 months)
Preferred design	Cohort study with control drug, self-controlled designs	Interrupted time trend, preferably with control group

Refinement

On an intermediate path between scaling up and abandonment are decisions to refine the program model (Models 1.1 and 1.2 in Figure 11.5). These might involve changes throughout the model (applying to all patients, all services, all products, and all settings) or changes to only part of the model. Figure 11.5 illustrates three major classes of decision after dividing the model based on differential success:

1) Scaling up the successful part and abandoning the unsuccessful part

2) Scaling up the successful part and refining the remaining part

3) Abandoning an unsuccessful part and refining the remaining part

This underscores the importance of understanding subgroup performance, especially locations of "positive deviants"—the rare but very creative clinicians and administrators who will discover better ways of implementing the policy. The locations (subgroups) where performance has been poorer are usually very keen to know what worked better elsewhere.

Additional cycles of RCE are needed to evaluate the refined models, but the evaluation need not start again at square one if the refinements are relatively small. However, if the changes are so large that the original intervention is essentially abandoned, then evaluation must start all over again. Although prior evaluation results should be combined with future evaluation results, to avoid confusion, it is appropriate to refer to a substantially refined program as a new model (Model 2 in Figure 11.5).

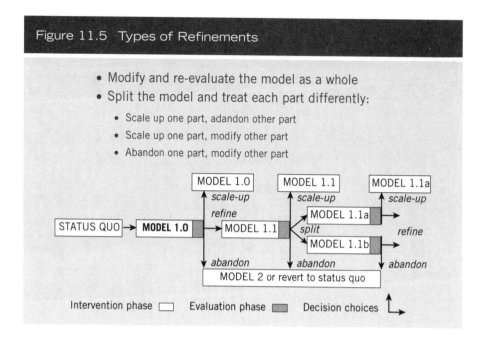

Figure 11.5 Types of Refinements

- Modify and re-evaluate the model as a whole
- Split the model and treat each part differently:
  - Scale up one part, adandon other part
  - Scale up one part, modify other part
  - Abandon one part, modify other part

Abandonment

A pilot failure will often be followed by a return to the *status quo*. But in today's climate of unsustainable health care growth, there will be pressure instead to try alternative innovations (Model 2 in Figure 11.3). In both cases, continuing RCE of the pilot sites might produce additional evidence for decision makers. RCE not only enables earlier detection of complete failures; it also is likely to reduce their number, because proponents of the pilot of a new funding model will react to disappointing preliminary results by increasing their efforts and creative solutions to their implementation problems. In other words, proper use of RCE can help even struggling models evolve rather than die.

Postpone Decisions and Continuing Evaluation

Because of the noted complexities of evaluating real-world health care programs (as compared with randomized efficacy trials of drugs), decisions about the fate of a funding model will be made by committees whose members often disagree. As evidence accrues through periodic RCE updates, the balance of opinion in the committee will gradually shift from "wait and see" to "time to decide." The option to postpone a decision on the program and continue evaluation can involve particularly strong differences of opinion. A substantial benefit of RCE is that it makes such differences of opinion more manageable, because proponents and opponents can often be persuaded to wait for another cycle of evidence. Merely discussing the measures of impact and anticipating results of an evaluation often helps bring consensus, by causing policymakers to focus more closely on how the program is intended to change behavior and improve results. The speed and assertiveness of decision making can sometimes be inversely proportional to the observed effect size.

Postponement may be particularly appropriate, either when unintended consequences are uncovered during the course of the evaluation that need more data to be understood, or when findings are ambiguous. For example, when there is evidence of heterogeneity, but the source remains undetected, collecting additional data on potential sources of variation may make delaying a directional decision a reasonable action. RCE provides the opportunity to hypothesize and test reasons for heterogeneity not afforded by *post hoc* black box summative evaluations.

One of the most basic decisions for information-overloaded policymakers and clinicians is "Should I spend time and energy on this issue?" Frequent interim results help answer this question. Preliminary findings that are inconsistent with a theoretically valid intervention reinforces the need for busy decision makers to spend time and energy understanding reasons for less than optimal results. Indeed, with multiple programs being continually studied by RCE, directing decision makers' attention to meaningful findings is becoming an important task for evaluators.

Like the first three decisions, postponement is also subject to the consequences of false decision making:

1) Incorrectly continuing or scaling up an ineffective program will not improve quality and/or will waste resources.

2) Incorrectly continuing or scaling up an ineffective program may inhibit progress, by curtailing or delaying research on and dissemination of truly effective programs.

3) Incorrectly discontinuing a program is a lost opportunity for saving costs and/or improving care.

Whether the decision is to scale up, abandon, or refine a model, the opportunity and need for RCE is likely to continue. Fortunately, many of the procedures for implementing RCE can usually be routinized, with only modest modifications to customize the RCE process to fit a specific intervention. The data and resources necessary to conduct RCE vary across interventions and likely co-vary with the complexity and scope of an intervention. Nonetheless, RCE represents an opportunity for rapid feedback, participation of managers and policymakers with the evaluation, and the engagement of stakeholders with all aspects of the evaluation. These attributes are associated with greater utilization of evaluation results and increase the value and potential of an evaluation to provide meaningful data for evidence-informed decision making.

Cases: Examples of Decisions

If a positive impact of a program is clear and desirable, does not increase costs or reduce scope, and has results that are generalizable to a broader population, the rational policy decision should be to scale up the program.

One example of such a decision is Medicare's prospective payment system, in which Medicare pays hospitals a prospectively determined amount for the hospital-specific costs of a hospitalization. This program was predated by a demonstration project in New Jersey in the early 1980s that tested the impact of prospective payments for hospitalizations. Substantial reductions in Medicare spending followed, without consequent reductions in quality or adverse clinical outcomes. The program was scaled nationally and is now widely believed to have reaped massive savings for the federal government.[6]

Another example is the Medicare Recovery Audit Contractor program. The program was tested as a demonstration that started in 2005, in which contractors were assigned to assess the medical necessity of hospitalizations. Hospital stays deemed unnecessary were not reimbursed at inpatient rates, leading to a substantial increase in rates of observation status utilization. While unpopular with hospitals, the program led to massive Medicare savings without directly impacting medical care, and was scaled nationally in 2010 *before* the end date of the demonstration.[7]

An example, in the commercial insurance business, of a case when the results of a program were not definitive, but the value appeared likely enough for scale-up is the MI-FREE trial. This RCT, conducted by Aetna, assessed the effect of eliminating copayments for essential medications for patients who experience a myocardial infarction. While no statistically significant ($p < 0.05$) benefit was seen in the primary outcome (a composite cardiovascular outcome), a significant improvement was seen in the secondary outcome (a reduction in subsequent vascular events). The study was powered on clinical events, not costs. Although a trend of cost reduction was seen, it was not statistically significant. While the results appeared to be mixed, Aetna found them sufficiently compelling to scale the program to their fully insured book of business. This is a typical example of multiple outcomes of a complex intervention being evaluated and, based on a mix of effect sizes, a decision being made to scale up. Part of such a consideration was likely the conviction that some of the "nonsignificant" findings would have become "statistically significant" if the pilot had run longer or the sample size been larger—something that cannot, of course, be proven *ex post*.

Certainly not all programs tested are successful, and demonstrations encounter similar pressure to identify failing programs and terminate them promptly to save precious resources. One example is a Medicare demonstration project evaluating the effect of expanded chiropractic services on total cost of care.[8] The demonstration found no evidence of reduced spending, and even suggested increased overall spending, leading Medicare to abandon the program for the *status quo*. Similarly, Medicare supported a national RCT to test the efficacy of a clinical intervention (lung volume reduction surgery) on clinical outcomes to inform an up or down coverage decision. The trial did not find improved outcomes, and Medicare determined not to cover the service.

Sometimes, programs are abandoned for a different model altogether. An example is the Medicare Electronic Medical Record (EMR) demonstration, which used an RCT to test the effect of physician incentive payments on EMR record use and overall cost and quality of care. A national program (HITECH) was subsequently enacted that applied a different payment incentive to providers and rendered the trial irrelevant; the trial was terminated early for that reason, without producing usable results.[9]

Frequently, the available evidence from a test is inconclusive, and that information is used to adjust or modify the program and continue it, allowing for re-evaluation. An example is the high-cost demonstration, which provided per beneficiary per month fees to primary care providers to better manage complex Medicare beneficiaries.[10] The results were promising but not overwhelming for Medicare beneficiaries, but substantial learning was available from participants who assessed their own health successes and failures. This program was then modified to become the Comprehensive Primary Care initiative, a multipayer approach to providing primary care providers with larger per beneficiary per month payments to reward improved quality of care and efficiency for the entire patient populations they serve.

An example of policymakers choosing to split up results, and scale part of a program while abandoning other parts is the Medicare plus Choice demonstration, a test of the ability of health plans and provider organizations to manage the health of populations with risk-adjusted capitated payments for the beneficiaries they serve. The evaluation of that demonstration found health plans to be more credible partners than provider groups, resulting in the Medicare Advantage program being scaled nationally in partnership with health plans alone.[11]

An example of policymakers choosing to scale part of a program and alter another part for continued study is the physician group practice demonstration, which tested the effect of a shared savings payment model for health systems and found mixed results. When programmatic decisions were made about expansion, only interim analyses were available. Those early results informed development of several shared savings approaches that were variations on the Physicians Group Practice. The Medicare Shared Savings Program, a national program for Accountable Care Organizations, was implemented, and new demonstration programs were implemented to test the effect of greater risk sharing on care (the Pioneer ACO program, discussed in earlier chapters) and the possibility of providing capital to rural providers who choose to start their own ACO (Advance Payment ACO program).

An example of policymakers choosing to abandon unsuccessful portions of a program and modify more promising parts is the Medicare Care Coordination Demonstration. The demonstration awarded to 15 applicants the opportunity to test care coordination approaches to improve care and reduce costs for Medicare beneficiaries with serious chronic diseases. Despite great enthusiasm for the program, only one awardee, Health Quality Partners (HQP), had promising results at the end of the demonstration period.[12] All other tests were terminated, but HQP was continued for 12 years and tasked with expanding to different regions and demonstrating sustainability.

Evidence Thresholds for Decision Making in Rapid-Cycle Evaluation

Setting Evidence Thresholds

Evidence thresholds are used in the first two steps of the R.A.P.I.D. decision-making process (see Box 11.1 above for the 5 steps of R.A.P.I.D.). The reason for trying to define thresholds in advance is to reduce the temptation to lower thresholds when results are tending toward decision makers' hopes (or to raise the bar against results that conflict with decision makers' beliefs). In general, engagement of decision makers in all stages of an evaluation is desirable. More importantly, as noted, thresholds defined in terms of statistical significance or nonsignificance reduce what should be complex decisions to binary up/down choices, which are conducive to disengagement by both evaluators and decision makers. Engaging stakeholders is also generally useful in setting meaningful thresholds for identifying improvement, and deciding how that improvement will be recognized creates trust. Such engagement improves organizational capacity for learning, and increases the maximum appropriate utilization of evaluation results. (See Box 11.2 for how statistical significance differs from practical/policy importance.)

Refining Evidence Thresholds

Effect size thresholds are used in the second stage, as decision makers contemplate options for action. The translation of evidence into policy, as already emphasized, is not a simple linear process. Decision makers take into account aspects of context not examined in the evaluation or may propose options only indirectly addressed by the evidence. For example, "We observed a modest improvement with an incentive fee. What about scaling up with double the fee? Would we get a bigger improvement?" The threshold for evidence concerning the impact of the incentive fee, for example, may contribute to assessing the possible effect of doubling the fee—but the discussion between the evaluator and the decision maker will involve determining how far the results can be generalized to options for action not tested in the evaluation. Each new data point in RCE, as well as trends in effect estimates and precision over time combined with contextual knowledge (see Chapter 12 discussion of Bayesian methods and priors to ease interpretation of interim findings), may lead to reconsidering evidence thresholds. And decision makers might

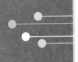

Box 11.2
Sample Size and Statistical Power Considerations

Selecting an optimal sample size is a concern in nearly all evaluations. Sample size, however, is only one of four components that determine the statistical results of an analysis. The other three are statistical power (1-beta or 1 minus the probability of a Type II error), the significance level (alpha or Type I error), and the effect size (the magnitude of the estimated effect). Fixing the values of any three of these components determines the value of the fourth.

In most program evaluations, analysts are confronted with one of two common scenarios. The first scenario is one in which it is feasible to draw a sample of study subjects prior to the evaluation. In this scenario, the investigator can fix the values for significance (at conventional levels such as 0.05 or 0.01) and power (0.80). After specifying the desired effect size, the sample size needed for both the treatment and control/comparison groups can be computed.

Deriving the effect size is one of the more challenging tasks in any evaluation. The effect size should represent the substantively important impact that would lead one to conclude that a treatment is worthwhile. There are several ways in which auxiliary information can be used to define the effect size. When costs are the primary outcome, one option is to set the effect size at a break-even point. For example, if a program costs $500 per patient to implement, then the desired effect might be set at $500 in savings for total health care costs to offset the treatment costs. Another approach is to use the Minimum Important Difference (MID) that has been established for some outcomes. MIDs are the changes that patients perceive when their health has improved (or declined). Finally, effect sizes can be based on clinical judgments of important differences.

The second common scenario is one in which the sample size is fixed in advance, usually because all available subjects have already been identified. In this situation, interest usually centers on the study's power to detect the desired effect size. If power is low (for example, less than the conventional level of 0.80), then the investigator may want to reconsider whether it is worthwhile to proceed with the study since the design is unlikely to detect substantively important findings.

Statistical significance should be the by-product of a carefully planned analysis. When a study has been appropriately powered with an adequate sample, the results will be significantly different from zero if the estimated treatment effect is equal to or greater than the desired effect size.

ask for new evidence sources about the processes that are producing unexpected impacts (or lack of impact).

Two alternative minimum requirements are often used to define success of a new program:

1. Improved effectiveness
2. No quality declines or cost increases

Figure 11.6 shows that different quantities of effect size/evidence are needed for different types of decisions, because the cost of being wrong differs between scaling up vs. abandonment vs. continuing with refinements. There are many examples of health care programs scaling up based on a Type I error (taking a positive result as true which is in fact false, a false positive). Type I errors in health care can be impossible to correct; after scaling up a program, it becomes difficult to dislodge or impossible to evaluate it, because that program is now regarded as "standard" care that cannot ethically be withheld from patients (even when that care is of demonstrated dubious worth). Thus, the opportunity cost of a false positive (in terms of lost opportunity for more rigorous evidence of program failure) can be exorbitant; as costs of ineffective programs keep on multiplying, such expenditures cannot be used for truly effective programs. Committing to an ineffective program also reduces the potential for effective programs to be identified and tested, as the "problem" may be considered "solved."

The lost opportunity for savings due to a Type II error (false negative) is not as great. Proponents are likely to continue to advocate for the program and may even come up with an improved version of the model and test it. Ultimately the cost of a false negative might be a delay in achieving potential gains; the cost of a false positive might be permanent losses year after year.

A common result of RCE will be a mixture of positive and negative impacts. Even if one wanted to set false positives and the resulting tradeoff in false negatives

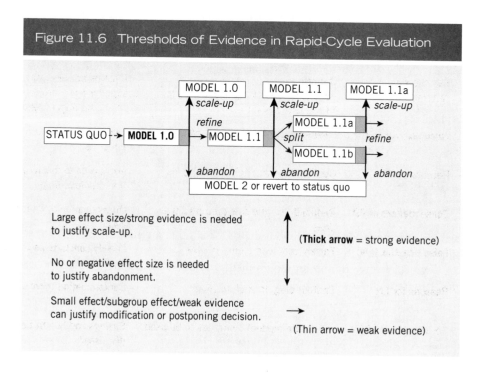

Figure 11.6 Thresholds of Evidence in Rapid-Cycle Evaluation

upfront, agreement from proponents and skeptics together is unlikely. Decision making on program continuation/discontinuation needs to consider more complex benefit-risk tradeoffs. Clear thresholds are defined for decision making on drug approval based on efficacy in a very narrow regulatory framework. For multi-faceted health care programs endpoints, such a framework does not exist. Instead, decision making has to be based on the preponderance of the entire evidence, mostly absolute effect sizes weighted by the clinical impact of harms and benefits.

The contrast between RCE and decision making in MS and CMMI is shown in Table 11.2. A key difference is that drugs evaluated in MS have already passed several hurdles and are considered efficacious in at least some patients and not harmful in the short term; otherwise, they would not have been approved by FDA. Therefore, MS is focused on accruing suggestive evidence of harm, not evidence of effectiveness. In contrast, a health care program such as a new funding model might not yet have passed even the first hurdle—showing some benefit—when RCE begins. The evaluation is focused initially on benefits (the reason for the new model), but it cannot neglect evaluation of harm.

Figure 11.7 illustrates accumulating evidence categorized into phases, where the model is initially "questionable" with highly variable effect estimates, then

	Mini-Sentinel Active Drug Safety Monitoring	Rapid-Cycle Program Effectiveness Evaluation
Table 11.2 Rapid-Cycle Evaluation-Based Decision Making Issues of Single Drug Safety in Mini-Sentinel vs. Program Effectiveness Evaluation CMMI		
Key decision after "alerting"	If a new drug might hurt patients, we need to do something about it (letters, REMs, withdrawal).	If a new delivery system produces superior outcomes or saves costs, it should be disseminated widely.
False positive (FP)	Falsely conclude a drug may *cause harm*	Falsely conclude an intervention is *effective*
Reasons for FP	Confounding, multiple comparisons	Regression to mean, co-interventions (i.e., *confounding*)
Consequences of FP	Reduced use of a safe (and effective) drug	Dissemination of an ineffective program, waste
False negative (FN)	Falsely conclude a drug is *safe*	Falsely conclude an intervention is *ineffective*
Reasons for FN	Confounding, lack of precision	Contamination (*confounding*), lack of precision
Consequences of FN	An unsafe product continues to be used.	Savings and health benefits will be dismissed.

Figure 11.7 Strength of Evidence Visualization and Explanation

'Strength' of evidence is due to the effect size of the impact and increasing narrowness of confidence intervals

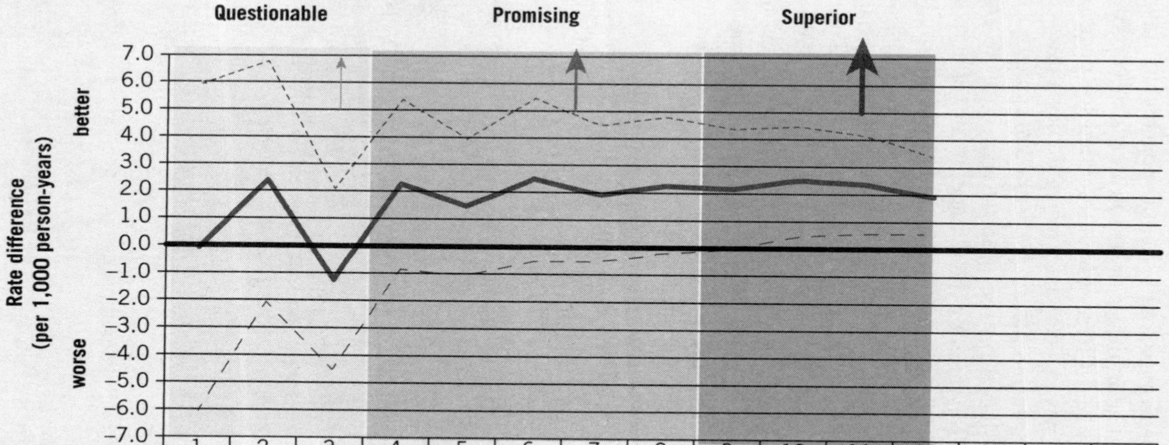

Questionable Promising Superior

Rate difference (per 1,000 person-years) — better / worse — scale 7.0 to -7.0

	1	2	3	4	5	6	7	8	9	10	11	12	13	14	15
Lower 95% confidence interval	-6.00	-2.00	-4.50	-0.80	-1.00	-0.50	-0.50	-0.20	0.00	0.50	0.60	0.60			
Cumulative rate difference	0.00	2.40	-1.20	2.30	1.50	2.50	2.00	2.30	2.20	2.50	2.40	2.00			
Upper 95% confidence interval	6.00	6.80	2.10	5.40	4.00	5.50	4.50	4.80	4.40	4.50	4.20	3.40			

- - - - - Lower 95% confidence interval
—— Cumulative rate difference
– – – Upper 95% confidence interval

Questionable:
- Investigate subgroup effects
- Continue evaluation

Promising:
- Continue program
- Continue evaluation
- Moderately expand program

Superior:
- Widely disseminate

"promising" with consistently elevated effect estimates, and finally potentially "superior" as the confidence limits around the elevated effect estimates increasingly narrow. Such a pattern might lead to a decision to scale up.

Evidence Thresholds in Light of Context

The following lists selected issues in benefit/harm assessment of drugs during rapid-cycle drug safety analyses of accruing data. These are analogues to issues evaluators and decision makers face whether doing traditional summative evaluation or RCE of health care programs. The list highlights how health care evaluation is influenced by aspects of the context that influence both benefits and costs.

Aspects of context that influence benefit:

Availability of an alternative drug

Comparative effectiveness of the new drug vs. alternative drug

Clinical value of benefits (lifesaving vs. cosmetic)

Number of potential life years lost by the user population aspects of context that influence harm:

Frequency of adverse effect (benefit/harm analysis is based on absolute risks)

Seriousness of adverse event (death vs. nose bleed)

Prevalence of the adverse event

In the setting of drug safety monitoring, many of these parameters are known or relatively well characterized. However, in health care, improvement programs may need to be evaluated simultaneously, as there is often little or no prior evidence to go on. Consequently, multiple parameters typically will contribute to success (e.g., several quality parameters, several cost parameters, and administrative burden of implementation) and the decision maker will need to determine the relative value (i.e., weight) of each—weights that must be factored with effect sizes of each outcome measure. It is in the nature of a multistakeholder environment that different stakeholders will have different weights. More often than not, such disagreements are due to diverse values on different outcomes (not due to disagreement about the direct evidence). It may be possible to mitigate the potential for disagreement. If these values can be explicated, and each parameter weighted in advance of the evidence becoming available, the potential for disagreement can sometimes be mitigated.

As stated earlier, the validity of the effect size of several key outcome parameters, and the weights attributed to them, are critical for decision makers. It is a specific advantage of RCE that precision can be extrapolated to some degree based on observed trends (see, technical discussion in Chapter 12).

Figure 11.8 Decision Making With Mixed Outcomes

Decisions are clouded if outcomes are mixed

- different strengths of evidence for different outcomes
- different opinions about relative value of different outcomes
- different opinions about what is clinical important change
- therefore, mixed threshold for decision making

	Data Quality	Data Quantity	Typical Impact
Cost	Solid	High	Moderate
Morbidity	Adequate	Medium	Low
Mortality	Solid	Low	Undetectable

SUMMARY

RCE is an evaluation method that takes advantage of the ever-more rapid availability of data to provide regular interim information (e.g., quarterly) on the likelihood of program success, failure, or something indeterminate in between. The opportunity for frequent updates using high-quality evidence provides an additional evaluation advantage, not a replacement of the more complete and rigorous findings available at the end of a summative evaluation.

DISCUSSION QUESTION

1. How can evaluators best decide if an intervention requires further evaluation or is simply ineffective? What are the rewards and potential pitfalls of each approach?

2. How quickly would you feel comfortable assessing an intervention's merits as a policymaker?

3. Is RCE different from doing traditional evaluation more frequently? If so, how?

NOTES

1. Hartzema A. G., C. G. Reich, P. B. Ryan, et al. "Managing Data Quality for a Drug Safety Surveillance System." *Drug Safety* 36 Suppl. 1 (October 2013): S49–S58. doi: 10.1007/s40264-013-0098-7.

2. Hartzema A. G., J. A. Racoosin, T. E. MaCurdy, J. M. Gibbs, and J. A. Kelman. "Utilizing Medicare Claims Data for Real-Time Drug Safety Evaluations: Is it Feasible?" *Pharmacoepidemiology and Drug Safety* 20 (2011): 684–88.

3. Avorn, Jerry, and Sebastian Schneeweiss. "Managing Drug-Risk Information—What to Do with All Those New Numbers." *New England Journal of Medicine* 361, no. 7 (2009): 647–49.

4. Langley G. L., R. Moen, K. M. Nolan, T. W. Nolan, C. L. Norman, and L. P. Provost. *The Improvement Guide: A Practical Approach to Enhancing Organizational Performance* (2nd ed.). (San Francisco: Jossey-Bass Publishers, 2009).

5. McCarney, R, et al., "The Hawthorne Effect: A Randomised, Controlled Trial," *BMC Medical Research Methodology* 7 (2007): 30. doi: 10.1186/1471-2288-7-30. Available at http://www.biomedcentral.com/1471-2288/7/30; Fox, N. S., "Clinical Estimation of Fetal Weight and the Hawthorne Effect," *European Journal of Obstetrics and Gynecology and Reproductive Biology* 141 no. 2 (2008): 111–14. doi: http://dx.doi.org/10.1016/j.ejogrb.2008.07.023.

6. Hsiao W. C., H. M. Sapolsky, D. L. Dunn, and S. L. Weiner, "Lessons of the New Jersey DRG payment system," *Health Affairs*, 5, no. 2 (1986): 32–45. doi: 10.1377/hlthaff.5.2.32.

7. "Recovery Audit Program," *CMS*, accessed 16 June 2016, https://www.cms.gov/Research-Statistics-Data-and-Systems/Monitoring-Programs/Medicare-FFS-Compliance-Programs/Recovery-Audit-Program/index.html.

8. "MMA Section 651 Expansion of Coverage of Chiropractic Services Demonstration," *CMS*, accessed 16 June 2016, https://innovation.cms.gov/medicare-demonstrations/mma-section-651-expansion-of-coverage-of-chiropractic-services-demonstration.html.

9. Electronic Health Records (EHR) Incentive Programs, *CMS*, accessed 16 June 2016, https://www.cms.gov/Regulations-and-Guidance/Legislation/EHRIncentivePrograms/index.html?redirect=/ehrincentiveprograms/.

10. "Care Management for High-Cost Beneficiaries Demonstration," *CMS*, accessed 16 June 2016, https://innovation.cms.gov/Medicare-Demonstrations/Care-Management-for-High-Cost-Beneficiaries-Demonstration.html.

11. "Health Plans—General Information," *CMS*, accessed 16 June 2016, https://www.cms.gov/Medicare/Health-Plans/HealthPlansGenInfo/index.html.

12. "Medicare Coordinated Care Demonstration," *CMS*, accessed 16 June 2016, https://innovation.cms.gov/initiatives/Medicare-Coordinated-Care.

12

Alternative Ways of Analyzing Data in Rapid-Cycle Evaluation

Thomas Nolan

Jerry Cromwell

Martijn van Hasselt

Nikki Freeman

Learning Objectives

To complement the theoretical rapid-cycle evaluation (RCE) decision making, this chapter presents and assesses analytic techniques to look at their relative strengths and weaknesses in bringing RCE from theory to practice.

A natural fit with looking at change over time is the statistical process control method. With its origins in the quality control world of product development, this approach shows change over time in an outcome, with prespecified boundaries that are calculated to correspond to meaningful differences. The relationship between the intervention and the outcome and its evolution over time is shown graphically.

Regression-based methods are well-known and can analyze the differences between treatment and comparison groups over time, usually in a difference-in-difference framework. This framework can include a number of covariates, in addition to the baseline data for both treatment and comparison groups. Its use in and RCE context shortens the time intervals of interest and provides a graphic interpretation for policymakers.

Bayesian methods are also used in these evaluations. They allow results to be more intuitively understood, as probabilities of different levels of change. They may also allow impact estimation with smaller samples than regression-based methods.

With the same data, each of these methods is used to assess the impacts of an intervention, how early the conclusion that was reached in the evaluation would have been reached, and what strengths each approach may demonstrate for policy.

This chapter outlines and applies three methods of analyzing quarterly data in an RCE using a standardized dataset. Of interest are the different strengths the three approaches demonstrate, in terms of ease of analysis, ease of understanding, and rigor. In an RCE world, extremely large volumes of data would be analyzed, reported, and acted upon each quarter (or other regular and frequent interval). For this reason, standardization of outcomes, specifications, and even analysis methods will help policymakers to know what they are seeing and what to make of it each quarter.

The three analytic approaches described and applied in this chapter are statistical process control (or Shewhart charts), and classical and Bayesian regression-based models. The extent to which, and conditions under which, results converge are of particular interest in keeping with the belief that results are most robust when they are consistent, regardless of the differing assumptions in the analytic techniques. There are also specific cases where one method may be more appropriate than another.

Statistical Process Control Methods

Statistical process control (SPC) methods have been used for almost one hundred years in industrial quality control situations. Developed by Walter Shewhart, this approach is intended to explain variation over time to support learning and improvement.[1] The approach relies on identifying an outcome of interest and plotting its rate over time (e.g., intensive care unit [ICU] complication rates). Specific types of charts for this purpose range from the very simple run chart to the more complicated and covariate adjusted Shewhart charts (see Table 12.1). They can be used to examine trends and predict future performance on a particular measure as well as incorporate interventions and comparison groups. Shewhart charts incorporate prespecified control limits that allow the evaluator to determine whether the process being examined is a stable process and when deviations from that process occur.

Table 12.1 Types of Control Charts		
Tool	**Attributes**	**Complexity**
Line chart Run chart	• Simple to construct • Can be used with little data to guide early learning • Identify signals of improvement	Low
Shewhart charts (basic)	• Distinguish common/special cause variation • Determine process stability • Predict future performance • Economic balance in decision making	Moderate
Shewhart charts (advanced)	• Can address issues such as overdispersion, rare events, transformations, autocorrelation, trend, O/E ratios, power, deviation from targets, seasonal adjustments, case mix, etc.	High
Planned experimentation	• Study influence of factors at different levels, interactions, background variables, block designs, fractional factorials, random assignment of treatment, a priori design	Highest

At its simplest level, the method utilizes the binomial distribution[2] to model the likelihood of observing five, six, or more points in a row below the baseline level that would have a very low probability if generated from a random process. SPC can also work with a pre-/postdesign without a comparison group under the assumption that the evaluator is studying a process change from a stable baseline in a fairly controlled environment (e.g., reducing ICU infections, reducing ER wait times, or improving home medications compliance).

More advanced adjustments to Shewhart charts involve smoothing data points with moving averages, adjusting for sloping baselines, subgroup charts, multi-variate T2 charts that combine two or more related measures (e.g., admissions and readmissions), autocorrelation across data points, and risk adjustment of data points using logistic and other regression-based functional forms. The purpose of all of these adjustments is to make the run charts more visually interpretable to users, by factoring out systematic variance.[3]

Comprehensive evaluations of programs to improve complex systems gener-ally require other types of analysis methods to supplement formal statistical analy-sis. Analysis of data over time is, for example, vital to understand the evolution of interventions facilitated by the financial or other policy mechanisms introduced as part of the program. Basic time series displays of key outcome measures are a start. More sophisticated analysis can be performed using Shewhart control charts (more aptly called process performance charts or learning charts). Shewhart developed the approach to learning and improvement to provide an objective criterion for deciding when a pattern of variation in the time series should signal further inquiry.[4]

Figures 12.1 and 12.2 contain Shewhart charts created as part of the CMS-designed community-based care transitions project. CMS selected 14 communities to participate in the project; depending on the strengths and priorities in a given community, a set of interventions to smooth the transition from hospital to home or to another care setting was developed and implemented. Hospitalizations per 1000 Medicare beneficiaries living in a defined geographic area was one of the outcome measures. Twelve quarters in 2007–2009 were used as the baseline for the project; eight quarters in 2009–2010 were used as the intervention period.[5] Figure 12.1 contains the Shewhart chart for one of the 14 intervention communities. The chart shows a center line at the average of the data and an upper and lower control limit computed as the center line ± three standard deviations. A pattern in the time series (referred to as a "special cause" in quality improvement work) warranting further analysis is indicated by 1 point outside the control limits or a sequence of 8 points in a row above or below the center line.[6] Figure 12.2 shows that a special cause exists during the intervention period and persists for three more quarters. Any qualitative data collected about the community's set up of the project, the organi-zational capabilities for improvement, and the interventions chosen for improve-ment will assist the analyst in determining whether the special cause was a result of system change or a less beneficial administrative change or system distortion. The Shewhart method may be even more useful to understand the context of the com-parison sites. It is unlikely that the evaluation's resource allocation would allow for

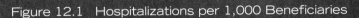

Figure 12.1   Hospitalizations per 1,000 Beneficiaries

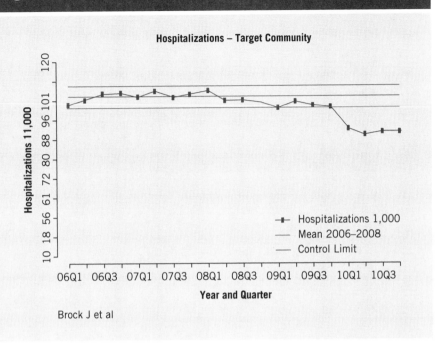

Brock J et al

an assessment of organizational capabilities for improvement in all the comparison sites. Use of the Shewhart chart can signal to the analyst when collecting qualitative data from a comparison site is likely to provide a good return on investment. For example, consider the charts in Figure 12.2 for the intervention site and its four comparison sites, all plotted on the same horizontal and vertical scales. The chart for the comparison site in the upper right corner in Figure 12.2 indicates a special cause reduction in hospitalizations during the intervention period. The question becomes, What mechanism–context combination produced this result?

The evaluator might pursue a line of inquiry for this comparison community like the following.

1. Was there intent to reduce hospitalizations either by community-based care transition improvements or some other system changes?

    - If answer to #1 is no, what accounted for the reduction: an administrative change or a system distortion? End inquiry. Take the answer into account in the formal statistical analysis.

    - If the answer to #1 is yes, were the basics of the program team set up followed?

2. Using the elements of the Consolidated Framework for Implementation Research framework (see Chapter 9) or an alternative, assess the organizational capabilities for system improvement.

3. What was the mechanism–context interaction that best explains the improvement?

4. How does the mechanism–context pair for this comparison community compare to that seen in the corresponding intervention community?

Figure 12.2   Hospitalizations per 1,000 Beneficiaries in One Intervention Community and Its Four Comparison Communities

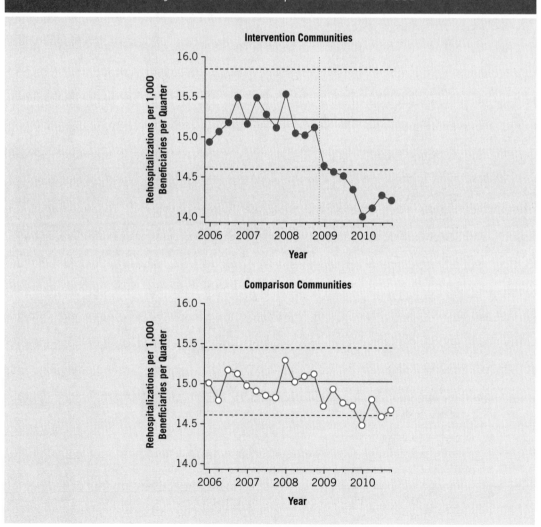

Note that the analysis using the time series and Shewhart charts adds some important insights that supplement the formal statistical analysis. In Figure 12.1, for example, suppose the data from the eight quarters during the intervention period actually occurred in reverse order (i.e., quarters 1, 2, 3, . . . occurred as 8, 7 ,6, . . .). With this sequence, the special cause would show up early in the intervention period and then disappear, perhaps indicating a weak or fragile process change; however, the formal statistical measures would be the same in both cases. This a good example of SPC's additional perspective on the process of change over time, which can provide enlightening additional information toward learning and evaluative objectives.

Regression Analysis for Rapid-Cycle Evaluation

Regression analysis is a flexible method for RCE because it allows us to isolate program effects, while simultaneously controlling for other factors that may also be at play. By using regression analysis, baseline trends can be teased out and quarter-by-quarter comparisons between the comparison group and intervention group can be estimated. In this section we discuss classical regression analysis; later in the chapter we discuss Bayesian estimation techniques and apply them to a regression model.

We begin our discussion of regression analysis by specifying a model that estimates program effects on a rolling basis. The regression specification used is the Quarterly Fixed Effects (QFE) model (using the patient-quarter as the unit of analysis):

$$y_{it} = \alpha_0 + \mu I_i + \sum_t^T \beta_t Q_t + \sum_t^T \theta_t Q_t \bullet I_{it} \bullet D_t + \sum_k \lambda_k X_{itk} + \varepsilon_{it} \qquad (12.1)$$

- y_{it} = a performance measure (e.g., cost per beneficiary per quarter) for the i-th beneficiary in period t

- I_i = a 0,1 indicator of the observation in the comparison (= 0) or intervention (= 1) group

- Q_t = 0,1 indicator of the observation in the t-th quarter

- D_t = a 0,1 indicator (= 0, base period, = 1, demonstration period)

- X_{itk} = a vector of k patient, practice, and/or other characteristics

- ε_{it} = regression error term

The I_i coefficient, μ, measures the average difference in performance between the intervention and comparison groups across all base and demonstration quarters. If intervention and comparison samples are well matched on baseline performance, $\mu = 0$. Separate quarter indicators (Q_t) are used from t = 2, the second baseline quarter (first baseline effects are in α_0) to the most current evaluation quarter (T). The β_t coefficients reflect the individual quarter-to-quarter changes in average comparison group performance through the entire baseline and intervention periods. Rising β coefficients in later quarters indicate greater spending per patient. During base period quarters, intervention performance would be ($\mu + \beta_t$), with the intercept ignored. To determine the marginal effects of the intervention during only the demonstration period, the quarterly indicators are interacted with an indicator representing a demonstration period quarter (D_t). The θ_t coefficients reflect the deviation from the intervention's baseline μ-effect in the demonstration quarters. Intervention performance averages ($\mu + \beta_t + \theta_t$) during the t-th demonstration quarter. A vector of patient, practice, and/or other relevant characteristics is also included to further explain variance in performance and improve the reliability of the estimated coefficients.

Statistical Tests of Intervention Effects

Standard regression software packages automatically provide t-values, p-values, and confidence intervals for each model coefficient, including each of the crucial θ_t estimates. In addition to quarterly effects, the evaluator may also be interested in the overall level of program performance through a given period (e.g., across the first four demonstration quarters or effects of the program-to-date). Software packages, such as Stata, SAS, and R, allow for a linear combination test of multiple coefficients. This means that sums of quarterly effects produced by the QFE model, say the sum of effects for the latest four quarters or the difference between the first and second quarter, can be estimated along with their standard errors and confidence intervals. In Stata, for example, a command of the following form can be used: lincom $\theta_1 N_1 + \ldots + \theta_T N_T$, level (90); where N_t = the number of observations in the intervention group in the t-th quarter, and level (90) generates a 90% confidence interval around the summative patient-weighted quarter effects.

Visual Tools for Policymakers

To assist the policymakers in evaluating future prospects of success, CMMI suggested four graphical representations of evaluation-regression results at each period of analysis. The four graphs involve two analyses at each period of analysis: (1) estimates of quarterly effects, and (2) estimates of program-to-date effects. For each of these regression formulations, there are two corresponding graphs. These graphs visualize the estimated effect sizes and the precision of the estimates. Additionally, they articulate the anticipated gains/losses of a particular program and the risks associated with them. We present the two types of graphs in Figure 12.3 for program-to-date effects. The graphs illustrate an example drawn from a Medicare payment reform demonstration and analyze program effects on cost. Quarterly cost data were available at the beneficiary level for individuals in an intervention group and a comparison group. The sample contained 67,390

Figure 12.3 Program-to-Date Effects on Costs and Strength of Evidence

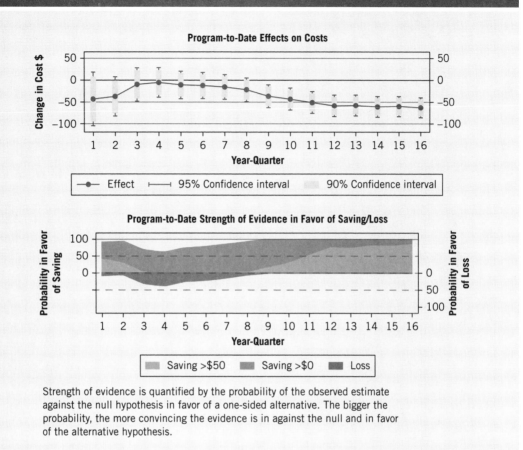

Strength of evidence is quantified by the probability of the observed estimate against the null hypothesis in favor of a one-sided alternative. The bigger the probability, the more convincing the evidence is in against the null and in favor of the alternative hypothesis.

individuals who were observed over a maximum period of 28 quarters. Quarters 1–12 represent the baseline period, and Quarters 13–28 represent the intervention period. The total sample contains 441,282 person-quarter observations.

The first graph plots the regression-generated point estimates—period by period—with 90 and 95% confidence intervals. After the 8th intervention quarter, program-to-date effects on cost indicate savings because the estimates and confidence intervals are decidedly below zero. The second graph plots the strength of evidence in favor of one-sided hypotheses of particular interest. These alternative hypotheses are (1) the estimate is greater than zero (dark blue); (2) the estimate is less than zero (medium blue); and (3) the estimate is less than $50 (light blue), indicating an estimated savings of at least $50. Technically, strength of evidence is computed by calculating and plotting the complement of the probability

(1 minus the probability) of observing, by chance, an estimate larger (smaller) than the estimate if the program actually had a zero (or other prespecified value) effect. Intuitively, the larger the probability for the desired effect shown in the graph, the more compelling is the evidence that the program has the desired effect.

Advantages and Disadvantages of Quarterly Fixed Effects Models

An obvious advantage of QFE modeling is its flexibility. It does not require prior specification of the functional form of intervention effects over the life of the intervention, or even the base period. For example, baseline trends in spending likely are not linear but exponential in nature from compounded volume and price effects. Similarly, it is not reasonable to expect intervention effects to be linear if interventions start slowly then produce accelerated effects.

Another advantage of QFE is that it reports intervention performance, relative to a comparison group, quarter-by-quarter. This enables the evaluator and policymaker to see any trends in performance that might be lost in a linear slope estimate of effects. How quickly a decision can be made to abandon, scale up, or refine an intervention depends on the observed pattern of θ_t coefficients? A more minor advantage is the fact that QFE modeling does not require season adjustors, because each quarter's effects are estimated separately, thereby "controlling" for season.

While QFE represents a very flexible approach to program testing, a disadvantage is that it adds considerably to model complexity. The fact that QFE estimation can involve many more coefficients could be considered a computational disadvantage. Another potential disadvantage is that one or two large quarters of "savings" or "losses" could result in an incorrect policy decision to expand or abandon a new program. This concern is heightened when estimating the model on small datasets with just a few hundred intervention observations, particularly for volatile spending information. Large savings one quarter can turn into large dissavings the next quarter. In both cases, the estimates may not be statistically significant at common levels of significance (10%, 5%), which makes inferences difficult. This problem is addressed to some degree by aggregating quarter-specific estimates by taking linear combinations of them, but it becomes an (unknown) trade-off between working with smaller samples and the number of quarters of data. Generally, smaller samples require more quarters of consistently better (worse) performance in the intervention group. Trade-offs also exist between how often to "look" at performance (monthly, quarterly, annually) and how significant short-period coefficients will be. More "looks" will show more volatility.

In Box 12.1, we provide two alternative QFE specifications. Readers who are not methodologically oriented may skip Box 12.1.

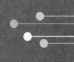

Box 12.1
Alternative QFE Specifications

Two alternative specifications to QFE invoke linear modeling (without or with discontinuity) to "smooth" the data across reporting periods (ignoring subscripts):

Linear (without discontinuity):

$$y = \alpha_0 + \alpha_1 I + \beta D + \delta_1 D \bullet I + \Sigma_k \lambda_k X_k + \eta \qquad (12.2)$$

Linear (with discontinuity, also known as "piecemeal"):

$$y = \alpha_0 + \alpha_1 I + \beta_1 Q + \beta_2 Q \bullet I + \delta_0 D + \delta_1 D \bullet I + \gamma_1 Q \bullet D + \gamma_2 Q \bullet D \bullet I + \Sigma_k \lambda_k X_k + \rho \qquad (12.3)$$

The δ_1 coefficient in Equation 12.2 represents the *change* in intervention mean performance minus the *change* in comparison performance for the demonstration and base period, controlling for other covariates. While estimated in linear form, no functional relation between changes and time period is presumed (as discussed later), but base trends are assumed equal between the two groups; otherwise, the estimated intervention effect is confounded with baseline differences. Nor is any information provided in the regression on the RCE performance of the intervention quarter-by-quarter. The linear discontinuity trend model, Equation 12.3, does allow for different baseline (β_2) and intervention (γ_2) trends between the intervention and comparison groups. It also allows for the intervention and comparison groups to be moving along a new discontinuous trend level (δ_0, δ_1).

A Bayesian Approach to Program Evaluation

In many recent and current evaluations of health care programs and interventions, RCE makes outcomes and other effectiveness data increasingly available during program implementation, and data are refreshed with higher frequency. For example, Medicare and Medicaid claims data can be compiled and extracted quarterly, and in some programs, participating organizations are required to provide progress reports and other performance indicators on a quarterly (or even monthly) basis. While analyzing data and calculating program effectiveness estimates more frequently does not present any special problems, it is harder to draw conclusions from a sequence of estimates. Statistical hypothesis testing procedures are more involved if testing is done repeatedly, for example, and it is harder to understand the probabilities of falsely rejecting a null hypothesis (Type I error) and not rejecting a null hypothesis when it is false (Type II error).

A Bayesian approach to inference and decision making is particularly useful in this context. It provides a consistent mechanism for updating program effectiveness estimates that does not require adjustments to account for repeated hypothesis testing. A second, and perhaps more important, advantage of this approach is that it provides policymakers directly with a probabilistic assessment of program effectiveness. A Bayesian analysis would enable us to answer questions such as, "What is the probability that the program yielded savings per patient of more than $100?" or "What is the probability that the program reduced ER utilization by 10% or more?" Strictly speaking, such questions cannot be answered by a non-Bayesian, "classical" statistical analysis in the same direct and straightforward way. In this section, we provide a brief introduction to Bayesian analysis and then consider a regression model estimated using Bayesian techniques.

Before we further discuss the Bayesian approach, Box 12.2 outlines the main ingredients of Bayesian inference for methodologically interested readers. Other readers are encouraged to skip Box 12.2.

Box 12.2
The Bayesian Paradigm
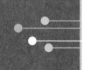

We first introduce some notation. Let θ denote the program effectiveness parameter, and D_t the data available from the first time of observation through time t. Distribution and density functions are denoted by $p(\cdot)$, where $p(y)$ is the distribution (density) of y and $p(y|x)$ is the conditional distribution (density) of y given x.

A Bayesian model consists of two components. The first, more familiar component is the *likelihood* function $p(D_t|\theta)$, which is a function of the parameter θ. This function relates the observed data D_t to the parameter θ and is also used in classical maximum likelihood estimation. The second component is the *prior* distribution of the parameter, $p(\theta)$. This is unique to a Bayesian model. The prior distribution (prior for short) reflects the degree of uncertainty or the beliefs about the parameter *before* observing the data. The prior can be specified as "vague," assigning probability to a wide range of parameter values, or more informative by concentrating probability over a narrower range of possible values. The latter case arises when information about program effectiveness outside of the data D_t, which may come from qualitative data or previous evaluations of similar programs, is leveraged to guide the specification of the prior.

In a Bayesian model, prior beliefs are updated after observing the data. This leads to the *posterior distribution* $p(\theta|D_t)$, which is calculated from the prior and likelihood using Bayes' rule:

$$p(\theta|D_t) = \frac{p(D_t|\theta)\,p(\theta)}{p(D_t)} \qquad (12.4)$$

The posterior distribution (posterior for short) reflects the parameter uncertainty that remains after the data have been observed. The denominator $p(D_t)$ is a normalizing constant, ensuring that probabilities add up to 1. It does not depend on θ and therefore does not determine the shape of the posterior. Thus, the previous equation is, instead, often written as a proportionality relation:

$$p(\theta|D_t) \propto p(D_t|\theta)\, p(\theta) \tag{12.5}$$

In words, the posterior distribution is proportional to the product of the prior distribution and the likelihood function. It is also the basis for Bayesian inference, and from it the Bayesian analogues of point estimates and credible intervals can be computed (these are discussed later in this chapter).

Finally, it is straightforward to generate predictions from a Bayesian analysis. Let X_{t+1} be a new, unobserved data point. The posterior predictive distribution for the new data point is

$$p(X_{t+1}|X_t) = \int_\theta p(X_{t+1}|\theta)\, p(\theta|X_t)\, d\theta. \tag{12.6}$$

The posterior predictive distribution utilizes the posterior and the likelihood function and averages over the parameter space to yield a distribution for the unobserved data point. Unlike classical prediction, which typically yields a point estimate and standard error, Bayesian prediction yields an entire distribution. The posterior predictive distribution describes the probability of seeing a particular data value dependent upon the data already observed and one's beliefs about the parameters.

Example: HIV Antibody Testing[7,8]

In Box 12.2, we presented the "main ingredients" of Bayesian inference. Before further discussing the Bayesian approach, we present a simple example to illustrate the role of the prior, the likelihood function, and the posterior.

Suppose that we randomly select a person from the United States. We are interested in whether this person is HIV positive, and we represent this with the parameter θ (rigorously, θ = {the individual is HIV positive}). Without further information, our best guess about whether the patient is HIV positive is the population prevalence, $p(\theta) = 0.005$, which in this example is our prior.

Enzyme immunoassays are an inexpensive diagnostic tool for HIV testing. The sensitivity of the test, the probability that the test is positive given that the patient tested is HIV positive, is 99.7%. The specificity of the test, the probability that the test is negative given that the patient tested is not HIV positive, is 98.5%. Symbolically, we can write the sensitivity as $p(\text{positive test}|\theta) = 0.997$ and the specificity as $p(\text{negative test}|\text{not } \theta) = 0.985$. In this example, the sensitivity and specificity together constitute a likelihood function.

We make two calculations that will be used to apply Bayes' rule. First, from specificity, we can determine the probability of a false alarm, the probability of a positive test given that a person is not HIV positive, by the straightforward calculation:

$$p(\text{positive test}|\text{not } \theta) = 1 - p\big(\text{negative test}|\text{not } \theta\big) = 1 - 0.985 = 0.015. \tag{12.7}$$

Second, we can use this and the law of total probability to calculate the probability of a positive test:

$$p(positive\,test) = p\left(positive\,test \middle| not\,\theta\right) \times p\left(not\,\theta\right) + p\left(positive\,test \middle| \theta\right) \times p(\theta) \quad (12.8)$$
$$= 0.015 \times 0.995 + 0.997 \times 0.005 = 0.02.$$

Suppose now the individual has been tested for HIV using an enzyme immunoassay and the test returns with a positive result. Given this new information, we want to answer: What is the probability that the individual is actually HIV positive? Symbolically, we want to find p(θ|positive test), which is exactly the posterior. We can find the posterior by using Bayes' rule:

$$p\left(\theta \middle| positive\,test\right) = \frac{p\left(positive\,test \middle| \theta\right) p\left(\theta\right)}{p\left(positive\,test\right)} \quad (12.9)$$

$$= \frac{0.997 * 0.005}{0.02} = 0.25.$$

By using Bayes' rule, we updated our prior belief with the new data (the test result) and conclude that given the positive test result, the probability that the individual is HIV positive is 25%. Hence, observing a positive test result makes it substantially more likely that a person is HIV positive. The fact that the posterior is "only" 25% might seem surprising. Some would (mistakenly) think the test is quite poor. However, this result arises because the population prevalence (prior) is very low. In other words, a positive test result is much more likely to be a false positive than a true positive. Finally, we emphasize that all Bayesian analyses rely on this logic of updating the prior data to yield the posterior. In the next section, we use the intuition about the prior, likelihood, and posterior gained in this simple example to discuss the Bayesian approach in more detail. We do this in the context of an empirical case study.

Case Study: A Payment Reform Demonstration

We now highlight some aspects of the process and outputs of a Bayesian evaluation. Throughout this discussion, we will utilize an example drawn from a Medicare payment reform demonstration, which was described earlier in the classical regression section of this chapter.

Model Specification

A Bayesian analysis, like a classical analysis, begins with model specification. We are interested in estimating the effect of the intervention on health care costs during each quarter. To this end, we use the following linear regression model:

$$\text{Cost}_{it} = \alpha_t + \beta_1 \text{Treated}_i + \beta_2 \text{Health}_{it} + \sum_{s=1}^{16} \gamma_s \text{Treated}_i \times I\{\text{Postqtr}_t = s\} + \mu_{it} \quad (12.10)$$

Here, $Cost_{it}$ is the cost for patient i in quarter t, α_t is a quarterly fixed effect, $Treated_i$ is a dummy variable equal to 1 if the patient is in the intervention group, $Health_{it}$ is a measure of health status, and $I\{Postqtr_t = s\}$ is an indicator, equal to 1 if quarter t is the s-th postintervention quarter and 0 otherwise (thus, $s = 1$ when $t = 13$, $s = 2$ when $t = 14$, etcetera). The set of coefficients γ_s are the intervention effects for each quarter. They measure if and how the cost difference between the intervention and comparison group changes during the intervention period. If the intervention is successful in lowering health care costs, then we expect to see $\gamma_s < 0$ in at least some of the postintervention quarters.

Equation 12.10 and the assumption that the errors (ε_{it}) are jointly normally distributed determine the likelihood function, which describes the relationship between the data and the parameters. This is the first component of the model. The second component is the prior distribution. It expresses the uncertainty about the parameters in a probabilistic form and is unique to the Bayesian approach. In this case, the parameters are the regression coefficients $\alpha_t, \beta_1, \beta_2, \gamma_1, \ldots, \gamma_{16}$, and σ_ε, the standard deviation of ε_{it}. We select independent normal prior distributions with mean 0 and standard deviation 1,000 for each of the coefficients and select the prior $\frac{1}{\sigma_\varepsilon}$ for σ_ε. These priors are standard choices in applied Bayesian work and carry little information as they are essentially "flat" or uniform for most values of the model parameters. Because of the scant amount of information in the priors, the likelihood function, the way by which the data enter the model, will largely determine the shape of the posterior.

Obtaining the Posterior

We estimate the model using PROC GENMOD in SAS version 9.4 although packages such as WinBUGS/OpenBUGS, JAGS, and Stan which also implement Bayesian analyses can be utilized through SAS, R, and Stata. All of these programs implement procedures to approximate the posterior distribution. Specifically, these procedures generate samples of parameter values that look like draws from the posterior. We avoid the details of Markov chains and sampling strategies (i.e., the specifics of how the sampling is done) and instead focus on why one would sample from the posterior and what exactly sampling from the posterior yields.

We first consider why one would sample from the posterior. Sometimes the posterior is a well-known distribution like the normal distribution; sometimes, however, the posterior is very complicated and simulation methods are required to approximate it. Simulation is achieved using Markov chain Monte Carlo (MCMC), a class of simulation algorithms.

The yield from MCMC is a collection of samples with which the posterior distribution for the parameters can be characterized. To conceptualize how the samples are obtained, one can imagine the MCMC algorithm as exploring the set of possible parameter values (the "parameter space"). For each step, the parameter value is recorded (these are samples). The algorithm may start very far away from the likeliest parameter values, but eventually it ends up generating parameter values that are the most likely under the posterior. As the number of steps (or draws) increases, the algorithm stabilizes, spending more time visiting parameter values that are likely under the posterior and less time at those values that are unlikely under the posterior. Since the initial draws may be unlikely under the posterior, it is common practice to discard the early draws. This is called the "burn-in" period. The total number of draws made before terminating the algorithm is a decision up to the evaluator. Diagnostics and a rich literature exists to inform the evaluator of the behavior of the chains and to assess when a sufficient number of draws has been generated.

Bayesian Inference

Once a sample from the posterior is obtained, the Bayesian analogues of point estimates and confidence intervals can be calculated. Point estimates for the parameters can be obtained by taking the mean of the posterior distribution of the parameter of interest. "Bayesian confidence intervals" are called credible intervals. A 95% credible interval is an interval that contains 95% of the simulated posterior values, a 90% credible interval is an interval that contains 90% of the simulated posterior values, and so on. In the example, the quarterly intervention effect sizes are the parameters of interest. For each of these parameters, Figure 12.4 presents

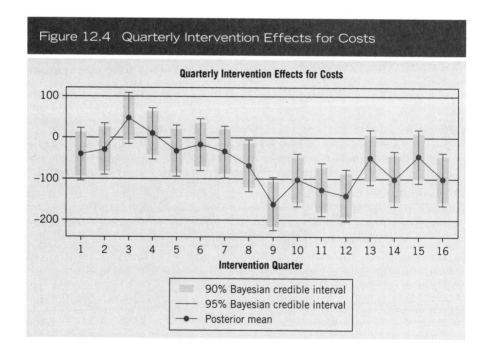

Figure 12.4   Quarterly Intervention Effects for Costs

(1) the means of the simulated values, (2) a 90% Bayesian credible interval, and (3) a 95% Bayesian credible interval. There is fairly strong evidence that, after postintervention Quarter 7, health care costs started to decline in the intervention group relative to the comparison group.

Unlike a classical confidence interval, Bayesian credible intervals are not uniquely defined. There are many ways to construct an interval that contains a certain fraction of the simulated values. Naturally, the question arises: How does one pick a particular credible interval to report? A common choice is the (90% or 95%) highest posterior density interval (HPDI). This is the interval that (1) contains a given percentage of the simulated values and (2) contains values with the highest posterior density. The HPDI does not need to be symmetric, centered in a particular way, nor contiguous. Hence Bayesian credible intervals and in particular, HPDIs, are highly flexible and useful when the posterior is multimodal or highly complex.

Accumulation of Evidence

To illustrate how Bayesian analysis can be used to track how evidence accumulates over time, we use a somewhat simpler regression model (12.11) and estimate it repeatedly, as more data become available. This approach mimics the situation that policymakers face in practice, when early evaluation findings are updated as more data become available.

$$Y_{it} = \alpha_t + \beta_1 \text{Treated}_i + \beta_2 \text{Health}_{it} + \gamma(\text{Treated}_i \times \text{Post}_t) + \varepsilon_{it} \qquad (12.11)$$

In Equation 12.11, $Post_t$ is an indicator for the intervention period, equal to 1 if quarter t is postintervention and 0 otherwise. The remaining variables are defined as before. The coefficient of primary interest is γ, which is a measure of the average intervention effect over a given number of postintervention quarters. We first estimated γ using data from Quarters 1 through 13. Since the intervention started in Quarter 13, that estimate of γ is based on only a single postintervention quarter. We then added data from Quarter 14 and re-estimated γ. This process was repeated until all quarters of data were used.

With the same prior distributions as before, we obtained 5,000 sample values of the model parameters. The posterior mean and 90% and 95% Bayesian credible intervals were then calculated for γ. The results are depicted in Figure 12.5.

Note two aspects of the results. First, the credible intervals get narrower as more quarters of postintervention data are used. This simply reflects the accumulation of information over time. Second, while the posterior means are always negative, suggesting that the intervention lowered health care costs, the credible intervals contain the value 0 up to the point where eight quarters of postintervention data are used. After that, the intervals dip decidedly below zero, and the posterior mean stabilizes somewhere around –$60. Thus, two years after the start of the intervention, the evidence has become very convincing that, on average, the intervention has been effective.

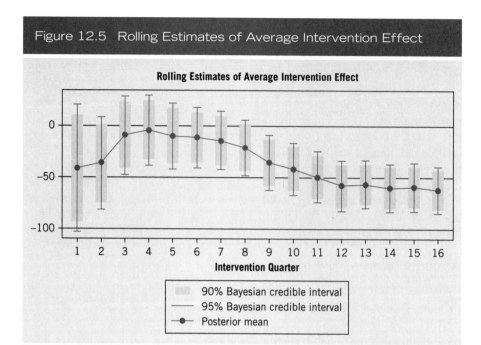

Figure 12.5   Rolling Estimates of Average Intervention Effect

Rolling Estimates of Average Intervention Effect

Intervention Quarter

90% Bayesian credible interval
95% Bayesian credible interval
Posterior mean

Probabilistic Interpretation

Bayesian analysis stands out from classical analyses in the ease with which the results can be interpreted in probabilistic terms. In classical hypothesis testing, results are binary: Do the data support or fail to support the null hypothesis that there is no evidence of savings? A more natural question might be, "What is the probability that the effect size is negative (shows savings)?" This question cannot be answered in the classical framework because parameters are fixed and thus do not have probabilities associated with them. In the Bayesian framework, because parameters are random and posterior distributions are distributions on parameters, these questions can be answered easily.

Another example of easier interpretation comes from the credible intervals produced in Bayesian analysis. One can recall from their introductory statistics class the ubiquitous warning about the confidence level not being the probability that a parameter falls within the interval, but rather, the confidence level is the probability that the method used to create the confidence interval will capture the true value of the parameter of interest. Credible intervals are considerably easier to interpret; the probability of a parameter falling in a 95% credible interval is 95%.

Probabilistic evidence for the reform payment demonstration example using Equation 12.11 is shown in Figure 12.6. The graph depicts (1) the probability (in medium blue) that the intervention is associated with average savings ($\gamma < 0$), (2) the probability (in light blue) of average savings in excess of \$50 per patient

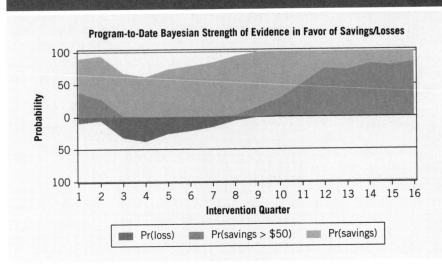

Figure 12.6   Program-to-Date Bayesian Strength of Evidence in Favor of Savings/Losses

Program-to-Date Bayesian Strength of Evidence in Favor of Savings/Losses

Intervention Quarter

■ Pr(loss)   ■ Pr(savings > $50)   ■ Pr(savings)

($\gamma < -50$), and (3) the probability (in dark blue) of an average loss or increase in costs per patient ($\gamma > 0$). At early assessment points, there is still quite a bit of uncertainty about whether the intervention increases or decreases health care costs: using four quarters of postintervention data reveals the probabilities of savings and losses at around 60% and 40%, respectively. However, as additional quarters of postintervention data are used in estimation, the probability of savings rapidly approaches 1 (at the same time, of course, the probability of losses goes to zero). Three years or more after the start of the intervention (postintervention Quarters 12 through 16), there is also strong evidence that the savings were in excess of $50 per patient, with the probability of this hovering around 75%–80%.

Potential Advantages of Including a Bayesian Approach in an Evaluation

A Bayesian analysis can be a useful complement to most program evaluations, because it allows evaluators to make probabilistic statements about program effectiveness—rather than having to rely only on repeated sampling arguments and classical hypothesis tests. Bayesian inference can estimate the probability that the program has a positive effect, or that it has an effect of a certain magnitude. Such probabilities factor prominently into risk calculations for decision making. A related advantage is that a Bayesian model lends itself naturally to making predictive statements, which are important to understanding the likely impact of scaling or modifying the program.

Another potential advantage of Bayesian analysis is estimation stability. In complicated models, classical maximum likelihood estimation can be numerically difficult. Bayesian computation does not require maximization, and thereby avoids these difficulties.

Bayesian models can readily incorporate information into the model from other data sources, both internal and external to the program. The prior distribution provides the mechanism for doing so. Moreover, information or assumptions can be incorporated into the statistical model with varying degrees of confidence, rather than having to make binary, true/false choices.

In the context of hierarchical models, a Bayesian analysis allows for the "borrowing of strength" and can yield "shrinkage" estimators. Suppose a sample of observations from a program is available that can be divided into a number of groups. An evaluator may be interested in both group-specific effects as well as overall program effects. The Bayesian framework allows for information to flow up from the group-level inferences to the overall parameters. Additionally, since the overall and group-specific parameters are being estimated simultaneously, the updates to the overall parameters flow down to the various group-parameters. Thus as in classical models, Bayesian estimation utilizes the borrowing of information across groups, which is often referred to as borrowing strength. Furthermore, in the hierarchical context, Bayesian analyses can yield shrinkage estimators. When a particular group is small, its group-level effect estimate is pulled (shrunk) toward the overall grand mean (borrowed strength), whereas when a particular group is large, it will exhibit less shrinkage (less borrowed strength).

Challenges of Including a Bayesian Approach in an Evaluation

As in traditional statistical modelling, Bayesian analyses require careful thought about the model. An incorrectly specified model may have poorly identified parameters or parameters that are not identified at all. The textbook example of this situation is (near) multicollinearity in a set of explanatory variables in a linear model. Goodness-of-fit tests, information criterion (statistics of parsimony), and model diagnostics are available and should be used along with the expertise of the evaluator to find the best model for the evaluation.

In addition to the likelihood function, the choice of prior for a Bayesian model needs to be considered carefully. In the absence of strong prior information about θ, default vague priors are often used in practice. Examples are distributions that are (locally) uniform, such as a normal distribution with a large variance. However, in certain situations, seemingly vague priors can strongly affect the shape of the posterior and the resulting Bayesian inferences. This likely arises because of two reasons. First, this may be a symptom of the likelihood being misspecified, which we discussed above. Second, the sample size may be too small to reliably inform us about θ. In this case, the prior distribution will dominate the likelihood function and different prior choices are likely to have a large effect on the posterior.

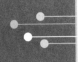

Box 12.3
When to Use a Bayesian Analysis

Bayesian inference presents an entirely different paradigm for thinking about data and statistical modeling. In some cases, Bayesian and classical inference yield similar answers. However, in the following contexts, a Bayesian approach may have added value to an evaluation.

- Bayesian analyses can be used in situations when little data is available.

- When data are accumulating over time, Bayesian estimation does not require corrections (such as a Bonferroni correction) for repeated testing.

- Bayesian estimation yields probabilistic inference, which in some cases is more informative than results from classical hypothesis tests.

- Bayesian estimation allows for the borrowing of strength and shrinkage, which are considered middle ground between fixed effects and random effects hierarchical models.

- In a Bayesian analysis, it is straightforward to generate predictions and an associated measure of uncertainty.

In evaluations based on small samples, a careful and defensible choice of prior is critical. However, if a "good" prior can be found, Bayesian analysis can be implemented with very little data, which is a huge benefit over classical analyses which overwhelmingly rely on asymptotic theory. In large-scale evaluations (for example those based on analyzing large medical claims databases), in contrast, the data and the likelihood function will dominate the information contained in the prior, and the resulting posterior distribution will be robust to the choice of prior.

SUMMARY

During the course of an evaluation, administrators and funders face a number of options for making programmatic changes: (1) discontinuing the program if there is clear evidence it is not reaching its intended goals; (2) continuing to monitor the program in its current form; (3) implementing changes to improve quality and enhance program effectiveness; and (4) scaling up the program to other organizations, settings, and target populations if there is clear evidence of effectiveness. With RCE, the data on which these decisions are based are collected and analyzed on a quarterly basis. In this chapter, we presented three ways in which the wealth of information afforded by quarterly impact data can be used in an optimal way. SPC and regression cannot only be used to analyze frequently collected data, but also have corresponding graphs that assist decision makers in visualizing and intuiting the analyses. Regression models can be estimated using classical or Bayesian techniques; sometimes one estimation strategy, such as when prior information is available, may be more favorable to the other. The methods introduced in this chapter, SPC, classical regression, and Bayesian regression, are flexible tools that can accommodate data collected on a rolling basis, provide clear estimates of program effects, and whose outputs can be visualized and understood in a clear way.

DISCUSSION QUESTIONS

1. What are some of the disadvantages of using Bayesian as opposed to classical techniques?

2. When might SPC be a good method to use?

3. Are these methods applied differently because of the RCE context?

NOTES

1. Walter Shewhart, *The Economic Control of Quality of Manufactured Product*, 1931 (Milwaukee, WI: reprinted by ASQC, 1980).

2. "Shewhart references Tchebycheff's inequality to put probability bounds on the limits. Tchebycheff's inequality can be used to show that the probability for making a mistake of identifying a special cause for a stable process . . . each time the three-sigma limits are used, regardless of the distribution of the data, is less than 11%." Provost, L. P. and S. K. Murray, *The Healthcare Data Guide: Learning From Data for Improvement* (San Francisco: Jossey-Bass, 2011), 115.

3. For more methodological specifics, see Provost, L. and S. Murray, *The Healthcare Data Guide: Learning from Data for Improvement* (San Francisco: Jossey-Bass, 2011). Software is also available to create these charts, notably Chartrunner. We turn now to an example of SPC in a health care delivery setting.

4. Shewhart W. A, *Statistical Methods from the Viewpoint of Quality Control* (Washington, DC: Graduate School, Department of Agriculture, 1939).

5. Brock, J. et al. "Association Between Quality Improvement for Care Transitions in Communities and Rehospitalizations Among Medicare Beneficiaries," *JAMA* 309 no. 4. (2013): 381–91.

6. Wheeler D. J., and D. S. Chambers. *Understanding Statistical Process Control* (2nd ed.). (Knoxville, TN: SPC Press Inc., 1992).

7. Chou R., L. H. Huffman, R. Fu, A. K. Smits, and P. T. Korthuis, "Screening for HIV: A Review of the Evidence for the U.S. Preventive Services Task Force." *Annals of Internal Medicine* 143 (2005): 55–73. doi:10.7326/0003-4819-143-1-200507050-00010

8. Centers for Disease Control and Prevention (CDC). "Prevalence of Diagnosed and Undiagnosed HIV Infection—United States, 2008–2012." *MMWR. Morbidity and Mortality Weekly Reports* (2015, June 26).

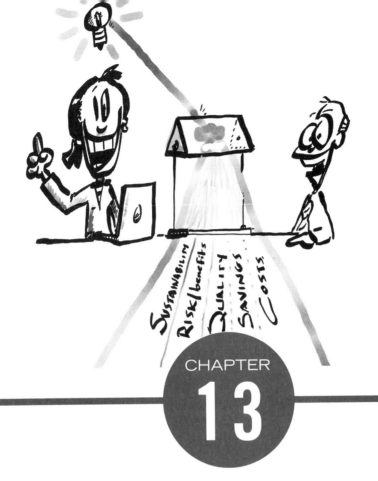

Synthesizing Evaluation Findings

Anupa Bir

Kevin Smith

Jim Derzon

Martijn van Hasselt

Nikki Freeman

Learning Objectives

This chapter proposes an extension of meta-analysis to help policymakers to understand the vast array of information available as a result of evaluation research. This may require a culture shift in the way analysts present findings, rather than any particular methodological innovation. Meta-analysis offers some distinct advantages to those in policy-making positions including standardized outcomes across studies, the ability to understand the strength of findings from different studies, and a way to navigate the age old challenge of what to do when three studies find positive, negative, and null effects of the same intervention.

Finally, as a result of these efforts to standardize outcomes and some inputs, Centers for Medicare and Medicaid Innovation has begun to explore meta-analysis of outcomes across evaluations. These meta-analytic efforts do more than explain variation in outcomes, as they can also synthesize implementation data and build on a careful and systematic categorization of intervention components. The results from these efforts can be presented using an interactive dashboard, which allows policymakers to get a sense of the data and find the aspects of the results that are most germane to the questions they need to answer.

The ultimate objective of the array of program/intervention evaluation methods discussed in this book is to inform the policy process. This can only happen, of course, if the evaluation findings that are presented to policymakers answer the policy question of most interest in a way they trust. Trust requires knowing enough about the methods used to balance the implications of the findings with the caveats attached. Use in policymaking requires that the findings can indeed answer the questions at hand. If those questions cannot be answered with the analytically most appropriate or most rigorous findings, the findings may not get used appropriately. But policy decision making must, and will, proceed.

The advances made in illustrating the probability of savings over time in response to an intervention, as demonstrated in Chapter 12, allow a clear and uniform understanding of the likelihood of positive, neutral, or negative results. With consistent measures and approaches, these data displays serve a real purpose for the policy process. They show the results from the application of rigorous methods without constraining policy decisions, allowing policymakers to bring their own risk tolerance or other information to bear in the decision making.

Meta-analysis is helpful in clarifying the overall results of a large number of studies, instead of leaving policymakers to decide which of conflicting study results to believe. Bayesian analysis and inclusion of priors also incorporates additional evidence from earlier studies. Examining the strength of evidence for different policy questions, or building on the existing literature using meta-analytic methods, is not new. This general approach of understanding the connection between current work to the related studies that came before is a foundational element of research.

Although meta-analytic methods are used frequently to synthesize what is known and how reliable this knowledge is for policy purposes, there have been recent developments in this facet of policy research. CMMI has funded several studies which purpose is to look across prior evaluations to seek new information that individual evaluations may not provide. These efforts have led to the development of tools and techniques that go beyond traditional meta-analysis, allowing a broader understanding of the features that relate to larger and smaller intervention impacts. Three studies of this nature are currently under way. One of the studies examines more than 100 awardees funded through the Health Care Innovation Awards (HCIA). The HCIA awardees are implementing a variety of innovations that test payment models and service delivery models. Throughout our discussion, we will use this application and extension of meta-analysis as an example, however the ideas presented here apply broadly. This chapter describes the tools developed for applying meta-analytic techniques to evaluation findings, demonstrating how they can analyze and synthesize lessons across numerous programs in a way that is maximally useful for policy. A resource for more information on traditional meta-analytic methods is *Practical Meta-Analysis* by Mark Lipsey.

Meta-analysis

Meta-analysis uses quantitative findings across a number of studies, or in our case, evaluation findings, along with the codification of program components. It begins with transforming the summary evidence from a study, the result(s), to a common metric known as an effect size. By extracting evidence from multiple studies and placing the results on a common scale, meta-analysis produces a best estimate of the true relationship being estimated. Furthermore, meta-analytic techniques can be used to analyze the differences between studies, quantify the inconsistency of results between them, and evaluate which program or program components have the biggest impact on outcomes. Pooling results from multiple studies through meta-analysis improves the power to detect a true effect, particularly when the body of evidence is characterized by small or underpowered studies.

One limitation of meta-analysis is that it is only as good as the data that go into it—the inputs are drawn from reported study findings rather than actual study data, and those data may not accurately reflect actual study procedures or the full study findings. Many studies are never published; if, as has been claimed, journals bias their study selection toward those with statistically significant findings, the selection of study findings available for review may introduce bias. Furthermore, published descriptions of the intervention are often limited, with typically no information about the services members of the counterfactual comparison group may have received. Lastly, meta-analysis is based on a nonexperimental model of variation in study findings, limiting findings to observed associations and leaving questions about causal influence unanswered.

In the context of extending the meta-analysis approach to synthesize findings from CMMI programs, the inputs are evaluation findings rather than studies. The evaluation findings are of known quality, use published methods for determining causality, and share a number of intervention components, implementation processes, and outcomes. Furthermore, they enable the categorization and coding of the research design used in an individual program, which can be of great help in identifying whether or not the research design itself had an impact on the program's findings. Meta-analysis extended in this way takes advantage of natural variation to get inside the so-called black box of the actual intervention. To the extent that inputs and outcomes are commonly defined across studies, these approaches can provide powerful new understanding.

Meta-evaluation Development for Health Care Demonstrations

The development of meta-analytic techniques has ushered in the application of methodological techniques in novel ways. We highlight three areas of note in which innovation has taken place and together provide the foundation to our application of meta-evaluation to health care demonstrations:

1. The careful and systematic descriptions of interventions that can incorporate qualitative data

2. The standardization of outcome variables and analytic approaches

3. The use of interactive data dashboards to investigate factors related to impact

4. The use of Bayesian methods to translate findings to more easily interpreted probabilities

We describe the first two developments here and save our discussion of the data dashboard for later in this and subsequent chapters.

Features of each awardee's innovations were systematically collected and coded to identify innovation components and implementation characteristics. We call this "structured coding" to distinguish it from coding that characterizes traditional qualitative research, which seeks to identify "themes" across awardee reports. Structured coding begins with well-defined, predetermined uniform data elements and an associated coding scheme that a trained team of coders applies to each innovation to result in a standardized dataset that characterizes each innovation's target population (children, adults, elderly, etc.), setting (ambulatory, postacute, long-term care facility, etc.), and components (use of health information technology, provision of care coordination, use of community health workers, etc.). Data for the structured coding came from evaluators' reports as well as

Figure 13.1 How Well Did Awardees Execute Their Plan?

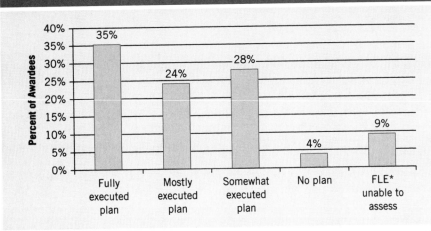

Note: **Stands for** *frontline evaluator,* or those who calculate the treatment effects that are used in the meta-analysis.

annual awardee surveys completed by the evaluation site-visit teams. Collecting data in this well-planned, theory-driven way, enables data collected on a large scale, such as for the 108 diverse HCIA awardees, to be organized, summarized, and compared. Figure 13.1[1] displays the implementation characteristics of the interventions from the awardee summary forms.

The standardization of outcome variables and analytic approaches is an advantage in the application of meta-analysis to evaluation. For example, CMMI has set priority evaluation outcome measures, such as the "core four": total cost of care, hospitalizations, hospital readmissions, and emergency department use. This is important because by prioritizing these outcomes, not only are the primary evaluations guided toward these measures, but their availability across all studies enables those outcomes to be meta-analyzed. When it is possible, coordination and cooperation between the evaluator and meta-evaluator can ease the process of outcome standardization.

Once qualitative and quantitative data are collected, standard meta-analysis techniques may be implemented. By using the program features identified through intervention component coding, subgroup analyses can be done; for example, programs taking place in an ambulatory setting may be analyzed separately from those taking place in a postacute care setting, or programs targeting children may be analyzed separately from those targeting elder adults. Additionally, the heterogeneity, or dissimilarities, between programs can be quantified using measures such as I^2 and the Q test statistic. I^2 quantifies the percentage of variation attributable to study heterogeneity, and the Q test provides a formal statistical test for the presence of heterogeneity. Although these statistics are important in quantifying the amount of heterogeneity present or not present between programs, they do not explain which program characteristics are associated with better or worse outcomes. Meta-regression, which we discuss next, relates qualitative program characteristics with program outcomes, highlighting which features correlate with better outcomes.

Meta-regression Analysis

Meta-regression is a technique for explaining heterogeneity among programs when it has been determined that the overall program effects are not homogeneous (i.e., the variation between programs is greater than would be expected from sampling error). The regression model may be based on either a fixed or a random effects approach.[2]

Fixed-effects meta-analysis assumes that all samples contributing to the analysis share a common population parameter and that the only differences among program estimates are attributable to sampling error. In fixed-effects modeling, the outcomes of each program are weighted by their inverse variance and pooled, and an overall grand mean is calculated. Standard errors and confidence intervals are produced so as to provide the degree of confidence in the weighted mean level of portfolio performance. Two forms of mean deviation exist: the first arising from sampling error that occurs within sampling units (called within-sample variance), and the second for design/implementation differences that "move the observed performance" away from the true underlying mean level of intervention success (called between-sample variance).

Random effects modeling, in contrast, assumes that each sample is drawn from its own distribution (i.e., there is no common parameter underlying the different program estimates). Random effect models estimate this random component and then reweight the inverse variance estimates so that programs are more equally weighted. That is, mean performance of smaller programs is given greater weight than when using the fixed effects approach. The reason for this is that, as independent "windows" on intervention performance, they bring added information to the policy decision beyond their meager size. As with fixed effects, overall awardee performance is calculated as the grand mean but with the revised inverse weights. The weighting method has two implications relative to the fixed effects method. First, because the estimates are more equally weighted, random effects confidence intervals tend to be wider than confidence intervals calculated using fixed effects. This generally means that findings based on random effects are more conservative (i.e., less likely to reach statistical significance) than those obtained using fixed effects. The second implication is that, because random effects do not assume homogeneity of effect, results from random effects models are more likely to generalize beyond the program sample.

It is important to recognize that much of the variation in program effect sizes can be due to factors other than the intervention itself. Lipsey, for example, conducted a variance components analysis of effect sizes from more than 300 juvenile justice programs.[3] He found that only approximately 25% of the overall variation was attributable to characteristics of the intervention, another 21% was contributed by features of the methods used to conduct the analysis, and the remaining variation was due to either sampling error or residual sources. Thus, meta-regression approaches generally used forced entry regression, isolating methods effects before estimating substantive program effects. A core goal of the meta-evaluation efforts has been to compare the effectiveness of different interventions, *while controlling for the confounding factors*. This is possible with well-specified meta-regression models.[4]

For methodologically interested readers, Box 13.1 includes the details of meta-regression model specification and estimation. Other readers are encouraged to skip Box 13.1.

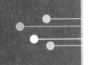

Box 13.1
Meta-regression Estimation

Meta-regression can be estimated based on the following general equation that explicitly accounts for heterogeneity across awardees:

$$Y_i = \alpha + \Sigma_j \beta_j X_{ji} + \Sigma_k \lambda_k Z_{ki} + \mu_i + \varepsilon_i \qquad (13.1)$$

where

- Y_i is the outcome variable for the *i*-th program,

- α is an average baseline level of performance (depends on how X and Z are measured),

- X_{ji} is a set of j characteristics of the *i*-th program (e.g., duration in quarters),

- Z_{ki} is a set of k features of the research design of the *i*-th program (e.g., pre/post),

- μ_i is unexplained (unobserved) variation in the *i*-th program from "true" program effect, and

- ε_i is residual sampling error in the *i*-th program.

The vector of X characteristics adjusts for differences in the way the program was implemented across awardees, including type of treatment, intensity or duration, and who participated.[5] For example, the HCIA awardee participants likely will be exposed to the intervention for varying numbers of months. The β coefficient for duration of intervention will adjust the predicted outcome up or down,

(Continued)

(Continued)

depending on the duration of exposure. Ideally, we would also have information by awardee on the frequency of intervention contacts to further adjust for variation in intensity of treatment.

The vector of Z features is used to adjust for systematic effects of study design. These features can include evaluation design type (e.g., randomized trial or not, pre-/post- versus difference-in-difference), comparison group selection and matching, study sample size, and quality of data sources.

This leaves potentially two error variance terms in the model: one (ε_i) is the usual result of the samples chosen for study (which could have been different at another time), and another (μ_i) is the result of failing to capture in X and Z all other reasons why awardee performance differs in a systematic way. The ε_i error is called the within-study (i.e., awardee) variation, while μ_i represents between-study variation. Without adjusting for X and Z, the between-study variation is likely to be large given the heterogeneous collection of awardees. After adjusting for X and Z in the meta-regression, the expectation is that the residual between-study variation is trivial, and only random sampling error remains with an expected value of zero with unbiased coefficients.

If we assume that between-study variation is reduced to a minimum, and expected error is zero, then the expected mean intervention outcome for the i-th awardee is

$$Y* = \alpha + \Sigma_j \beta_j X_{ji} * + \Sigma_k \lambda_k Z_{ki} * \qquad (13.2)$$

where * equals mean values averaged across awardees. Suppose the outcome variable is cost savings per beneficiary, and the estimated equation is

$$y_i = 10 + 3 \cdot \text{Duration}_i - 15 \cdot \text{PS}_i \qquad (13.3)$$

where duration equals the number of quarters the intervention was evaluated on, and PS equals 1 if propensity score weighting of comparison beneficiaries was used to derive cost savings, and it equals 0 otherwise. For an awardee evaluated over six quarters with propensity score weighting, the expected cost savings are $13 ($10 + $18 – $15) per beneficiary-quarter. If another awardee's intervention ran 12 quarters, but without propensity weighting, its predicted cost is $46 ($10 + $36 – $0). An overall portfolio estimate of cost savings is derived by inserting portfolio mean values for X and Z. If the mean duration is 10 quarters, and 50% of awardees used in the meta-regression were propensity score weighted, then the overall average cost savings is $32.50 ($10 + $30 – .5 x $15).

Equation 13.2, when estimated, also is of value if some of the X and Z coefficients are statistically significant. For example, the duration coefficient informs policymakers as to the sensitivity of performance to how long the intervention is run, and patients are exposed. However, it must be remembered that, like all studies, the results of a meta-analysis are only as good as the data contributing to the analysis. If the mix of awardees included in the analysis is not representative of the mix of the eventual target population, the means of X and Z variables may not generalize.[6]

Random effects, sometimes referred to as multilevel or hierarchical linear modeling, explicitly recognize the heterogeneity of studies by proposing a two-stage estimation process. This method is particularly relevant to CMMI as it addresses the heterogeneity present in many quality improvement initiatives. Ignoring the problem of heterogeneity, that is considering Equation 13.2 without X and Z, regression estimates could be found using weighted generalized least squares (GLS) methods. Operationally, this involves multiplying both left- and right-hand sides of Equation 13.2 by $(1/\sigma_i)$, thereby factoring out any heteroskedastic differences in within-awardee sample variance due to varying sample sizes. Although it is known that heteroscedasticity does not produce inconsistent estimates of intervention effects, at least for larger samples, the estimated coefficients are inefficient with confidence intervals that are too wide. GLS methods put all observations on a "standard variance" basis that makes the estimates more reliable. This approach is insufficient, however, when dealing with heterogeneity.

There are two approaches to adjusting for heterogeneity. It is standard in meta-analysis to use a non-regression method of moments approach with formulas for calculating τ^2 or between-study variance. The alternative approach applies random effects regression in estimating the Equation 13.2 parameters. Our approach first addresses awardee heterogeneity directly by the inclusion of X and Z variables. This approach could adjust completely for heterogeneity simply by using inverse-variance weights because intervention and methodological features are "fixed" by X and Z at the awardee level. In this case, any residual μ_i becomes trivial and can be ignored. Unfortunately, the researcher does not know ex ante whether the proxies used for sample and design features have controlled enough for cross-study differences, hence, the use of random effects estimation.

Assuming residual heterogeneity in Equation 13.2, even after including X and Z, what is required to efficiently estimate Equation 13.2 is to weight by $(1/\text{sqrt}\{\sigma_i^2 + \sigma_\mu^2\})$, or both the sampling variation (σ_i^2) and the residual between-awardee variation (σ_μ^2) that may remain even after controlling for X and Z. This weight reduces equation standard errors for two kinds of residual errors. But because we do not know how large σ_μ^2 is until Equation 13.2 is estimated, a two-step approach is required. In the first step, the GLS method is used using the simple inverse-variance weights. Then an estimate of σ_μ^2 is derived and used in a second-round estimation of the same equation, but using the $(1/\text{sqrt}\{\sigma_i^2 + \sigma_\mu^2\})$ weight.

Bayesian Meta-analysis

In Chapter 12, we discussed the Bayesian framework for analysis and its application to rapid-cycle evaluation. Bayesian analysis can also be used in meta-analysis. As in all Bayesian analyses, Bayesian meta-analysis incorporates beliefs about the effect size and variance parameters *before* observing the data through the prior. Data are introduced into the model through the likelihood function, and the prior and likelihood functions together yield the posterior distribution. The posterior reflects parameter uncertainty that remains after observing the data from the programs included in the analysis.

The advantages and challenges associated with a Bayesian approach to statistical inference were discussed in detail in Chapter 12. In this section, we highlight a few potential advantages that are particularly relevant for meta-analysis.

Because the posterior is approximated using Markov chain Monte Carlo (MCMC) techniques, complex data relationships can be modeled with relative ease. This is important because the data included in a meta-analysis may come from a variety of sources with complicated data structures. In the CMMI meta-evaluations, clustering, multilevel (hierarchical) relationships, and correlated data have been encountered. Although the inherent difficulty of dealing with these is not assuaged by Bayesian meta-regression, the burden of estimation can be reduced. Additionally, data models utilizing a nonnormal distribution, such as the t-distribution or mixture distributions, can also be readily estimated using Bayesian computation.

In our discussion of classical meta-regression, we elucidated key differences between fixed effects and random effects models. We highlight a few advantages of estimating a meta-regression model using Bayesian techniques. First, classical random effects meta-analysis relies on point estimates that feed into different stages of the analysis, which implicitly assumes that these estimates accurately represent the real impact and are not subject to any uncertainty. In contrast, the Bayesian approach does not rely on single point estimates. Instead, it uses prior probability distributions that express the range and likelihood of various parameters and thus fully captures the uncertainty associated with each of the model parameters. As such, a Bayesian meta-analysis properly propagates uncertainty about unknown parameters throughout the entire random effects model.[7,8] Furthermore, it is relatively straightforward to incorporate additional layers of uncertainty into a Bayesian model. Thus, it is useful if the programs on which a meta-analysis is based vary in evaluation design. A three-level Bayesian random-effects model can then be specified that accounts for uncertainty due to (1) within-program variation, (2) between-program variation, and (3) between-program variation in design.[9]

Finally, a Bayesian meta-analysis naturally lends itself to making predictive statements. The posterior distribution and the likelihood function can be combined to calculate a (posterior) predictive distribution for the effect size in a future program. Such distributions provide information about the potential impacts of future programs and can be used to inform decisions about replicating or scaling up programs in different settings.

Putting It Together

Extending meta-evaluation is pioneering work that combines not only evaluation findings across programs, but also combines qualitative and quantitative findings to characterize entire portfolios of programs. It can answer who's doing what, when, and at what level on an unprecedented scale. By aggregating the answers to these questions, decision makers can find the common themes among successful programs, compare implementation effectiveness, and identify key components in health care innovation. They can also tease out whether observed effects are real or due to evaluation design.

Although meta-evaluation is a powerful tool that provides a plethora of information, the presentation of this information to policymakers is a serious challenge. In meeting this challenge, for the HCIA meta-evaluation, we have developed a data dashboard to organize and disseminate meta-evaluation findings in a timely manner; the data dashboard is the third major development resulting from applying meta-analysis to evaluation and completes our previous meta-analysis development discussion. For the HCIA meta-evaluation, a database has been developed that includes characteristics for each HCIA

Figure 13.2   HCIA Dashboard: Forest Plots of Intervention Impacts on Total Costs of Care

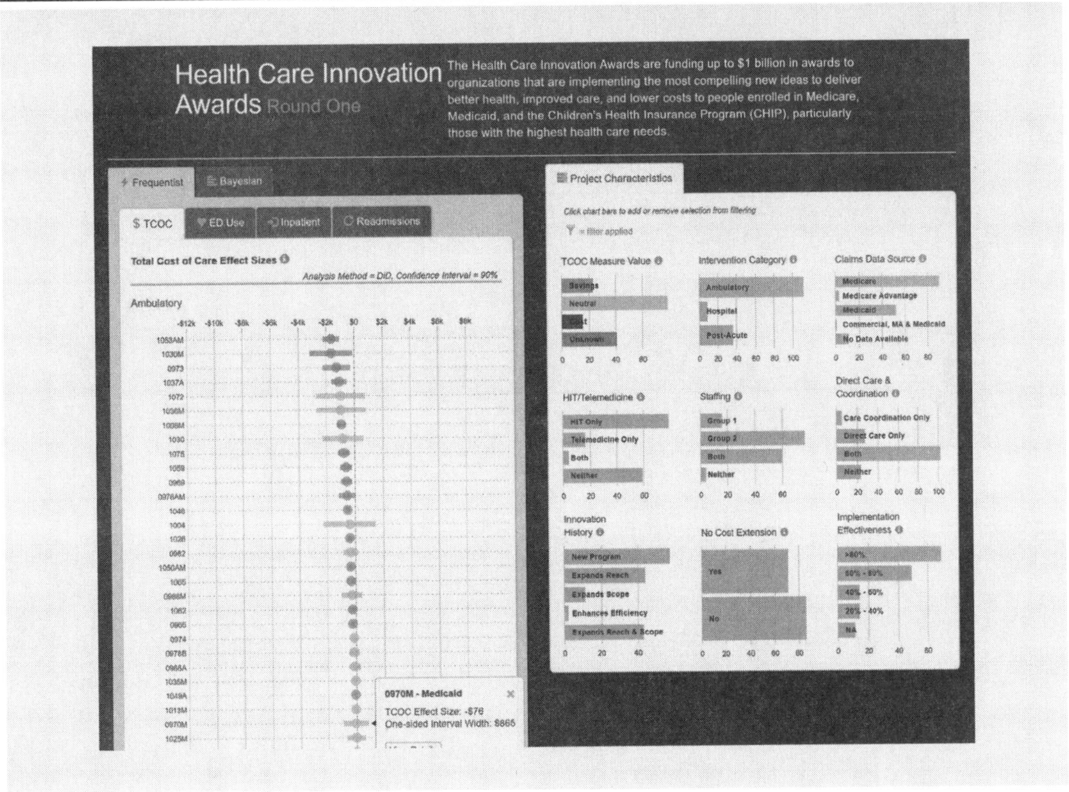

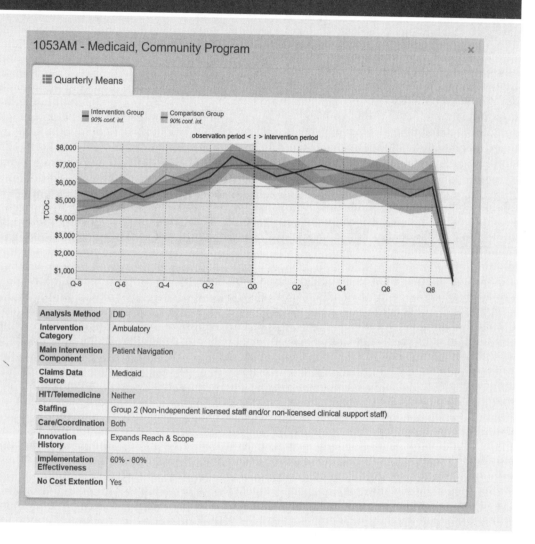

awardee. The database is presented as a data dashboard that allows others to
understand HCIA's clustering of implementation features and outcomes, and
to examine subgroups instantaneously through the use of interactive features
and filters (see Figures 13.2–13.5 and http://hciameta.rtidatascience.org/).
The characteristics displayed come from multiple data sources, including

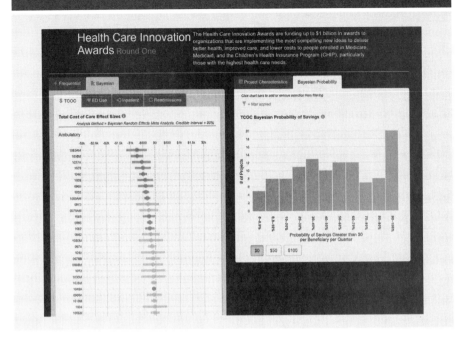

Figure 13.4 HCIA Dashboard: Forest Plots of Intervention Impacts on Total Costs of Care (Bayesian Probabilities)

coded qualitative data, awardee monitoring data, annual awardee summary forms, and quantitative outcomes based on claims analysis for intervention and comparison groups. As additional data are gathered throughout the life of the evaluation, the dashboard, linked directly to the database, can be updated to reflect the most recently available information. As a Web-based tool, the dashboard is a convenient and immediate way to display new data as they become available.

For policymakers, the dashboard allows policymakers to select the characteristics by which to sort and visually compare awardees, empowering them to explore answers to their own questions as they arise without the need for programming and statistical expertise. It also provides a way for them to manage data from a vast number of sources; rather than keep track of volumes of technical reports from a myriad of evaluators and sources, meta-evaluation and the dashboard create a sleek, unified, and responsive tool to quickly examine evaluation findings. Furthermore, it provides decision makers timely information about which characteristics are associated with promising outcomes and may inform decisions about which programs should be scaled up or modified.

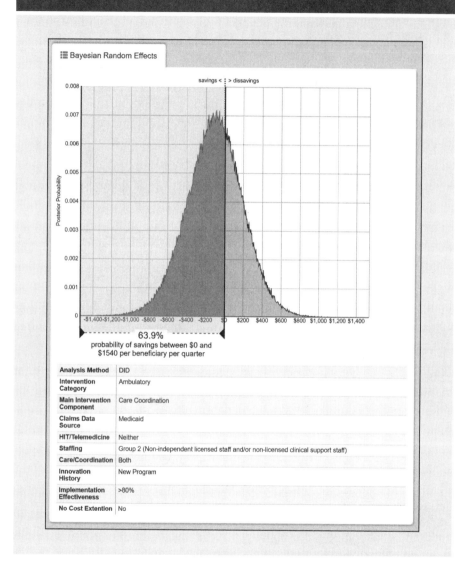

Analysis Method	DID
Intervention Category	Ambulatory
Main Intervention Component	Care Coordination
Claims Data Source	Medicaid
HIT/Telemedicine	Neither
Staffing	Group 2 (Non-independent licensed staff and/or non-licensed clinical support staff)
Care/Coordination	Both
Innovation History	New Program
Implementation Effectiveness	>80%
No Cost Extention	No

SUMMARY

Meta-evaluation is a potent methodology that can enhance the statistical power to detect effects among programs. Its implementation has affected change in how information is collected and brought together qualitative and quantitative data to fully describe programs across vast portfolios. Standard meta-analysis techniques can quantify the heterogeneity among programs. Meta-regression can provide explanatory power and help explain heterogeneity by relating program features and components to outcomes. Meta-evaluation can be done via a classical or Bayesian framework. Through innovative delivery systems such as the data dashboard, synthesized information can be accessed by policymakers with ease and readily updated quarterly in the RCE framework.

DISCUSSION QUESTIONS

1. How can meta-analysis account for the possibility of biased data? Is there an advantage to meta-analysis relative to individual evaluations in this regard?

2. What information can meta-analysis provide policymakers that is not otherwise available or accessible?

3. Are there additional qualitative, contextual elements that could be included in these HCIA analyses?

NOTES

1. This type of form can be used to support qualitative comparative analysis (QCA), which was discussed in Chapter 9.

2. Hedges, L. V., and T. D. Pigott, "The Power of Statistical Tests for Moderators in Meta-Analysis," *Psychological Methods* 9 no. 4 (2004): 426–45. https://doi.org/10.1037/1082-989X.9.4.426. The authors outline a series of tests to determine the statistical power of moderators in both fixed and random effects models. They also outline how to assess the goodness of fit associated with these models. See also Wooldridge, Jeffrey M. 2002. *Econometric Analysis of Cross Section and Panel Data* (Cambridge, MA: MIT Press, 2002).

3. Lipsey, M. W., "The Primary Factors that Characterize Effective Interventions with Juvenile Offenders: A Meta-Analytic Overview," *Victims and Offenders* 4 (2009): 124–47. doi:10.1080/15564880802612573.

4. If sample sizes are very different and estimates not very precise, then it is possible to run a weighted least squares regression using t-values as the left-hand side variable. This method has several advantages in terms of dealing with heteroscedasticity of effects (Stanley, T. D., and Stephen B. Jarrell, "Meta-Regression Analysis: A Quantitative Method of Literature Surveys." *Journal of Economic Surveys* 19 no. 3 (2005, July): 299–308. However, the size of the estimator is not easily interpretable. Becker and Wu write that t-values do not necessarily correspond with "estimators of effect magnitude." See, Becker, Betsy Jane, and Meng-Jia Wu. "The Synthesis

of Regression Slopes in Meta-Analysis." *Statistical Science* 22 no. 3 (2007): 414–29. doi: 10.1214/07-STS243. http://projecteuclid. org/euclid.ss/1199285041.

5. Lipsey, M., and D.Wilson, *Practical Meta-analysis* (Thousand Oaks, CA: Sage, 2001).

6. Rhodes, William, "Meta-Analysis: An Introduction Using Regression Models," *Evaluation Review* 36 (2012): 24–71. doi: 10.1177/0193841X12442673.

7. Higgins, Julian, Simon G. Thompson, and David J. Spiegelhalter. "A Re-evaluation of Random-effects Meta-analysis." *Journal of the Royal Statistical Society: Series A (Statistics in Society)* 172, no. 1 (2009): 137–59.

8. Sutton, Alex J., and Keith R. Abrams, "Bayesian Methods in Meta-analysis and Evidence Synthesis," *Statistical Methods in Medical Research* 10, no. 4 (2001): 277–303.

9. This is useful when modeling binary outcomes—see, Thompson, S. E., Bayesian Model Averaging and Spatial Prediction. PhD thesis, Colorado State University, 2001; Warn D. E., S. G. Thompson, D. J. Spiegelhalter, "Bayesian Random Effects Meta-Analysis of Trials with Binary Outcomes: Methods for the Absolute Risk Difference and Relative Risk Scales," *Statistics in Medicine* 21 (2002):1601–23—or when a normality assumption for effect sizes is unreasonable, for example, to describe between-study variation with a very small number of studies. Burr D., and H. A. Doss, "Bayesian Semiparametric Model for Random-effects Meta-analysis." *Journal of the American Statistical Association* 100 (2005): 242–51; Prevost T. C., K. R. Abrams, and D. R. Jones, "Hierarchical Models in Generalized Synthesis of Evidence: An Example Based on Studies of Breast Cancer Screening." *Statistics in Medicine* 9 (2000): 3359–76. doi: 10.1002/1097-0258(20001230)19:24<3359:: AID-SIM710>3.0.CO;2-N.

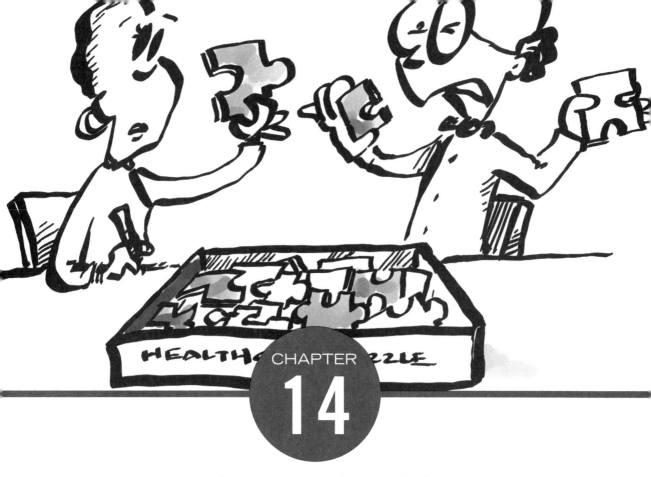

14

Decision Making Using Evaluation Results

Steven Sheingold

Learning Objectives

The previous 13 chapters have described the context and methods for producing rigorous evaluations and a variety of ways to present the results to
make them useful for decision makers. The key objective for these efforts is to
provide better information for decision making about programs and policies.

(Continued)

It is important to understand, however, that many important program and policy decisions will not solely be determined by evaluation results. Whether in the public or private arenas, making important decisions can be a complex and multifaceted process. While results from high-quality evaluations are critical to making good decisions, other factors also play key roles and must be integrated with evaluation results. Adding to decision-making complexity is that program and policy decisions are seldom binary; there are typically multiple courses of action that might be chosen by decision makers. These factors are discussed in the Chapter, with the presentation of a framework for decision making and a recent policy example to which it has been applied.

In the past, there have been obstacles to using evaluation results for policy decision making, including timeliness and relevance and ability to provide adequate quantitative results. To the extent that evaluations can be prospectively planned and integrated with program design and implementation as discussed in this primer, these obstacles can be significantly reduced. Evidence still does not inevitably translate into policy.

For a number of reasons, it is important that researchers and evaluators fully understand the decision-making environments in which their products will be considered. Understanding the decision-making processes will be helpful in terms of developing evaluation methods. It will be especially helpful for researchers in terms of choosing and developing strategies for presenting the results. Finally, knowledge of factors that must be balanced with research evidence can help dampen potential disappointment about how these results are used. In this chapter, we discuss a framework for evidence-based or evidence-informed decision making that describes how evaluation evidence and other important policy factors may interact with each other. In doing so, and in providing a recent example, we provide guidance for researchers/evaluators relevant to making their results most useful for policy and their interactions with policymakers as productive as possible.

Research, Evaluation, and Policymaking

There has been a considerable amount of literature written about whether research and evaluation are distinct from one another, whether they overlap, or whether one is a subset of the other. To the extent that evaluation is heavily weighted toward the impact evaluation—that is, where research is directed toward the impact of a program or policy rather than general knowledge—the overlap would be substantial: "However, in deference to social science research, it must be stressed again that without using social science methods, little evaluation can be done."[1] In terms of understanding the relationship of the two to policy therefore, they can be treated similarly.

As mentioned in Chapter 1, researchers have long hoped that their work could be more relevant to policy but have often been disappointed. This has been particularly true in health services research where there have been notable successes in the past,[2] but in general, there has been disappointment and frustration. Thirty years ago, Marion Ein Lewin wrote:

> In the world of policymaking and politics, the discipline of health services research has often experienced rough sledding. Not as widely acclaimed or well understood as biomedical research, this field, along with many other of the social sciences, has had to struggle for recognition and support.[3]

> Twenty-six years later:

> Of all the ways to influence health policy, using research to inform change has the dual appeal of sounding both straightforward and rigorous. However, reality intrudes in many forms to disrupt the otherwise common-sense connection between what we know, what we consider as policy and what we are doing. Different languages (academic versus political), disparate timeframes (deliberate versus opportunistic), and contrasting priorities (most rigorous versus good enough) often make translating research into policy an exercise in frustration.[4]

Recently, AcademyHealth has stressed the need for researchers to understand policymaking:

> Despite years of study and many efforts in this country and internationally to document the policymaking process, the research community is not always aware of the political, social, and economic contexts in which policymakers view research findings. Translation and dissemination will fail if the content of research findings does not fit the needs of the policy community.[5]

The ACA and subsequent legislation has opened an era in which the link between research, evaluation, and policy can be strengthened. But to be successful in this new environment, researchers and evaluators cannot conduct business as usual. They must increase their understanding of the policy decision-making processes, and how to conduct their research and present findings in ways consistent with these processes. The following sections provide a conceptual model and an example of how evaluation results might be used for a real-world policy issue.

To place the subsequent discussion in the proper context, it is important to note that research can affect policy in different ways. Previous work on evidence-informed policy has provided detail on the types of change related to research and the manner the change was related to the research.[6] Types of change are classified as follows:

- Capacity changes are changes in the knowledge, skills, and/or attitudes of researchers, policymakers, or others involved in the research activity.

- Conceptual changes are changes in the way people conceptualize a given issue including changes in people's general awareness of a given topic.

- Instrumental changes are concrete, specific changes to a policy or program.

The manner in which research has led to that change is classified into the following categories:

- Symbolic use of evidence is when evidence is used to legitimize a decision that had already been made.

- Indirect use of evidence is when research leads to a change in some intermediate variable, which in turn leads to a policy/program change.

- Direct use of evidence is when a specific research finding is applied to change something.[7]

For the remainder of this chapter, the discussion will focus on the direct use of evidence in the decision-making process concerning a specific program or policy. That is, an evidence-informed decision-making framework that is consistent with what has been called the "interactive model" of research utilization in which evidence is "introduced into a complicated process that also encompasses experience, political insight, pressure, social technologies and judgement."[8,9]

Program/Policy Decision Making Using Evidence: A Conceptual Model

Figure 14.1 summarizes the multiple factors that may affect decision making and potential decision points. Decision making may be called for in a variety of situations that reflect different phases of a program or policy. At the initial phases, there is a need for evidence and assessment that informs that best strategies for development and implementation of a policy or program in a way that increases its chances for success. Thus, evidence collected and analyzed is typically from studies and other sources that are as closely related as possible to the

Figure 14.1 Conceptual Framework for Evidence-Informed Decision Making

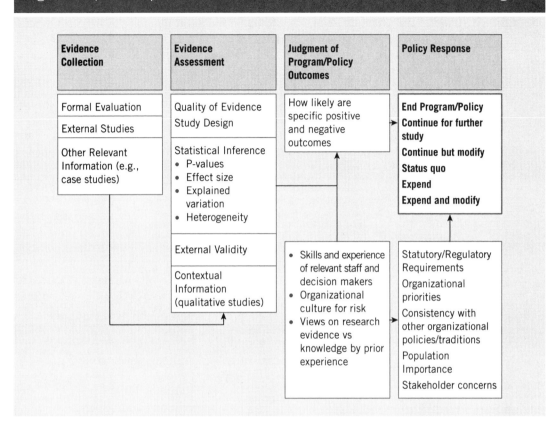

current decision. For purposes of this chapter, we focus on decision making after a program or policy has been in effect for a sufficient period of time to have its own data formally analyzed and evaluated.

The second step on the figure is empirical factors the decision makers might use (often based on reports and briefings from evaluators or information provided by staff) in assessing the evidence. As also indicated on Figure 14.1, a number of factors specific to the decision makers and the organization play a key role in how these factors are assessed, and in what conclusions might be drawn about the outcomes of the policy or program, the level of uncertainty that should be attached to these findings, and the potential specific outcomes that might occur from changing or expanding the program. Making the actual decision among the various options available also takes into account a number of important factors that affect the organization, its policies, and programs. These factors play a role in how the decision is shaped given the evidence assessment that has been made.

Collection of Evidence

The initial phase for any evidence-based policy-making framework is the collection of the evidence. To the extent that a formal evaluation has been conducted for the program or policy in question, particularly if it was prospectively planned and integrated, a significant share of the evidence is conveniently available to decision makers. Nonetheless, evidence-based decision making may be enhanced by assessing all relevant information. For example, an evaluation might focus on a particular Medicare payment model, but evidence on similar efforts by private insurers may be instructive for assessing the results. Assessing evidence from a particular education or training program might better be assessed within the context of evidence from similar programs implemented elsewhere. Likewise, a variety of qualitative and contextual information about organizational and individual behaviors, although not directly related to the model/decision at hand, may provide important information for assessing evaluation results for a decision.

It is important to realize that while we use evidence hierarchies based on the design and quality of studies, valuable evidence for decision making can be any source of information policymakers find useful. Depending on training, experience, and preferences of particular decision makers, information coming from case studies or even anecdotes may help them in assessing the totality of evidence relevant to a particular decision, and how to structure a decision based on that assessment. Indeed, some decision makers may rely on their own experiences for insight into choices before them. Depending on these experiences, some decision makers might give less weight to even high-quality research and evaluation evidence relative to other types of information and even their own intuition.

Assessing the Evidence

As described below, there are a number of aspects of evaluation results that must be assessed and transmitted to decision makers in a way that makes them useful.

Study Design

There is a considerable amount of literature on how to systematically assess the quality of evidence once it is all collected. Systematic reviews are enormously helpful in this regard, although the ability to assess the quality and usefulness of individual studies is critical. In many situations, evidence-based policymaking means examining the strength of evidence that has been generated external to the particular organization, population, or policy area. Essentially, an assessment is made as to the strength of the overall evidence in predicting how likely specific outcomes of implementing a program are to occur, that is, assessment of the internal and external validity of those studies.

When a formal evaluation has been planned and commissioned for a particular program or policy, the questions remain the same, but the assessment activities differ to some degree. Presumably, the best study design possible has been built into the program evaluation. Nonetheless, the evaluation results must be carefully assessed as to the relevance for policy within the context of that study design. That is, how much uncertainty does the design leave regarding potential positive and negative outcomes of the program? Moreover, the design and the results must be assessed within the context of learning about the implementation and operation of the program itself. For example, did the characteristics of program participants differ from those expected? Did participants implement the program interventions as expected? Did the time trajectory of activities and outcomes follow the expected path? Finally, even evaluations designed for a particular program or policy may leave some questions about external validity (i.e, would we achieve the same results by expanding the program to new participants?).

Statistical Inference

Most evaluations will rely totally or heavily on quantitative methods to inform the key questions about the impacts of a program or policy. A combination of data availability, capacity to store and process large quantities of data, and the ability to easily employ an increasing array of sophisticated statistical techniques means that assessing results becomes a complex process for both evaluators and decision makers. Along with the study design, these methods must be assessed with regard to their appropriateness for the task at hand and for the uncertainties left to consider in decision making using the results. In addition, more sophisticated techniques may require greater efforts and more attention paid by evaluators in how to present and explain results to the decision makers. In the next chapter, we provide a discussion of how to communicate research and evaluation results to policymakers.

Factors Other Than
Evidence That Affect Policy Decisions

Once evaluation evidence is available and presented in the best manner possible, decision makers need to assess the information, judge the likelihood of outcomes, and then use that assessment to choose a policy position. A number of factors are likely to influence both how the relevant evidence is accepted and assessed by decision makers and how important that assessment is relative to other policy-making criteria.

Factors That Affect Judgments About Outcomes

Based on the evidence assessment, decision makers will make judgements about the implications for policy: Is there a problem to address, and how large? What are the implications of the findings for how current programs or policies are performing? What do these results tell them about the magnitude of risks associated with the status quo versus alternative courses of action?

Even the highest-quality research leaves uncertainties with regard to these questions. The culture of each organization, as well as the skills, preferences, and experiences of its individual decision makers, are all likely to have a significant effect on how evidence is used and interpreted for decision making. These factors may be influential as decision makers assess the empirical evidence provided by evaluators to draw conclusions about program/policy outcomes. In particular, they will likely influence the weight given to the evaluation evidence vs. decision makers' past experience with similar policies and programs, and anecdotal evidence and interactions with stakeholders in drawing such conclusions.

A critical consideration is that even the best of evaluations leave uncertainties with regard to outcomes. Decision makers need to assess those uncertainties as they are considering the likelihood of certain outcomes flowing from particular decisions. The uncertainties, whether related to a particular measure such as the p-value, or what is explained versus unexplained by the statistical model used, means that other information must be used and filtered through a lens of decision makers' comfort with empirical methods, views on anecdotal evidence, and sensitivity to staff positions on what might occur. Lastly, organizations differ in terms of their attitudes and preference toward risk. That is, the extent to which organizations may be willing to foster experimentation and accept the risk of failure to seek the possibility of significant gains. The same set of evidence might be viewed by one organization as highly likely to produce desirable effects from a particular policy decision, while another might view moving forward as too risky based on that same set of evidence.

Other Important Factors
That Affect the Policy Decisions

Once decision makers have assessed the evidence—that is, made judgments about its quality and likelihood key outcomes would occur, including how much weight is placed on what is known versus unknown from the evidence—these results become part of an often complex decision process. Indeed, the evidence is considered along with a variety of factors that affect organizations' programs and policies. As shown on Figure 14.1, these can include both internal and external influences. Policy and program decisions may require a tradeoff between these factors, and the evaluation evidence can often inform the terms of these tradeoffs.

For public policy, statutory and regulatory requirements are often critical to choosing among policy alternatives. These requirements can set bounds on the choices that can be made and can provide directives as to how these choices are made. For example, the Center for Medicare and Medicaid Innovations' initiatives can only be scaled to beyond their original scope if it can be demonstrated that the expanded model will either reduce costs without impairing quality or be cost neutral while improving quality. If these thresholds are not met, CMMI may terminate the initiative, modify it, or continue it if there is an expectation the results will improve with more data or a longer period of time. Clearly, the judgment about the quality of evaluation evidence for predicting key outcomes under an expanded model is critical to any of these choices.

Regardless of the program or policy area considered, statute and regulation may limit choices in other important ways. For example, policies or programs authorized by statute cannot in many cases be eliminated by program officials even if the evaluations are negative. In these cases, officials responsible for implementing the policy can either follow processes to change the statute, make changes to how it is implemented, or both.

In any of the above situations, using evidence alone, even within the bounds set by statute and regulation, is seldom sufficient to derive policy choices. For example, even if the cost and quality thresholds described above for the health delivery system initiatives are met, CMMI still has choices to make about whether to expand the initiative and how much to expand. Beyond the evidence, organizations are likely to weigh several other factors that are critical to the decision-making process. These include budgetary considerations, population importance, policy traditions, consistency with other policy priorities and objectives, and stakeholder views and concerns. All of these factors may play a role to varying degrees depending on the exact program and policy being considered. Indeed, the findings derived from the assessment of the evaluation evidence (e.g., the program was effective, ineffective, harmful) may influence how these other factors are brought to bear in the decision-making process. For example, if the program or policy is considered very important to the population served and views of stakeholders are very supportive, less weight might be given to the results of high-quality evaluations that suggest very weak or modest positive effect of a program.

Budgetary limitations often play a significant role in decision making and interact with the other policy-relevant factors. Limitations in funding as well as staffing and other administrative resources may limit an organization's ability to maintain or expand some programs that may have strong evidence of success. It is for this reason that other policy factors such as the importance to the population served of the program, and consistency with other organizational goals and policies, become critical.

Attention to other goals and objectives of the organization, and how they might interact with and policy decisions occasioned by the evidence, is also important. Most organizations or public policy agencies have multiple goals in their strategic plans. Any one program or policy established or modified to achieve a particular objective, or reflect evidence, may conflict with others. For a hypothetical example, an agency may have a stated objective of providing training to the most disadvantaged individuals, but well-designed program evaluations suggest that it is more cost effective to target less-disadvantaged individuals. Another agency may have goals of providing adequate financial assistance to individuals and is strongly encouraging seeking employment and training opportunities. An evaluation might demonstrate that certain level of financial assistance provide disincentives for job seeking. In both cases, strong evidence may suggest one policy direction, but the decision may take another, depending on how the agency assesses the tradeoff between its objectives. Undoubtedly, the values and beliefs of the organization and those of its decision makers would play a key role.

Particularly for public agencies, what might be called policy traditions and precedents may be important in any decision. Policy traditions may be thought of the ways an organization has historically reached decisions, that is, chosen among alternatives and preferences for implementing these decisions. Most policy decisions can be thought of as having two types of effects: the immediate impact on the program and those it serves and precedent it might set that will affect the agency's ability to make decisions in the future. In particular, decisions that depart from policy traditions without strong rationale may set precedents that restrict flexibility to make evidence-informed choices in the future.

A good example is how differences in costs are treated for purposes of Medicare's prospective payment systems for health care providers. Policy tradition has been to pay single rates based on a measure of central tendency (e.g., mean, median) from a national distribution of relevant provider costs. Providers are financially accountable for variations in costs around that payment rate that are considered within the providers' control (e.g., improving efficiency). Differences in costs that are considered legitimate and beyond the immediate control of providers are recognized by adjustments to the single national rate (e.g., for teaching and local wage cost for hospitals, local practice cost variations for physicians) rather than creating separate rates for the various provider groups. These adjustments have generally been based on statistical models in which a direct relationship between the adjustment factor and the policy standard (cost in this case) have been estimated. Any new payment systems or overhauls of existing ones that created separate payment groups for providers would need to have a strong rationale for departing from tradition, or risk setting new precedents that could affect future payment policy.

Multiple Alternatives for Decisions

As displayed on Figure 14.1, many policy decisions are not binary; there are many possible outcomes. An evaluation of a specific program might inform decisions on whether to continue or end the program, expand it, or modify it to make improvements or modify it to collect more information for future decisions. Within each of these possible outcomes, there might be several alternatives. For example, a decision to expand a program may choose among several methods of expansion (e.g., nationally, regionally, and locally).

The variety of policy choices available to decision makers, in addition to the policy factors described above, increases the responsibility and complexity for evaluators in preparing and presenting their results. At the risk of being repetitive, evaluators must recognize that their results will not automatically lead to yes/no decisions. Indeed, empirical results must be suitable for use throughout a complex process in which they will help navigate tradeoffs and weigh alternatives. An example is provided in the next section.

A Research Evidence/Policy Analysis Example: Socioeconomic Status and the Hospital Readmission Reduction Program

Medicare's Hospital Readmissions Reduction Program (HRRP) was implemented on October 1, 2012. Under this program, which was created as part of the Affordable Care Act (ACA), hospitals face payment penalties if they have higher-than-expected readmission rates for a key set of conditions common in the Medicare population. The program initially focused on acute myocardial infarction, heart failure, and pneumonia, but has now expanded to include chronic obstructive pulmonary disease, and total knee or hip arthroplasty. Program penalties are applied to Medicare base-operating diagnosis-related group (DRG) payments, across hospitals' total Medicare book of business.

The HRRP follows a specific methodology to calculate risk-standardized readmission rates for each hospital in the program. This methodology adjusts for age, sex, and medical comorbidities and uses the statistical technique of multilevel modeling with hospital-specific intercepts so that the model compares a particular hospital's performance on the readmission measure to the average performance of a hospital with the same case mix. The HRRP penalty is based on payments for these higher-than-expected readmissions as a proportion of total payments for all admissions. Thus, the proportion of all admissions for the five conditions currently included in the excess readmission calculation is a significant driver of the size of penalties.

In the 1st year of the program, the maximum penalty was 1% of base DRG payments; in 2014 this maximum penalty rose to 2%, and in 2015 to 3%, where it will remain. Evidence suggests that the program has been successful: from 2007 to 2015, readmission rates for targeted conditions declined from 21.5% to 17.8%, with the majority of the decline seen shortly after the passage of the ACA and announcement of the HRRP, followed by a slower decline from 2013 to 2015. Though decreases in readmission rates were seen for both targeted and non-targeted conditions, the declines for targeted conditions were larger.

The appropriateness and desirability of accounting for socioeconomic status (SES) factors (also called social risk factors) in the HRRP has been the source of significant debate. Some have suggested altering the program to reduce the impact of HRRP penalties on safety-net providers, but these suggestions have been controversial. Proponents of including a measure of SES in the HRRP argue that safety-net hospitals face penalties for outcomes that are beyond their control, pointing out that factors such as the availability of primary care, housing stability, medication adherence, and mental health and substance use disorders impact readmission rates, are not evenly distributed between hospitals, and are not accounted for when judging hospital performance. On the other hand, some worry that accounting for SES in the HRRP program will institutionalize poor performance in the safety net, sending the implicit message that worse clinical outcomes at these hospitals are acceptable.

The impacts of HRRP and the role of SES factors in determining readmissions have now been carefully evaluated. Consistent with a variety of early studies, recent research has shown that patients in safety net hospitals are more likely to be readmitted, even after controlling for the clinical risk adjustment factors used by the program. Measures of patients' SES (dual eligibility for both Medicare and Medicaid), hospital, and community characteristics explained a relatively small amount of the remaining differential between safety net and other hospitals. Approximately one half of the differential could not be explained by the measured factors used in the study. Moreover, the study conducted an impact analysis and found that safety net hospitals were slightly more likely to be penalized for excess readmissions, but that penalty amounts as a percent of Medicare inpatient payments was nearly identical between the two sets of hospitals. A mandated report to Congress found similar results for HRRP as well as for a variety of other value-based pricing programs.[10]

Should policymakers consider a change to HRRP for recognizing SES, there might be two decisions: (1) should a change be made, and (2) if yes, what specific policy option among many available should be adopted. For example, both direct risk adjustment for social risk factors and stratification (comparing hospitals only to those similar to them in terms of low-income-patient load) have been proposed.

Based on the research and impact results described above, researchers should make clear to officials who might be considering SES related changes to HRRP the following key results:

- Patients treated in safety net hospitals were more likely to be readmitted

- Dual eligible were more likely to be readmitted than other patients in either set of hospitals

- These results were statistically significant by conventional standards

- After accounting for the clinical risk adjustment made by the program, SES factors, as well as other patient and hospital characteristics, about half of the differential between safety net and other hospitals could not be explained by measured factors

- HRRP's method for calculating excess readmissions reduces disparities in raw readmission rates so that the safety net hospitals were slightly more likely to be penalized, but the penalties realized by them were virtually the same as for other hospitals

As described by Sheingold et al., these results for HRRP (and the other programs) were consistent and significant by traditional statistical standards. Despite the apparent high quality of the results, and the research that produced them, the other policy factors that were considered made for a complex decision-making process.[11] Members of the policy team differed in factors such as their experience with past payment policies, their expectations about the likelihood of unanticipated consequences, and their sensitivity to stakeholder concerns. Reflecting these differences, some members of the team thought there was a strong rationale for risk adjustment, whereas other members viewed the impacts as small enough to merit careful monitoring in moving forward, but not significant enough to take action.

Other Policy Factors Considered

A range of policy objectives came into play as the policy team evaluated policy alternatives. These policy objectives included (1) protecting safety net providers from unfair financial harm, (2) preserving payment equity by accounting for cost/quality factors beyond the control of providers, (3) providing strong incentives to both improve overall quality of health care and reduce disparities, and (4) maintaining transparency of information. Moreover, the secretary of Health and Human Services had recently established goals for the share of Medicare payment that would flow through alternative payment models.[12] Thus, encouraging providers to join new delivery system models that provide patient-centered, coordinated care across the full range of services was an additional objective.

Policymakers pay close attention to the way Medicare payment policy impacts providers that disproportionately serve low-income or vulnerable populations. Maintaining payment equity in a way that reflects the greater clinical or access needs of low-income or vulnerable populations has been a central tenant across Medicare's prospective payment systems. Policies such as the disproportionate share adjustment to hospital inpatient rates and the accommodations provided for many rural hospitals recognize the unique challenges that providers face related to their patient population and environment. Similar models could be used to account for social risk in payments or quality measures. The rationale for these policies to achieve payment equity is that they are necessary when deviations from a national standard (such as a group of providers whose costs are above national payment rate) are beyond providers' control, but that providers should be financially accountable for variations resulting from factors considered within their control.

Although it was one of the policy objectives, existing data did not fully clarify the extent of disparities that were and were not under providers' control. The Report to Congress's research used measures of explained and unexplained variation as a guide. The explained variation decomposed into within-provider and between-provider variations, with the former used as a proxy for the portion of the estimated impact that was beyond providers' control. The assumption was that each provider rendered the same care to all of its patients, so differences in outcomes were due to differences between patients, particularly their social risk profiles. This proxy is imperfect at best, as it is quite possible that there were differences in care provided to patients within the same setting. Furthermore, it is not possible to assess whether the unexplained variation was due to quality differences that could be addressed by providers or unmeasured factors beyond their control.

These uncertainties have potential implications for assessing adjustment options. For example, direct risk adjustment for the social risk factor(s) based on the statistical models would reflect explained variation and carry less risk of accounting for factors within the providers' control.

Maintaining incentives for quality improvement, and reducing disparities in quality, was also important. There is growing evidence that value-based payment has resulted in quality improvements, particularly for providers that faced the largest penalties when programs began.[13] So, an important consideration was ensuring that the financial consequences of these programs did not reduce safety net providers' ability to care for patients, while also maintaining the incentives for continued quality improvement. Providers serving socially at-risk patients clearly fared worse in value-based pricing programs, but the overall adverse financial impact was limited. For some decision makers, the positive response to program incentives, combined with less threatening financial impacts, seemed to support taking a more conservative approach. That is, maintaining the status quo, while monitoring current programs to ensure that any one of them, or the cumulative impact of several, did not significantly or unfairly impact safety net providers.

Another key policy objective in current law and policy implementation is transforming the delivery system to improve value. Currently, innovative payment models being tested are designed to encourage providers to be responsible for providing high-quality, well-coordinated care across the full range of health care services. Under these models, providers are financially accountable for both cost and quality. One concern about accounting for social risk is that reducing financial consequences for some providers would lessen incentives for them to join the new delivery models. To the extent that the most productive way to improve care for patients at social risk is creating networks of providers to coordinate care, reducing the incentive to enter these models might be harmful to socially at-risk patients.

Based on all of these factors, the Report contained a nuanced set of policy considerations rather than strong recommendations concerning whether to adjust or not adjust for social risk. Thus, the case provides a good window into how high-quality research and other factors may enter into the policy process. Researchers and evaluators must respect that beyond the results, decisions depend on organizational culture, values, stakeholder concerns, and the cost of making program changes. Researchers/evaluators' key role would be to present the results as cleanly as possible to inform the tradeoffs that might be considered in this decision.

Advice for Researchers and Evaluators

The discussion and case study in this chapter is meant to remind evaluators that even the clearest results from well-designed studies are just one answer to a puzzle that has many pieces. The generic model of evidence-informed decision making described here is intended to increase awareness of the role research and evaluation results can play in policy analysis. The exact machinery for decision making will likely vary considerably between organizations, and even within organizations, depending on the exact nature of the policy or program issue at hand. The bottom line is that there is no simple pathway from a *p*-value to a policy decision. Being aware of the complexities of policy decision making can help researchers to structure their analyses in more useful ways, as well as in ways to package and present their results to make them most useful. It may also prevent disappointment and frustration when decisions do not reflect results in a way that might seem apparent to researchers.

DISCUSSION QUESTIONS

1. Should evaluation methods change based on the organizational decision-making process of policymakers? Why, or why not?

2. Select a recent policy change in health policy, ideally from a recent Report to Congress. Discuss what evidence you can find that contributed to the policy change.

3. What suggestions do you have for improving the connection between evidence and policy?

NOTES

1. Scriven, M. "Michael Scriven on the Differences Between Evaluation and Social Science Research." *The Evaluation Exchange* 9 no. 4 (2003/2004). Available at http://www.hfrp.org/evaluation/the-evaluation-exchange/issue-archive/reflecting-on-the-past-and-future-of-evaluation/michael-scriven-on-the-differences-between-evaluation-and-social-science-research.

2. Etheredge, L. "Government and Health Care Costs: The Influence of Research on Policy," In *From Research Into Policy: Improving the Link for Health Services,* edited by M. E. Lewin (Washington DC: American Enterprise Institute, 1986).

3. Ein, Lewin M. *From Research into Policy: Improving the Link for Health Services* (Washington, DC: Aei Press, 1986).

4. Davis M. M., C. P. Gross, and C. M. Clancy, "Building a Bridge to Somewhere Better: Linking Health Care Research and Health Policy," *Health Services Research* 47 no. 1 pt. 2 (2012): 329–36. doi: 10.1111/j.1475-6773.2011.01373.x.

5. Gluck M. E., and J. Hoadley, *Moving Health Services Research Into Policy and Practice: Lessons from Inside and Outside the Health Sector* (Washington, DC: AcademyHealth, 2015).

6. Department of International Development, *What is the evidence on the impact of research on international development?: A DFID Literature Review.* UKAID Department for International Development, July 2014.

7. Ibid.

8. Ibid.

9. Weiss, C., "The Many Meanings of Research Utilization," *Public Administration Review* 39 no. 5 (1979): 426–31.

10. Department of Health and Human Services, Office of the Assistant Secretary for Planning and Evaluation, "Report to Congress: Social Risk Factors and Performance Under Medicare's Value-BasedPurchasing Programs, December 21, 2016, https://aspe.hhs.gov/system/files/pdf/253971/ASPESESRTCfull.pdf.

11. Sheingold, S. H. et al., "Should Medicare's Value Based Pricing be Adjusted for Social Risk Factors? The Role of Research Evidence in Policy Deliberations," *JHPPL* 43 no. 3 (June 2018): 401–25.

12. Sylvia M Burwell, "Setting Value-Based Payment Goals—HHS Efforts to Improve U.S. Health Care." *New England Journal of Medicine* (March 5, 2015) 372, no. 10: 897–99. doi: 10.1056/NEJMp1500445

13. Rachael B., Zuckerman, Steven H., Sheingold, E., John Orav, Joel Ruhter, and Arnold M. Epstein. "Readmissions, Observation, and the Hospital Readmissions Reduction Program." *New England Journal of Medicine* 374, no. 16 (February 24, 2016): 1543–51. doi:10.1056/NEJMsa1513024.

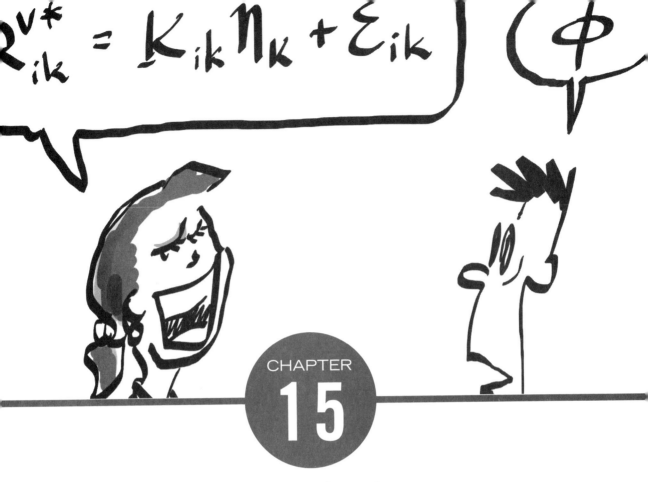

CHAPTER

15

Communicating Research and Evaluation Results to Policymakers

Steven Sheingold

Anupa Bir

Learning Objectives

In this book, we have provided explanations and examples of modern evaluation methods, alternative ways of summarizing and presenting complex results, and a

(Continued)

(Continued)

framework for understanding how these results might be used in a multifaceted policy process. In this final chapter, we discuss the important topic of communicating research and evaluation results to policymakers to increase the chances these results will be influential. As described in the previous chapter, there has at times been a gulf between the research community and policymakers that has meant good research has often not been useful for influencing policy. Fifteen years ago, a report by Canadian Institute for Health Information stated: "Still, it remains clear that researchers and policymakers do not always communicate clearly with each other, and that poor communication can hamper the uptake of research knowledge at the policy level. At the heart of this communication gap lies a lack of understanding by each group of the other's cultures, priorities, and processes."[1] In this chapter we suggest ways to reduce the gap.

There has perhaps never been a greater opportunity to narrow the gulf between researchers and policymakers, as evidence-based policy has become well accepted and codified in statute by the U.S. Congress. Nonetheless, researchers must address the issue of how to effectively communicate their results to policymakers. Whether your results are influential for policy may depend more on how well you can communicate them than on how rigorous your methods are or how publication worthy are the results. In this chapter, we discuss some considerations about how to best engage with policymakers by making sure your presentation of results is concise, clearly focused on answering the policy and research questions, and most importantly, understandable for the target audience.

A few key items that have been observed about policymakers and their willingness and ability to absorb and utilize research evidence in their deliberations follow:[2]

- Policymakers are typically busy and juggling many issues. The more highly placed in the organizational decision-making chain they are, the truer is this statement. If you are given a 1-hour meeting slot, it likely means you have 30–40 minutes of real time for engagement. Plan your message to take no longer than 10 minutes, and have supplementary materials prepared in case there is additional time and interest. It is far better to engage and generate questions than to give half of a very detailed presentation. Consider the simple three-part presentation structure: What? So What? Now What?

- In addition to your results, policymakers typically will receive a variety of information from multiple sources that they need to evaluate. To the extent that you can anticipate and situate your work in that context, it will help policymakers to not have to do all of the triangulation on the fly.

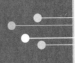

Box 15.1
Storytelling in Policy Research

The ubiquity of story is a testament to our collective ability to understand information in that particular structure. Stories do the work of synthesizing information for the audience and delivering it in a considered structure. Stories have a beginning with a hook to grab the audience's attention, a middle to communicate the study and its findings, an end that resolves tension, and situates the findings and implications in a broader context. Making the story personal and relatable, or using surprising statistics can engage the audience. The goal is to connect with the audience and ideally its emotions. The recent explosion in the study of story continues to offer new insights into the best ways to prepare and present messages. (More information is available at www.duarte.com/.)

- Based on training, experience, and personal preferences, policymakers vary in how they receive, interpret, and evaluate various sources of information. Research to know and understand your audience, the way you would in other situations.

- Policymakers want to jump to the end of the study and hear the results. Many policymakers do not love or understand the detailed methodological issues researchers face in conducting their study. They want results they can readily use, and not the detailed analytic plan. Because researchers love the analytic detail, they sometimes assume others do too.

- Policymakers want to know the magnitude of the problem they might address and have clear and defensible estimates to assess the consequences of various policy strategies. They tend to focus on high-level study limitations to understand the quality of the evidence so they can assess their risks in taking a specific policy proposal forward.

Suggested Strategies for Addressing Communication Issues

Researchers, whether in health services research, other social sciences or hard sciences, must decide on their benchmarks for success. If academic success, publication and recognition are the ultimate goal of research, then tailoring your results for the academic audience is sufficient. If you aim for having your research influence important policy issues and decisions, developing the right communications strategy is crucial. The lessons of Chapter 14 are that in most cases, your results can influence policy but do in concert with a number of other factors. Recognizing and studying those other factors and the unique policymaking environments in which they interact with evidence is a start to developing effective communication strategies.

The communication strategies discussed below are based on the literature cited in this chapter, as well as many years of experience of the authors at interacting with policymakers.

Carefully explain your policy and research questions. They are not the same questions and both are important to introduce and provide context for your research. Policy questions make clear to the audience what the policy issues are that your research will inform. The research questions specify what particular information your research will provide. To illustrate, consider the social risk factor case described in Chapter 14. The policy question was:

> *Should Medicare adjust its value-based purchasing programs to account for social risk factors?*

The research questions were:

> *Is there a relationship at the patient level between social risk factors and performance on the metrics in Medicare payment programs?*

> *Under current design, do providers that serve socially at-risk beneficiaries do more poorly under Medicare's value-based payment programs?*

The study was designed to answer these research questions in a way that could best inform deliberations about the policy question.

Recognize that time is limited for conveying your results. Written and oral presentation of research results must be concise and to the point. Briefings for high level decision makers typically have less presentation time than the scheduled time slot: They can start late or end early based on other demands for their time. Moreover, briefings can have interruptions as other matters are brought to policymakers' attention. Thus, a great deal of time and attention must be given to selecting the most important points to convey to the target audience and how to present them in the most concise way possible; and in a way that can keep on track despite interruptions.

It is important to have a backup plan for modifying the presentation in response to changing situations. Again, a late start or one or more interruptions can shorten the time you have to present. From any point in your presentation, you must be able to adjust your material to the remaining time you have in a way that still gets across those results and implications most important to the audience. Having a good grasp on the implications of your research will help you to cut to the chase.

Most policymakers will not read long technical papers or sit through very long briefings that contain very technical analytic details. So as part of selecting the most important information to convey, be continually aware of which analytic details that may be necessary (in a very brief manner) to set the context for understanding results from those that are best left for more technically oriented audiences. Discussions of fuzzy versus sharp regression discontinuity or many ways to deal with nonindependent data may be fascinating over lunch or martinis with colleagues but are not likely to be a big hit with most policymakers. Likewise, do not use jargon that may be acceptable or even facilitate discussion in research circles but that will have little or no meaning to many policymakers. Learn how to describe your technical terms in more meaningful ways. For example, consider research on the impact of the number of generic manufacturers entering a market on the price of the drug. One could use the technical concept and say that there is concern that the estimated effect would be biased due to endogeneity. Instead, one could say there is concern that manufacturers are attracted to markets in which the initial price is very high, which could overstate the relationship between the number of manufacturers and the decline in the drug price.

Focus on what best meets policymakers' information needs. In addition to modifying the technical detail of the presentation, considering the amount of information to include is important. As researchers, we can also spend significant time immersed in the programmatic and contextual details of our subject area. We can become experts in a way that makes us believe all of the details we know are important and necessary to convey in presentations. Researchers with little policy experience may learn the hard way that this is not true when they lose their audience well before they have gotten to the critical part of the presentation. There must be careful analysis and consideration by researchers about what are necessary pieces of information that support your critical message, and those that may take away time and attention but do not strengthen your ability to convey the message. For those with considerable expertise the process of parsing details may seem like choosing among your children, but it is necessary. In a following section, we have suggestions about getting to know the needs and preferences of your target audience to make this process more efficient.

Finding the optimal visual displays for your results is critical. Developing presentation display methods should be an ongoing process as the research progresses—not something first addressed shortly before the presentation. Results from statistical and simulation models can be complex, and policymakers may differ in terms of what display methods are most effective for their comprehending the results. Again, knowing the target policymakers is useful, but researchers should test different ways of presenting the same results—for example, what types of tables, charts, and other methods seem to convey the information most effectively. Infographics can be helpful and are easily shared in social media. Interactive dashboards can also be helpful. Figure 15.1 provides screenshots of an interactive Bayesian dashboard that allows users to select the range of savings desired to dynamically update the probability of saving. This is possible for any range of savings or dissavings that might be relevant to future decision making.

In Chapter 14, we used the issue of whether Medicare should adjust value based pricing programs for patients' social risk factors as an example of using evidence for policy deliberations. Table 15.1, which presents odds ratios estimated from logistic regressions, was used to brief the Department of Health and Human Services policymakers. At that time, many of the individuals in leadership positions had come from academic and research backgrounds and were comfortable with this format. It is often the case that leadership will have less research experience and alternative methods, such as bar charts, may be more effective at conveying the important relative magnitudes of the results.

Be ready to compare and contrast your results to the other sources of information. Policymakers often receive from stakeholders a variety of information including published and unpublished papers, contractor reports and briefs, news articles

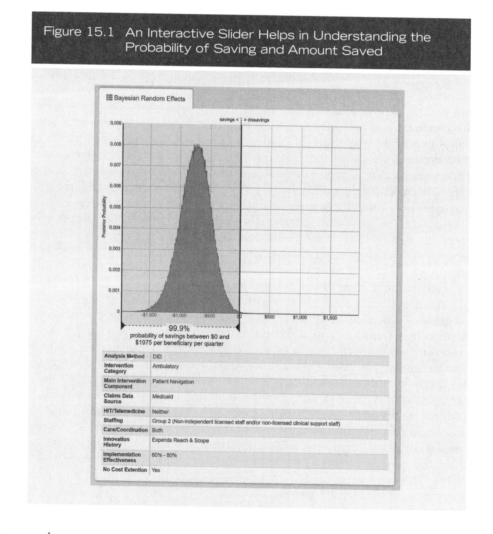

Figure 15.1   An Interactive Slider Helps in Understanding the Probability of Saving and Amount Saved

Figure 15.1 (Continued)

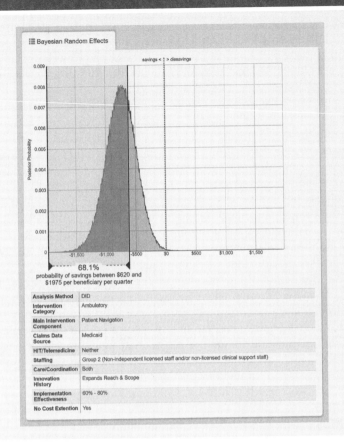

Analysis Method	DID
Intervention Category	Ambulatory
Main Intervention Component	Patient Navigation
Claims Data Source	Medicaid
HIT/Telemedicine	Neither
Staffing	Group 2 (Non-independent licensed staff and/or non-licensed clinical support staff)
Care/Coordination	Both
Innovation History	Expands Reach & Scope
Implementation Effectiveness	60% - 80%
No Cost Extention	Yes

Table 15.1 Odds of Readmission for Heart Failure, by Social Risk Factor

Social Risk Factor	Social Risk Factor Alone	Social Risk Factor, Adjusting for Comorbidities (age, kidney failure, heart failure, etc.)	Social Risk Factor, Adjusting for Comorbidities and Other Social Risk Factors**
Dual status	1.24	1.13	1.10
Low-income ZIP		1.00	1.00
Black	1.12	1.09	1.01
Hispanic	1.10	1.04	0.96
Urban	1.05	1.04	1.05

and anecdotes. Researchers should be prepared to discuss results and implications of these alternative sources whether they agree or disagree with their own. Busy policymakers may find it helpful for you to provide advice on how to evaluate and choose among these sources. Perhaps more importantly, your advice on how to stitch together your work with these other sources to create a comprehensive picture of the policy problem and the potential solutions may be appreciated. We strongly suggest therefore, that researchers make the effort to stay aware of all the information available in your topic area.

It is important that any disagreements between results be described in a respectful and evidence-based manner. Being overly critical of alternative analyses risks alienating those policymakers they may rely on or trust the alternative source. Of equal importance, contrasts can be more effective if put in policy relevant terms rather than technical ones. For example, your study of savings attributable to the medical home model uses intent to treat analysis, while an alternative study of the same model does not. It may be more useful to policymakers to cast this difference as our method assumes medical homes are responsible for the costs of patients even if they leave the model, while the alternative analysis only includes those who remain in the model. Policymakers can then decide which methods meet their objectives for the cost accountability of medical homes.

Characterizing Statistical Inference in Your Presentations. As described in earlier chapters, a critical issue for researchers and evaluators is how to present the results of statistical analyses in the best way possible for decision makers to interpret and make an assessment about potential program/policy outcomes. One controversial issue in presenting and interpreting research results is what weight to put on the p-value, and how it should be interpreted. The size of the p-value is often held up as the key criterion in evaluating the importance and significance of results and may influence what research gets published in high-level journals. More importantly, the p-value is often interpreted as a "walk off" criterion for decision making about a policy or program. In this approach, a p-value less than a commonly used threshold such as .05 is interpreted as statistically significant, while a p-value greater than that level is interpreted as not statistically significant. These findings can often be misinterpreted— statistically significant is often wrongly conflated with the existence of an important program effect, not statistically significant by the p-value criteria misinterpreted as meaning no program effect. Either misinterpretation can influence policy decisions in a way that may be inconsistent with an organization's goals and objectives, such as achieving health care value or improving public health. In addition, basing or heavily weighting the p-value as a decision criterion may ignore important information from the data analyses that reflect on program goals or objectives.

Indeed, the American Statistical Association recently published a position paper which emphasizes that p-values are not intended or appropriate as a sole criterion for decision making.[3] They represent one finding about your data relative to a specific hypothesis called the null. The null typically hypothesizes that there is a zero effect. A p-value less than a specified level simply means that if the null hypothesis were true, the research finding would be very unlikely.

That is, there is a small probability of obtaining the result due to random variation. It does not mean the effect is important in terms of magnitude or that it should translate into an automatic decision for program or policymakers. It does not imply anything about the probability that either the null or research hypothesis is true—both are common misinterpretations of the p-value. Some of these misinterpretations have led to greater interest in Bayesian statistics, purely for the relative clarity of presentation. Instead of the confusion about p-values, Bayesian findings are expressed as probabilities. Policymakers can readily understand and use information that says clearly that there is an 80% probability of saving $100 per person per quarter. They can decide whether that seems like a good bet given their other considerations and the context. P-values do not offer a similar interpretation.

Researchers should carefully interpret their results regarding p-values, both above and below a prespecified level such as .05. A value less than .05 does not necessarily translate into an important program effect. A p-value greater than the prespecified level does mean that there is no effect or that a policy or program has not met its objectives. It simply means there is a somewhat higher probability of observing the obtained result by chance. Put another way, the p-value might be considered as evidence against the null hypothesis. A higher p-value means there is weaker evidence against the null (no effect) than a lower one. Whether decision makers would accept p-values that are higher than .05 will likely be dependent on the specific values of the organization and the particular context of the program in question and its potential outcomes. For example, decision makers might accept a higher p-value for programs with a potential for positive outcomes and whose worst case is no effect and set stricter standards for programs whose worst case is negative outcomes or harms. Researchers must be very careful in characterizing these issues in a way that provides maximum information for policymakers to consider in their decisions, without biasing the message with words such as not significant or no effect.

Characterizing Magnitude and Uncertainty. Decision makers need to know both the magnitude of the estimated impact and the uncertainty around that estimate. In that regard, confidence intervals (CIs) may provide more complete information than p-values. The CI provides information simultaneously on estimated magnitude of the effect and the uncertainty around it. Decision makers can make judgements about estimates such as those that may have little uncertainty (small CIs) but around as estimated magnitude too small to be important, and those that may reflect estimates large in magnitude, but also with considerable uncertainty. At the same time, CIs also provide the needed information to assess evidence against a null hypothesis if so desired. Figure 13.1 illustrates the magnitude of the savings across a number of health care innovations, visually displaying the magnitude of the effects and the confidence intervals of each innovation. A glance allows one to interpret the body of evidence quickly, understanding which innovations have large effects and which of the effects deserve the most confidence.

Researchers should also be careful to distinguish statistical significance of the results from the magnitude of the implied effects of a program or policy. Policymakers care more about the actual effects on key stakeholders more than how large or statistically significant are coefficients from a model. For example, in the social risk deliberations, it was critical information that the seemingly much higher odds of dually eligible beneficiaries being readmitted to hospitals, the actual financial consequences under HRRP for hospitals that treated a disproportionate share of these patients was relatively small. Finding ways to add this extra information can be extremely important in some cases.

It is also important to provide decision makers with information to assess how much of the variation in key outcomes can be explained by the policy or program effect. Typical effect size measures standardize the magnitude of the estimate by the standard deviation or as a percent of total variation in the outcome explained. It is possible for statistical models to exhibit a highly significant effect of one or more variables but leave much of the variation in outcome unexplained. This would mean that predictions from the model would be imprecise—that is, the prediction interval would be wide. More importantly, while an r^2 of .4 or .5 along with some low p-values may be a great success for journal articles, they may be less useful for policy decision makers without further information and analyses. The possible content of the variation in outcomes not explained by the model may be as policy relevant as the explained variation. For example, was it due to random variation or unmeasured but important variables, such as differences in the capabilities of participants and fidelity of implementation?

Chapters 8, 9, and 13 described this issue in terms of how to assess and quantify variation in outcomes in a useful way to inform policy. While it is clearly essential to have credible estimates of average program impacts, it is just a part of the story helpful to program and policy decisions. What is also needed is an understanding of whether program impacts vary, by how much, and why. For example, we might learn a lot about the conditions under which findings may generalize from a randomized controlled trial by detecting and quantifying variation in program impacts.[4] Moreover, learning either in a quantitative or qualitative manner about program participants that had above-average impacts and distinguishing them from those who were less successful can be very informative for policy. For example, could what we learned about best practices from successful participants be disseminated to participants in a continued or expanded program to improve overall performance? Looking at the combination of impacts, populations, and patterns of variation is part of the advantage of meta-evaluation approaches for informing policy.

Getting to know policymakers and building relationships with them can be an effective way of learning how to best present information. In most relationships, communication improves when the parties get to know each other better. Communications between researchers and policymakers is no exception. Many of the suggestions for tailoring presentations described above are easily implemented if researchers have become familiar with the relevant policymakers' backgrounds, preferences for different types of information, listening/querying styles, and how they respond to different types of visual displays for research results. The question then becomes how do researchers build these relationships and develop interactions in a way that guides them to creating the most effective presentations of research results to inform policy deliberations?

In answering this question, it is useful to consider that in most organizations there are multiple layers of staff and managers involved in the process. While the staffing configurations and policy processes may differ in agencies responsible for public policy, a generalization may be useful. Final policy decisions are typically made, or at least approved, at the highest levels of the organization. Individuals at this level are often political appointees. Detailed technical and programmatic knowledge exists at the staff level where policy analysis and development typically occur. In between these two levels of the agency are usually mid-level managers, often responsible for communicating program knowledge, analyses, and policy issues to the higher-level officials.

Researchers are most likely to build working relationships at the technical staff level and have opportunities to learn how to tailor and present results to them. These staff members are often responsible for packaging and interpreting your results along with their own analyses to the higher levels. Whether your research influences policy can depend on these staff members understanding and accepting research results in a way that assists them with these tasks. There also may be cases in which researchers make presentations to the higher-level officials. In these situations, relationships with the technical staff can be enormously helpful. They can use their firsthand experience to provide guidance on how and what to present.

Other Considerations for Tailoring and Presenting Results

The suggested strategies above have focused more on oral communication than on written. Providing well-crafted briefings on progress of research and final results is critical. Nonetheless, written products can also be a crucial part of the process of translating research results into policy deliberations. Good written products can prepare technical/program staff for in person briefings in a way that makes the briefings more productive. More importantly, these products can be useful for the staff as they prepare briefings for higher-level decision makers. It is good practice for researchers to work with these staff members to develop the format and style of written products that convey the research results in the most helpful manner.

There are two basic policy situations that may be influenced by research: (1) using research to identify and quantify an issue to gain the interest of policymakers; and (2) informing policy deliberations on an issue already being addressed. The approach and presentation in these two situations should be somewhat different from

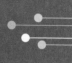
There are now extensive resources available to support the use of plain language. As a direct counter-blow to the overly wrought language sometimes encouraged in graduate programs, plain language guidelines suggest using short sentences and paragraphs with everyday words, avoiding jargon and paying attention to the structure of the presentation. One example developed for their training purposes illustrates the difference.

- **Before**

  This program promotes efficient water use in homes and businesses throughout the country by offering a simple way to make purchasing decisions that conserve water, without sacrificing quality or product performance.

- **After**

  This program helps homeowners and businesses buy products that use less water, without sacrificing quality or performance.

Checklists and examples are available at www.plainlanguage.gov/resources/checklists/.

each other. In the first situation, policymakers are being introduced to a potential policy issue and may deliberate on whether to take action and if so, what alternatives to pursue. Thus, background and context for the issue is important to present, along with the research results that provide the magnitude and other key features of the problem. In the second case, policymakers have already identified a potential problem and have decided to consider taking action—even if status quo is the eventual decision. In these cases, researchers should be careful not to use valuable presentation time with information that would be doing no more than convincing policymakers about a problem of which they are already aware. They are likely to most want to know what the consequences would be of taking different approaches to solving the problem.

Policymakers are likely to want to know your thoughts on the policy implications of your research findings. In these situations, it is useful to demonstrate your understanding of the policy process as described in Chapter 14. A safe response might be put in the context of what your results would imply for policy if there were no other relevant factors to consider. Demonstrating an understanding of these other factors, and the complexity of the policy-making process, may enhance the credibility of both the researchers and the results. In any case, preparing in advance for these types of questions is always a good idea.

Closing Thoughts on Communicating Research Results

To be most useful for the policy-making process, research and evaluation must be relevant, high quality, and timely. Tailoring written and oral communication of results to the relevant policymakers' needs increases the chances the research will be impactful. It is important to understand the organization for which you are providing the research and the nature of its decision makers. Listen carefully to questions that are asked and provide answers that demonstrate an understanding of the decision-making environment and its information needs. Decision makers must be convinced of the relevance of your results to their needs. For example, questions about underlying factors related to uncertainty in your results that are answered in purely technical terms may not bond decision makers to your research.

Be careful and thorough about presenting standard measures of statistical inference. It may be more useful to present p-values without the prejudgement of statistical significance. Allow decision makers to assess the values within the context of the appropriate meaning of the p-value and in the context of "typical" thresholds used for statistical significance. Likewise, emphasize magnitude and effect size of estimated program effects, preferably within a comparative context that makes them meaningful, that is, based on prior research related to similar programs or policies.

DISCUSSION QUESTIONS

1. What are the main obstacles policymakers and researchers face in effectively communicating with each other?

2. Assume you have just completed a large scale, potentially policy relevant research project. What steps would you take in preparing to communicate your results effectively to policymakers?

3. Examine the results in the Report to Congress "Report to Congress: Social Risk Factors and Performance Under Medicare's Value-Based Purchasing Programs" referenced in Chapter 14. How would you present the results and policy implications to policymakers?

NOTES

1. Susan Goldberg, "You say 'to-may-to(e)' and I say 'to-mah-to(e)': Bridging the Communication Gap Between Researchers and Policy-Makers." Canadian Institute for Health Information, 2004. Available at https://secure.cihi.ca/free_products/CPHI_Bridging_Gap_e.pdf.

2. Ibid.; Pittore, K., J. Meeker, and T. Barker, "Practical considerations for communicating evidence to policymakers: Identifying best practices for conveying research findings." Global Support Facility for the National Information Platforms for Nutrition Initiative, 2017. Available

ay http://www.nipn-nutrition-platforms.org/
IMG/pdf/communicating-evidence-to-policy-
makers.pdf; Hollander Feldman, P., P. Nadash,
and M. Gursen, "Improving Communication
Between Researchers and Policy Makers in
Long-Term Care: Or, Researchers Are From
Mars: Policy Makers Are From Venus." *The
Gerontologist* 41 no. 3 (2001): 312–21; Cairney,
P., and R. Kwiatkowski, "How to communicate
effectively with policymakers: Combine insights
from psychology and policy studies." *Palgrave
Communications* 3 no. 37 (2017). Available at

https://www.nature.com/articles/s41599-017-
0046-8.pdf.

3. Ronald L. Wasserstein, and Nicole A. Lazar,
"The ASA's Statement on P-Values: Context,
Process, and Purpose," *American Statistician* 70
no. 2 (2016): 129–33.

4. Raudenbush S. W., and H. S. Bloom,
"Learning About and From a Distribution
of Program Impacts Using Multisite Trials,"
American Journal of Evaluation 36 no. 4 (2015):
475–99.

Appendix A

The Primer Measure Set

The following table displays a set of measures for evaluators to consider. The measure set encompasses structural, process, and outcome measures listed by the National Quality Standard (NQF) priorities to use in assessing health care delivery interventions. Measures included represent differing units of measurement and supporting varying levels of analysis. Most of the measures are constructed from data that are routinely collected, such as administrative data and existing quality reporting programs to minimize the reliance on new data collection efforts.

The measures we list include measures endorsed by the NQF, to ensure the measures provided have been fully evaluated on the reliability, validity, and usability of the measures. Measure development entities, such as the National Committee for Quality Assurance, have additional measures that can be considered, particularly within the context of quality improvement and accreditation. In addition, a number of non-NQF endorsed measures are worthy of examination (e.g., measures from the Patient Reported Outcomes Measurement Information System), particularly when the included set is inadequate to meet the specific needs of a particular study.

Measures within the list are organized within the Donabedian framework, matched with the Institute of Medicine's six aims, and subcategorized by clinical condition or disease. While a single set of measures will not be appropriate or applicable to all evaluations, the consideration and use of measures from a standardized set offers many benefits. The chief advantage is that many of these measures are constructed using administrative and other commonly collected heath care data. Also, consistency in measurement across program evaluations allows researchers to readily build a body of evidence from the results of multiple interventions. This can be especially beneficial in payment or service delivery reforms where similar interventions are carried out across isolated geographic locations, service sectors, or populations. Having the ability to aggregate the results may increase the ability to understand an intervention's effects. Practically, alignment of measurement to evidence-based measure sets can be more efficient to the evaluator since she or he can rely on existing specifications and data collection protocols. Streamlining data collection reduces respondent burden, which may improve respondent retention in the study and increase data accuracy.

Table A.1   Primer Measures Set

Domain	National Quality Standard (NQF) Priority	Measure
Structure	Patient Safety	**1. Skill mix (Registered Nurse [RN], Licensed Vocational/Practical Nurse [LVN/LPN], unlicensed assistive personnel [UAP], and contract) (NQF 0204)** The measure includes the following components: NSC 12.1—Percentage of total productive nursing hours worked by RN (employee and contract) with direct patient care responsibilities by hospital unit; NSC 12.2—Percentage of total productive nursing hours worked by LPN/LVN (employee and contract) with direct patient care responsibilities by hospital unit; NSC 12.3—Percentage of total productive nursing hours worked by UAP (employee and contract) with direct patient care responsibilities by hospital unit; NSC 12.4—Percentage of total productive nursing hours worked by contract or agency staff (RN, LPN/LVN, and UAP) with direct patient care responsibilities by hospital unit.
Prevention		
Screening and Immunizations		
Process	Health and Well-Being	**2. Influenza Vaccination (NQF 0041)** Percentage of patients aged 6 months and older seen for a visit between October 1 and the end of February who received an influenza immunization OR patient reported previous receipt of an influenza immunization
Process	Health and Well-Being	**3. Pneumonia Vaccination Status for Older Adults (NQF 0043)** Percentage of patients 65 years of age and older who ever received a pneumococcal vaccination
Process	Health and Well-Being	**4. Colorectal Cancer Screening (NQF 0034)** Percentage of members 50–75 years of age who had appropriate screening for colorectal cancer
Process	Prevention and Treatment of Cardiovascular Disease	**5. Measure Pair: (A) Tobacco Use Assessment, (B) Tobacco Cessation Intervention (NQF 0028)** (A) Percentage of patients who were queried about tobacco use one or more times during the 2-year measurement period (B) Percentage of patients identified as tobacco users who received cessation intervention during the 2-year measurement period
Process	Health and Well-Being	**6. Adult Weight Screening and Follow-Up (NQF 0421)** Percentage of patients aged 18 years and older with a calculated body mass index (BMI) documented in the medical record AND if the most recent BMI is outside the parameters, a follow-up plan is documented

Domain	NQS Priority	Measure
Process	Health and Well-Being	**7. Screening for Clinical Depression and Follow-Up Plan (NQF 0418)** Percentage of patients aged 18 years and older screened for clinical depression using a standardized tool and following up plan documented

Children's Health

Domain	NQS Priority	Measure
Process	Health and Well-Being	**8. Childhood Immunization Status (NQF 0038)** Measure calculates a rate for each recommended vaccine and nine separate combination rates.
Process	Health and Well-Being	**9. Well-Child Visits in the First 15 Months of Life (NQF 1392)** Percentage of members who turned 15 months old during the measurement year and who had the following number of well-child visits with a primary care provider during their first 15 months of life.
Process	Health and Well-Being	**10. Well-Child Visits in the 3rd, 4th, 5th, and 6th Years of Life (NQF 1516)** Percentage of members 3–6 years of age who received one or more well-child visits with a primary care provider during the measurement year
Process	Health and Well-Being	**11. Weight Assessment and Counseling for Nutrition and Physical Activity for Children/Adolescents (NQF 0024)** Percentage children, 3 through 17 years of age, whose weight is classified based on BMI percentile for age and gender

Endocrine and Cardiovascular

Domain	NQS Priority	Measure
Outcome	Patient Safety	**12. Diabetes Long-term Complications (NQF 0274)** The number of discharges for long-term diabetes complications per 100,000 population age 18 years and older in a metro area or county in a 1-year time period. Measures 67–70 are used as part of the Centers for Medicare and Medicaid Services (CMS) Physician Feedback/Quality Resource Use Report "Diabetes ACSC Composite Measure."
Outcome	Patient Safety	**13. Diabetes Short-Term Complications (NQF 0272)** The number of discharges for diabetes short-term complications per 100,000 age 18 years and older population in a Metro Area or county in a 1-year period. Measures 67–70 are used as part of the CMS Physician Feedback/Quality Resource Use Report "Diabetes ACSC Composite Measure."
Outcome	Patient Safety	**14. Uncontrolled Diabetes Admission Rate (NQF 0638)** The number of discharges for uncontrolled diabetes per 100,000 age 18 years and older population in a metro area or county in a 1-year period. Measures 67–70 are used as part of the CMS Physician Feedback/Quality Resource Use Report "Diabetes ACSC Composite Measure."

(Continued)

Domain	NQS Priority	Measure
Outcome	Patient Safety	**15. Rate of Lower-Extremity Amputation in Diabetes (NQF 0285)** The number of discharges for lower-extremity amputation among patients with diabetes per 100,000 age 18 years and older population in a metro area or county in a 1-year period. Measures 67–70 are used as part of the CMS Physician Feedback/Quality Resource Use Report "Diabetes ACSC Composite Measure."
Outcome	Patient Safety	**16. Congestive Heart Failure Admission Rate (NQF 0277)** Percent of county population with an admissions for congestive heart failure
Pulmonary and Urinary		
Outcome	Patient Safety	**17. Chronic Obstructive Pulmonary Disease (NQF 0275)** This measure is used to assess the number of admissions for chronic obstructive pulmonary disease (COPD) per 100,000 population
Outcome	Patient Safety	**18. Bacterial Pneumonia (NQF 0279)** Number of admissions for bacterial pneumonia per 100,000 population
Outcome	Patient Safety	**19. Adult Asthma (NQF 0283)** Number of admissions for asthma in adults per 100,000 population
Outcome	Patient Safety	**20. Urinary Tract Infection Admission Rate (NQF 0281)** Number of discharges for urinary tract infection per 100,000 population age 18 years and older in a metro area or county in a 1-year time period
Treatment		
Endocrine		
Process	Affordable Care	**21. Proportion of Days Covered: Five Rates by Therapeutic Category (NQF 0541)** Percentage of patients 18 years and older who met the proportion of days covered threshold of 80% during the measurement year. Rate is calculated separately for the following medication categories: beta-blockers, angiotensin-converting enzyme inhibitor/angiotensin receptor blocker, calcium-channel blockers, diabetes medication, statins

Domain	NQS Priority	Measure
Process	Effective Communication and Care Coordination	**22. Comprehensive Diabetes Care: Eye Exam (NQF 0055)** Percentage of adult patients with diabetes aged 18–75 years who received an eye screening for diabetic retinal disease during the measurement year
Process	Effective Communication and Care Coordination	**23. Diabetes: Foot Exam (NQF 0056)** Percentage of adult patients with diabetes aged 18–75 years who received a foot exam (visual inspection, sensory exam with monofilament, or pulse exam)
Process	Effective Communication and Care Coordination	**24. Comprehensive Diabetes Care: Medical Attention for Nephropathy (NQF 0062)** The percentage of members 18–75 years of age with diabetes (Type 1 and Type 2) who received a nephropathy screening test or had evidence of nephropathy during the measurement year.
Process	Prevention and Treatment of Cardiovascular Disease	**25. Angiotensin-Converting Enzyme (ACE) Inhibitor or Angiotensin Receptor Blocker (ARB) Therapy for Left Ventricular Systolic Dysfunction (LVSD) (NQF 0066)** Percentage of patients aged 18 years and older with a diagnosis of cardiovascular disease (CAD) seen within a 12-month period who also have diabetes or a current or prior LVEF <40% and who were prescribed ACE inhibitors or ARB therapy.
Cardiovascular		
Process	Prevention and Treatment of Cardiovascular Disease	**26. Antiplatelet Therapy (NQF 0067)** Percentage of patients aged 18 years and older with a diagnosis of CAD seen within a 12-month period who were prescribed aspirin or clopidogrel.
Process	Prevention and Treatment of Cardiovascular Disease	**27. Beta-Blocker Therapy—Prior Myocardial Infarction or Left Ventricular Systolic Dysfunction (NQF 0070)** Percentage of patients aged 18 years and older with a diagnosis of CAD seen within a 12-month period who also have prior myocardial infraction (MI) or a current or prior LVEF <40% and who were prescribed beta-blocker therapy.

(Continued)

Domain	NQS Priority	Measure
Process	Prevention and Treatment of Cardiovascular Disease	**28. Beta-Blocker Therapy for Left Ventricular Systolic Dysfunction (NQF 0083)** Percentage of patients aged 18 years and older with a diagnosis of heart failure with a current or prior LVEF < 40% who were prescribed beta-blocker therapy either within a 12-month period when seen in the outpatient setting or at hospital discharge
Process	Prevention and Treatment of Cardiovascular Disease	**29. Use of Aspirin or Another Antithrombotic (NQF 0068)** Percentage of patients 18 years and older with ischemic vascular disease (IVD) who were discharged alive for acute myocardial infarction, coronary artery bypass graft, or percutaneous coronary intervention from January 1 to November 1 of the year prior to the measurement year, or who had a diagnosis of IVD during the measurement year and the year prior to the measurement year and who used aspirin or another antithrombotic during the measurement year.
Process	Prevention and Treatment of Cardiovascular Disease	**30. Fibrinolytic Therapy Received Within 30 Minutes of Hospital Arrival (NQF 0164)** Percentage of AMI patients with ST-segment elevation or left bundle branch block on the electrocardiogram closest to arrival time receiving fibrinolytic therapy during the hospital stay and having a time from hospital arrival to fibrinolysis of 30 minutes or less
Process	Prevention and Treatment of Cardiovascular Disease	**31. Fibrinolytic Therapy Received Within 30 Minutes of Emergency Department Arrival (NQF 0288)** Emergency room AMI patients receiving fibrinolytic therapy during the emergency department (ED) stay and having a time from ED arrival to fibrinolysis of 30 minutes or less
Process	Prevention and Treatment of Cardiovascular Disease	**32. Median Time to Transfer to Another Facility for Acute Coronary Intervention (NQF 0290)** Median time from ED arrival to time of transfer to another facility for acute coronary intervention
Outcome	Prevention and Treatment of Cardiovascular Disease	**33. Controlling High Blood Pressure (NQF 0018)** Percentage of patients >18 years of age with a diagnosis of hypertension in the first 6 months of the measurement year or any time prior with last blood pressure measurement <140/90 mm Hg

Domain	NQS Priority	Measure
Pulmonary		
Process	Effective Communication and Care Coordination	**34. Pharmacologic Therapy for Persistent Asthma (NQF 0047)** Percentage of all patients with mild, moderate, or severe persistent asthma who were prescribed either the preferred long-term control medication (inhaled corticosteroid) or an acceptable alternative treatment
Behavioral and Mental Health		
Process	Effective Communication and Care Coordination	**35. Initiation and Engagement of Alcohol and Other Drug Dependence Treatment (NQF 0004)** The percentage of adolescent and adult members with a new episode of alcohol or other drug (AOD) dependence who received the following: a) Initiation of AOD treatment: The percentage of members who initiate treatment through an IP AOD admission, outpatient (OP) visit, intensive OP encounter, or partial hospitalization within 14 days of the diagnosis b) Engagement of AOD Treatment: The percentage of members who initiated treatment and who had two or more additional services with a diagnosis of AOD within 30 days of the initiation visit
Process	Effective Communication and Care Coordination	**36. Postdischarge Continuing-Care Plan Created (NQF 0557)** Patients discharged from a hospital-based inpatient psychiatric setting with a continuing care plan created overall and stratified by age groups
Process	Effective Communication and Care Coordination	**37. Postdischarge Continuing Plan Transmitted to Next Level of Care Provider Upon Discharge (NQF 0558)** Patients discharged from a hospital-based inpatient psychiatric setting with a continuing care plan provided to the next level of care clinician or entity overall and stratified by age groups
Process	Effective Communication and Care Coordination	**38. Follow-up After Hospitalization for Mental Illness (NQF 0576)** Percentage of discharges for members 6 years of age and older who were hospitalized for treatment of selected mental health disorders and who had an outpatient visit, an intensive outpatient encounter, or partial hospitalization with a mental health practitioner. Two rates are reported: (1) the percentage of members who received follow-up within 30 days of discharge, (2) the percentage of members who received follow-up within 7 days of discharge

(Continued)

Domain	NQS Priority	Measure
Care Coordination		
Process	Effective Communication and Care Coordination	**39. Three-Item Care Transition Measure (NQF 0228)** Unidimensional patient self-reported survey that measures the quality of preparation for care transitions
Process	Effective Communication and Care Coordination	**40. Care Transition Record Transmitted to Health Care Professional (NQF 0648)** Percentage of patients, regardless of age, discharged from an inpatient facility to home or any other site of care for whom a transition record was transmitted to the designated health care provider for follow-up care within 24 hours.
Process	Effective Communication and Care Coordination	**41. Documentation of Current Medications in the Medical Record (NQF 0419)** Percentage of visits for patients aged 18 years and older for which the eligible professional attests to documenting a list of current medications using all immediate resources available on the date of the encounter
Outcome	Patient Safety	**42. Hospital All-Cause Unplanned Readmissions, Risk Adjusted (NQF 1789)** Hospitalwide, all-cause, risk standardized readmission rate following hospitalization for all conditions and procedures
Outcome	Patient Safety	**43. Skilled Nursing Facility 30-Day All-Cause Readmission Measure (NQF 2510)** This measure estimates the risk-standardized rate of all-cause, unplanned, hospital readmissions for patients who have been admitted to a skilled nursing facility within 30 days of discharge from a prior inpatient admission to a hospital, CAH, or a psychiatric hospital
Outcome	Patient Safety	**44. Rehospitalization During the First 30 Days of Home Health (NQF 2380)** Percentage of home health stays in which patients who had an acute inpatient hospitalization in the 5 days before the start of their home health stay were admitted to an acute care hospital during the 30 days following the start of the home health stay

Domain	NQS Priority	Measure
Outcome	Patient Safety	**45. All-Cause Unplanned Readmission Measure for 30 Days Postdischarge From Inpatient Rehabilitation Facilities (NQF 2502)** This measure estimates the risk-standardized rate of unplanned, all-cause readmissions for patients (Medicare fee-for-service [FFS] beneficiaries) discharged from an inpatient rehabilitation facility (IRF) who were readmitted to a short-stay acute-care hospital or a long-term care hospital (LTCH), within 30 days of an IRF discharge. The measure is based on data for 24 months of IRF discharges to nonhospital postacute levels of care or to the community.
Outcome	Patient Safety	**46. Pediatric All-Condition Readmission Measure (NQF 2393)** This measure calculates case-mix-adjusted readmission rates, defined as the percentage of admissions followed by 1 or more readmissions within 30 days, for patients less than 18 years old. The measure covers patients discharged from general acute care hospitals, including children's hospitals.
Outcome	Patient Safety	**47. Emergency Department Use Without Hospital Readmission During the First 30 Days of Home Health (NQF 2505)** Percentage of home health stays in which patients who had an acute inpatient hospitalization in the 5 days before the start of their home health stay used an emergency room but were not admitted to an acute care hospital during the 30 days following the start of the home health stay
Mortality		
Outcome	Prevention and Treatment of Cardiovascular Disease	**48. Hospital 30-Day Mortality Rate, HF (NQF 0229)** The measure estimates a hospital-level risk-standardized mortality rate (RSMR), defined as death from any cause within 30 days after the index admission date, for patients 18 and older discharged from the hospital.
Outcome	Prevention and Treatment of Cardiovascular Disease	**49. Hospital 30-Day Mortality Rate, AMI (NQF 0230)** The measure estimates a hospital-level RSMR, defined as death from any cause within 30 days after the index admission date, for patients 18 and older, discharged from the hospital
Outcome	Health and Well-Being	**50. Hospital 30-Day Mortality Rate, COPD (NQF 1893)** The measure estimates a hospital-level RSMR, defined as death from any cause within 30 days after the index admission date, for patients 18 and older discharged from the hospital

(Continued)

Domain	NQS Priority	Measure
Outcome	Patient Safety	**51. Hospital 30-Day Mortality Rate, PN (NQF 0468)** The measure estimates a hospital-level RSMR, defined as death from any cause within 30 days after the index admission date, for patients 18 and older discharged from the hospital
Perinatal and Reproductive Health		
Process	Health and Well-Being	**52. Frequency of Ongoing Prenatal Care (NQF 1391)** Measure examines the percentage of Medicaid deliveries that received various numbers of expected prenatal visits.
Outcome	Affordable Care	**53. Elective Delivery Prior to 39 Completed Weeks Gestation (NQF 0469)** Percentage of babies electively delivered prior to 39 completed weeks gestation
Outcome	Affordable Care	**54. Cesarean Rate for Low-Risk First-Birth Women (NQF 0471)** Percentage of low-risk first-birth women (aka NTSV CS rate: nulliparous, term, singleton, vertex) with a Cesarean rate that has the most variation among practitioners, hospitals, regions, and states
Outcome	Health and Well-Being	**55. Healthy Term Newborn (NQF 0716)** Percentage of term singleton live births (excluding those with diagnoses originating in the fetal period) who DO NOT have significant complications during birth or the nursery care
Functional Status		
Outcome	Effective Communication and Care Coordination	**56. Change in Basic Mobility as Measured by the AM-PAC (NQF 0429)** The AM-PAC is a patient-reported functional status assessment instrument developed specifically for use in facility- and community-dwelling postacute care patients.
Outcome	Effective Communication and Care Coordination	**57. Change in Daily Activity Function as Measured by the AM-PAC (0430)** The AM-PAC is a patient reported functional status assessment instrument developed specifically for use in facility- and community-dwelling postacute care patients.

Domain	NQS Priority	Measure
Complications and Health Care Associated Infections		
Outcome	Patient Safety	**58. Patient Safety for Selected Indicators (NQF 0531)** A composite measure of potentially preventable adverse events for selected indicators including pressure ulcers, iatrogenic pneumothorax, central venous catheter-related bloodstream infections, postop hip fracture, postop hemorrhage or hematoma, postop physiologic and metabolic derangements, postop respiratory failure, postop pulmonary embolism or deep vein thrombosis, postop sepsis, postop wound dehiscence, accidental puncture or laceration
Outcome	Patient Safety	**59. National Healthcare Safety Network Catheter-Associated Urinary Tract Infection Outcome Measure (NQF 0138)** Standardized infection ratio (SIR) of health care-associated catheter-associated urinary tract infection calculated among patients in inpatient locations. Data from these locations are reported from acute care general hospitals (including specialty hospitals), freestanding long-term acute care hospitals, rehabilitation hospitals, and behavioral health hospitals. This scope of coverage includes but is not limited to all IRFs, both freestanding and located as a separate unit within an acute care general hospital. Only locations where patients reside overnight are included, that is, inpatient locations.
Outcome	Patient Safety	**60. National Healthcare Safety Network Central Line-Associated Bloodstream Infection Outcome Measure (NQF 0139)** SIR of health care-associated central line-associated bloodstream infection calculated among patients in inpatient locations. Data from these locations are reported from acute care general hospitals (including specialty hospitals), freestanding long-term acute care hospitals, rehabilitation hospitals, and behavioral health hospitals. This scope of coverage includes but is not limited to all IRFs, both freestanding and located as a separate unit within an acute care general hospital. Only locations where patients reside overnight are included, that is, inpatient locations.
Patient Experience		
Outcome, Process	Person- and Family-Centered Care	**61. Consumer Assessment of Healthcare Providers and Systems (CAHPS) Clinician/Group Surveys (NQF 0005)** CAHPS surveys ask consumers and patients to report on and evaluate their experiences with health care.
Outcome, Process	Person- and Family-Centered Care	**62. CAHPS Health Plan Survey (NQF 0006)** CAHPS surveys ask consumers and patients to report on and evaluate their experiences with health care.

(Continued)

Domain	NQS Priority	Measure
Outcome, Process	Person- and Family-Centered Care	**63. CAHPS Health Plan Survey v 3.0 Children with Chronic Conditions Supplement (NQF 0009)** CAHPS surveys ask consumers and patients to report on and evaluate their experiences with health care.
Outcome, Process	Person- and Family-Centered Care	**64. CAHPS Hospital Survey (NQF 0166)** Twenty-seven-items survey instrument with seven domain-level composites including communication with doctors, communication with nurses, responsiveness of hospital staff, pain control, communication about medicines, cleanliness, and quiet of the hospital environment, and discharge information
Outcome, Process	Person- and Family-Centered Care	**65. CAHPS Home Health Care Survey (NQF 0517)** CAHPS surveys ask consumers and patients to report on and evaluate their experiences with health care.
Outcome, Process	Person- and Family-Centered Care	**66. CAHPS Nursing Home Survey: Discharged Resident Instrument (NQF 0691)** CAHPS surveys ask consumers and patients to report on and evaluate their experiences with health care.
Outcome, Process	Person- and Family-Centered Care	**67. CAHPS Nursing Home Survey: Long-Stay Resident Instrument (NQF 0692)** CAHPS surveys ask consumers and patients to report on and evaluate their experiences with health care.
Outcome, Process	Person- and Family-Centered Care	**68. CAHPS Nursing Home Survey: Family Member Instrument (NQF 0693)** CAHPS surveys ask consumers and patients to report on and evaluate their experiences with health care.
Outcome, Process	Person- and Family-Centered Care	**69. CAHPS In-Center Hemodialysis Survey (NQF 0258)** CAHPS surveys ask consumers and patients to report on and evaluate their experiences with health care.
Cost and Resource Use		
Outcome	Affordable Care	**70. Medicare Spending per Beneficiary (MSPB), Risk-Adjusted and Price Standardized (NQF 2158)** MSPB measure evaluates hospitals' efficiency relative to the efficiency of the median hospital. Specifically, the MSPB measure assesses the cost to Medicare of services performed by hospitals and other health care providers during an MSPB episode, which comprises the period immediately prior to, during, and following a patient's hospital stay

Domain	NQS Priority	Measure
Outcome	Affordable Care	**71.** **Total Cost of Care Population-Based PMPM Index (NQF 1604)** Total cost index (TCI) is a measure of a primary care provider's risk adjusted cost effectiveness at managing the population they care for. TCI includes all costs associated with treating members, including professional, facility inpatient and outpatient, pharmacy, lab, radiology, ancillary, and behavioral health services.
Outcome	Affordable Care	**72.** **Relative Resource Use for People With Asthma (NQF 1560)** The risk-adjusted relative resource use by health plan members with asthma during the measurement year. This measure addresses the resource use of members identified as having asthma. Both encounter and pharmacy data are used to identify members for inclusion in the eligible population, and the results are adjusted to account for age, gender, and Hierarchical Condition Category–Relative Resource Use (HCC-RRU) risk classifications that predict cost variability
Outcome	Affordable Care	**73.** **Relative Resource Use for People With Chronic Obstructive Pulmonary Disease (NQF 1561)** The risk-adjusted relative resource use by health plan members with COPD during the measurement year. This measure addresses the resource use of members identified with COPD. Clinical diagnosis of COPD during the measurement year is used to identify members for inclusion in the eligible population, and the results are adjusted to account for age, gender, and HCC-RRU risk classifications that predict cost variability.
Outcome	Affordable Care	**74.** **Relative Resource Use for People With Cardiovascular Conditions (NQF 1558)** The risk-adjusted relative resource use by health plan members with specific cardiovascular conditions during the measurement year. This measure addresses the resource use of members identified with significant cardiovascular disease. Major cardiac events (AMI, CABG, PCI) and/or cardiovascular-related diagnoses (ischemic vascular disease) are used to identify members for inclusion in the eligible population, and the results are adjusted to account for age, gender, and the HCC-RRU risk classifications that predict cost variability

(Continued)

Domain	NQS Priority	Measure
Outcome	Affordable Care	**75. Relative Resource Use for People With Diabetes (NQF 1557)** The risk-adjusted relative resource use by patients 18–75 years of age with diabetes (Type 1 and Type 2) during the measurement year. This measure addresses the resource use of members identified with diabetes (Type 1 and Type 2). Diagnosis of the disease or use of anti-diabetic medications is used to identify members for inclusion in the eligible population and the results are adjusted to account for age, gender, and HCC-RRU risk classifications that predict cost variability.

Appendix B

Quasi-experimental Methods That Correct for Selection Bias

Further Comments and Mathematical Derivations

Propensity Score Methods

Here we present several methods to estimate the average treatment effect (ATE) and average treatment effect (ATT) on the treated in consideration of the propensity score (PS). The following discussion is a general overview of the methods in question.

Estimating PS. An unconfounded analysis assumes that the set of observable characteristics, *X*, *completely adjusts* for treatment-comparison differences, so that no material selection bias remains. It is therefore critical that the range of X values in the comparison group be very similar to the range in the treatment group. This is referred to as "overlap" between the two groups, and the PS plays a central role in estimating treatment effects and evaluating the quality of the assignment scheme.[1] The PS is the conditional probability, $e(x)$, of an observation (e.g., patient, hospital, medical home) receiving treatment conditional on the covariates:

$$e(x) = Pb[W = 1 | X = x],$$ (B.1)

or the likelihood that a subject with a value of x (e.g., low income, uninsured) is receiving treatment in the intervention. For all possible outcomes x of X, it is necessary that each unit in the defined population has some chance of being treated and some chance of not being treated; hence, $0 < e(x) < 1$. Analyzing the overlap assumption and changing the sample, if necessary, to achieve "good overlap," have become important steps in any program evaluation that assumes unconfounded assignment. Unfortunately, unless the PS is known to be 0 or 1 for certain values of x, PS cannot be used to determine whether overlap holds. This is because all parametric regression models for the scores—such as logit and probit—ensure that estimated probabilities are strictly *between* 0 and 1 for all x. For this reason, the evaluator must eliminate observations where the estimated PSs are "too close" to 0 or 1.[2]

Typically, the *PS* is modeled using a flexible logit or probit including squares, interactions, and in some cases, log-levels of the covariates.[3] For example, if there are three covariates, a general logit model would look like

$$e(x_1, x_2, x_3) = \Lambda[\gamma_0 + \gamma_1 x_1 + \gamma_2 x_2 + \gamma_3 x_3 + \gamma_4 x_1^2 + \gamma_5 x_2^2$$
$$+ \gamma_6 x_3^2 + \gamma_7 x_1 x_2 + \gamma_8 x_1 x_3 + \gamma_9 x_2 x_3],$$ (B.2)

where $\Lambda (x) = \exp(x)/(1+\exp(x))$ is the logistic function. Once the model is specified, obtaining PSs is easily done in statistical software such as Stata or R.

Assessing Overlap. It is common to study the full distributions of the PS scores in the treatment and comparison groups. This is usually done using a histogram or smoothed density curve; in Stata, it can be done with the psmatch2 command (see Figure B.1 for a graphical example). We should see sufficient overlap in the histograms of the estimated PSs to justify continuing the analysis of treatment effects. Intervention group subjects will often have higher PSs than those in the comparison pool, which is not surprising because they are, by design, in the treatment group to begin with. But there has to be overlap. One can infer causal effects only for regions of overlap in the scores.

Two simple approaches have proven useful in assessing overlap. One is to compute the normalized differences for each covariate j,

$$Normdiff_j = \frac{X_{1j} - X_{0j}}{\left[S_{1j}^2 + S_{0j}^2 \right]^{1/2}}, \tag{B.3}$$

where X_{1j} and X_{0j} are the means of covariate j for the treated and comparison subsamples, respectively, and S_1j and S_0j are the sample standard deviations. For

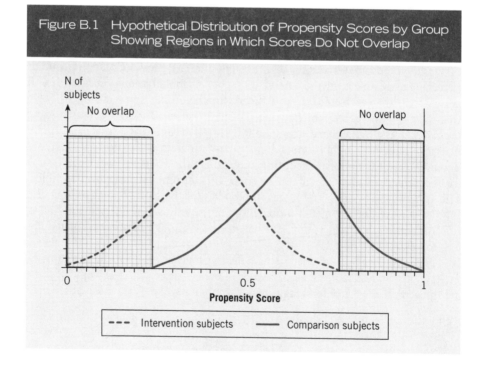

Figure B.1   Hypothetical Distribution of Propensity Scores by Group Showing Regions in Which Scores Do Not Overlap

example, normdiff = (.20 – 10) / [(.1^2 + .15^2)] = 0.55 implies that the treatment rate of 0.20 is slightly more than one-half a standard error above the control group (0.10). Notice that this is not the same as the t statistic for testing equality of the means in the two populations. *Statistical significance is not the critical issue here.* We are interested in the size of the difference in means when standardized by a measure of variability in the population distributions. While there are no firm rules, values of normdiffj that exceed 0.2 in absolute value are cause for concern. See Imbens and Wooldridge (2009) for further discussion.[4]

A second approach to assessing overlap is based on the PS rather than a particular covariate. Let e(x) be the estimated PS. Because e(x) is a function of X_i, its distribution should be *balanced* if overlap holds. So, rather than look at the normalized differences of each covariate, we can compute the normalized difference of e_i. Because e_i is bounded on the unit interval, it may be beneficial to use the predicted log-odds transformation, $log\left[\frac{e(x)}{1+e(x)}\right]$.

Balancing Study and Comparison Groups. If, after studying the normalized differences or estimated PSs overlap appears a problem, it must be adjusted before applying estimators of average treatment effects. This adjustment is often called "balancing the sample." Note that balancing has nothing to do with the outcomes Y_i; we use only the data on the treatment assignments, W_i, and covariates, X_i, for the initial sample of size N (including both groups). The two most common balancing methods are based on estimates of the PS, depending on the parameter of interest:

1) *When the parameter of interest is the ATT,*[5] Rubin (2006) summarizes a useful method that relies on the comparison sample being (considerably) larger than the treated sample.[6] Having estimated a model of the PS for treated cases (possibly a subset of the entire intervention) versus comparison group, scores are ordered by decreasing values. The highest treated unit is matched to the nearest comparison unit based on the smallest absolute difference in their PSs. The match should continue 1:1 without replacement until each treated unit is paired with a comparison unit. This leads to a new sample of 2N1 distinct units, where N1 is the size of the original treated subsample.

2) *When the outcome of interest is the ATE,* which includes the untreated who were assigned to the intervention group (sometimes called nonparticipants), the previous matching method does not work. In this case, the evaluator can drop observations for which the PS is close to 0 or 1—a common practice in evaluation studies that have initially unbalanced covariate distributions.[7] Intervention or comparison PSs near 0 or 1 indicate either (1) rare cases among the intervention group or (2) comparison cases only seen in the intervention group. Both are likely not to be treated. This method is generally applicable and does not require that the comparison sample be larger than the treated sample (also described in Imbens and Wooldridge, 2009).[8] The CHIM procedure drops units with $ê_i < α$ or $ê_i > 1 − α$, where α

is a value in the 0,1 interval suggested by the data. The trimming procedure usually drops *both* comparison and treatment units. In many cases, a simple rule-of-thumb works well: drop an observation if $\hat{e}i < .1$ or $\hat{e}i > .9$. With the resulting smaller but balanced sample, the evaluator can use any estimation method that relies on PSs to derive the ATE.

We should note here that any method used to balance the sample has two drawbacks. The first is that it changes the parameter being estimated. For example, instead of estimating the ATE in the original population, the CHIM approach estimates the conditional ATE *restricted to the subpopulation* with, say, $.1 \leq e(Xi) \leq .9$. Consequently, estimates using the restricted data have less external validity. The extent of the restriction is unknown, however, which makes it difficult to extrapolate to general populations of interest. But that is a price that is often worth paying to improve internal validity of the analysis.

The second drawback is that PS can be sensitive to particular outcomes. The most straightforward application of PSs occurs when the outcome is a single measure that applies to all patients (e.g., Medicare costs per beneficiary). But most quality indicators in an evaluation are relevant only for select subgroups of patients (e.g., mammograms for women aged 50 or older, hemoglobin A1c tests for persons with diabetes). Technically, the PS approach requires a separate comparison group for each outcome, with each requiring separate propensity models as well. One way to address this complexity is to use PSs to identify a single overall comparison group. The evaluator can then proceed under the assumption that any subgroups within the intervention and comparison groups (e.g., diabetic patients) were comparable for analysis purposes.

An Alternative to Propensity Score Methods

Matching on Covariates. A common alternative to creating PS groups is to select a comparison group with characteristics similar to those of the intervention group. Abadie and Imbens (2006) studied matching estimators that match on the full set of covariates.[9] In the simplest case, each unit is matched to one other unit (in the opposite treatment group). In the case of a tie, simple averaging is used.

One measure of closeness that is common and seems to work well is the Mahalanobis distance using the diagonal of the variance-covariance matrix. Choose a subject i from the comparison group for a given treated subject that minimizes $\Sigma_j (X_{ij} - X_{hj})^2/\eta_j^2$, where η_j^2 is the sample variance of the j-th covariate. Covariate matching has the benefit of avoiding functional form restrictions implied by parametric PS regression adjustments or choosing tuning parameters if we use nonparametric regression adjustment. The cost of this flexibility, other than computational, is that the matching estimator can have substantial bias, especially when the number of covariates is large.[10] Perhaps even more common than covariate matching is PS matching, because it matches on the one-dimensional estimated PS.[11]

Assessing Unconfoundedness

Unfortunately, the unconfoundedness assumption cannot be tested. The evaluator can never be sure that any set of covariates and weights completely eliminate biases introduced by nonrandom selection into the intervention and comparison groups. Superior leadership, an unobservable characteristic believed to influence intervention success, for example, is unlikely to be proxied by measured covariates. Consequently, any assessment of unconfoundedness is necessarily indirect. For example, Heckman, Ichimura, and Todd (1997) studied a situation with three groups: ineligibles, eligible nonparticipants, and eligible participants.[12] To assess unconfoundedness, the authors compare ineligibles in the comparison group with eligible nonparticipants in the treated group. If there is no treatment effect difference between them, then we can have more faith in unconfoundedness for the actual treatment.

Alternatively, suppose there are several pretreatment outcomes for the intervention and comparison groups (say, cost per beneficiary: $Y_i,-1$, $Y_i,-2$, and $Y_i,-3$). Suppose controls consist of time-constant characteristics, Z_i (say, physician practice size). Assuming an unchanged process linking covariates with outcomes (see Imbens and Wooldridge [2009] for discussion[13]), then if there is no confounded selection bias, $Y_i,-1$ should be uncorrelated with the treatment indicator, W_i, holding $Y_i,-2$, $Y_i,-3$, and Z_i constant. Unfortunately, a zero correlation of $Y_{i,-1}$ and W_i is neither necessary nor sufficient to guarantee unconfoundedness, because we can never rule out the possibility that all three lagged outcomes are needed to ensure unconfoundedness.

Nonetheless, we suggest the following approach to analyzing a dataset when assuming unconfounded treatment assignment:

1) Select a potential pool of comparison group candidates.

2) Use the normalized differences and PS estimates to determine the quality of overlap between intervention and comparison groups.

3) If necessary, use the PS to balance the sample by dropping outlier intervention and comparison subjects.

4) Apply (a) PS blocking, (b) covariate matching with regression adjustment, or (c) PS weighting of intervention and comparison subjects with regression adjustment to estimate ATEs.

5) If possible, provide an assessment of unconfoundedness after following all the above steps.

Using Propensity Scores to Estimate Treatment Effects

Blocking on the Estimated Propensity Score. Rather than use the PS to *weight*-treated and comparison observations, some approaches are less sensitive to small changes in the estimated PSs. A particularly useful method is to use the estimated

PSs form G strata ("blocks") of observations. Justification is based on a key result in Rosenbaum and Rubin (1983).[14] With proper balance, each block includes both treated and comparison units, and we estimate an average treatment effect *for each interval*; call these τ_g, g = 1, . . . , G. The estimate of ATE is then derived as the weighted average

$$\tau_{ate} = \Sigma_g \left(N_g / N \right) \tau_g, \tag{B.5}$$

where Ng is the number of observations in block g. The method of blocking based on the PS is mechanically similar to estimation of ATEs with stratified randomization, except that the stratification is *ex ante* on the basis of one or more covariates (say, age, and Medicaid coverage, but *never* on outcome, Y_i). Blocked PS regression, by contrast, has the strata determined *ex post*—that is, after having observed the nonrandom sample on the covariates and assignments.

Before choosing the blocks, it is important to understand that the blocking estimator is not consistently unbiased for the ATE, even if we consistently estimate the ATE within each block. Theoretically, the number of blocks needs to increase as the size of each block shrinks to 0. However, some simple rules of thumb have been used in the literature, such as choosing five blocks so that each block roughly contains $(N_g/N) = 20\%$ of the observations. But then how should we estimate the ATE within each block? Because we do not have random assignment *within* each block, it is better to use regression adjustment within each block, that is,

$$Y_{ig} = \alpha_g + \beta_{1g} W_{ib} + \beta_{2g} X_{ig} + \varepsilon_{ig}, \tag{B.6}$$

with β_{1g} representing the block-specific ATE. Squares and interactions among the elements of Xig can also be used, and there is probably no need to estimate separate regression functions for the control and treated groups, although this depends on the size of the blocks. Unlike using regression adjustment on the entire sample, regression adjustment *within* blocks does not suffer from having to predict across a wide range of cases unless there are only few (2–4) blocks. Imbens and Rubin (2015) contains a detailed argument for how regression adjustment can reduce bias.[15]

As before, the regression adjustment using X_i improves precision by reducing standard errors, especially if the covariates are still good predictors of the outcome within all or some of the blocks. Because estimation of the PSs and selection of the blocks can be automated,[16] one can carry out PS blocking without having to make functional form decisions (other than what to include in X_i).

The remaining issue is statistical inference. Obtaining a valid standard error for the overall ATE using blocks is complicated.[17] Fortunately, Imbens and Rubin show how to obtain standard errors for a broad class of estimators, including those based on PS blocking.[18]

In sum, on balanced samples, the combination of regression adjustment *and* PS weighting can yield reliable estimates. PS matching combined with regression adjustment, or PS blocking combined with regression adjustment, is preferred. In the first case, the PS matching is done on the full set of covariates. In the second case, blocking (or stratification) of the pooled sample is based on the estimated PSs.

Unconfounded Design When Assignment Is at the Group Level

When treatment assignment is at an aggregate level based on hierarchical sampling, the evaluator may still have to condition on covariates to ensure unconfoundedness. For example, schools with historically low funding or low test scores might be targeted by educational interventions. Very large integrated health networks may also be targeted for a demonstration that leads to a national program. In such cases, at a minimum, the evaluator may have to control for group-level covariates (such as funding level or group size) to ensure unconfoundedness. Group-level assignment of subjects generally requires clustering adjustments to ensure proper inference. This typically requires an evaluation regression model such as

$$Ygi = \alpha + \tau W_g + \gamma Z_g + \beta X_{gi} + \left(v_{gi} = C_g + \mu_{gi} \right), \qquad (B.7)$$

where W_g indicates that observations are assigned at the group level, Z_g are the g-group covariates, X_{gi} are the individual-specific covariates, and C_g is the (uncontrolled) cluster or group effect as part of the regression error term ($v_{gi} = C_g + \mu_{gi}$). Many statistical packages have an option to report standard errors, test statistics, and confidence intervals that are robust to adjustments for cluster correlation, as long as there are a reasonably large number of clusters.

Inference With a Small Number of Groups

With a small number of groups, and especially when the group sizes are large, the cluster-robust standard errors are not generally valid, because it is difficult to statistically isolate the group-selection process from the individual-specific random error. In such cases, there are alternative methods, but their applicability is somewhat limited when the number of groups is very small. Donald and Lang (2007) consider the simple equation above with a cluster effect in the error term:

$$v_{gi} = C_g + \mu_{gi}, \qquad (B.8)$$

assuming the mean values of C_g and μ_{gi} equal 0.[19] Averaging this equation, by rolling up subjects within groups, results in mean group averages on the treatment indicator, individual group indicators, and the mean errors of each group. Provided we have at least three groups, this equation can be estimated by ordinary least squares (OLS) to produce the treatment effect, at a serious reduction in degrees of freedom, of course. If treatment assignment is random across groups (i.e., W_g is independent of the error term with a normal distribution and constant variance), we can use the classical linear model setting, but with small G, the resulting inference is much less reliable with higher standard errors, than if the individual observations are treated as independent draws both within and across groups. Unfortunately, the individual observations are unlikely to be unrelated within groups. The combined between (σ^2_c) and within (σ^2_μ) group variance of v_g is $\sigma^2_c + \sigma^2_\mu / N_g$, where N_g is the number of individuals in group g. When group size is even moderately large, the regression error is dominated by group-level variance.[20] Constant variance (homoskedasticity) still is a reasonable assumption, but the normality assumption regarding the standard error requires C_g to have a normal distribution, which cannot literally hold with a discrete or binary outcome. Nonetheless, the inference obtained is likely much better than treating the errors as independent within cluster.

An alternative approach in Wooldridge (2003) assumes that individuals are random draws from a distribution so that the group sample average is unbiased, consistent, and approximate normally distributed.[21] In this case, the ATE is simply the difference in the overall average intervention and comparison group means.

Clustering Effects on Regression Standard Errors. The standard difference-in-difference (DiD) approach assumes observations are independently sampled from the different groups in different time periods. Recently there has been concern that the OLS standard errors for the DiD estimator may not be accurate in the presence of correlations between outcomes within groups and between time periods. This is a particular case of clustering, where the treatment indicator does not vary within clusters—for example, all individuals in a particular medical home are exposed to care management.[22,23,24,25,26,27,28] The starting point of these analyses is a particular structure on the error term U_i:

$$U_i = G_i, T_i + V_i, \tag{B.9}$$

where V_i is an individual-level idiosyncratic error term, and C_{gt} is a group-/time-specific component. The unit level error term, V_i, is assumed to be independent across all units, but *within* a group–time period pair; $C_{Gi,Ti}$ induces correlation in the errors among individual units. For example, patients in a medical home may show systematically lower ER use, even after controlling for covariates.

Suppose the C_{gt} are independent of treatment assignment and mutually independent, and the between group error, C_{gt}, is normally distributed with mean zero and constant variance. With two groups ($g = 0, 1$) and two time periods ($t = 0, 1$), and with large sample sizes in each group and time period, the predicted mean for the group–time period using Equation B.9 has the associated error, C_{gt}, so the ATE in a DiD format approaches the true treatment effect *plus* the difference between the treatment and nontreatment groups that are experiencing unequal time period changes. Thus, the conventional DiD estimator is not a consistent estimator of the true treatment effect in the usual sense. In fact, no consistent estimator exists, because there is no way to eliminate the influence of the four unobserved components of C_{gt}. In this two-group, two time period case, the problem is even worse than the absence of a consistent estimator, because one cannot estimate a between-group and time variance to determine if there is a clustering problem.

However, if there are data from more than two groups or from more than two time periods, one can typically estimate the between-group error variance, and thus, at least under the normality and independence assumptions for C_{gt}, construct confidence intervals for the ATE. One way to do this is, following Donald and Lang (2007), to aggregate individual data to the g and t levels.[29] These authors propose regressing the group/time–period average outcomes on period, group, and treatment indicators, assuming no temporal correlation of error terms (i.e., no autocorrelation). Unfortunately, with small G and T, the degrees of freedom in the resulting t distribution can be small. For example, two time periods and four groups yield eight observations in the regression available to estimate six parameters. So the inference would be based on a t distribution with two degrees of freedom. Because the Donald and Lang (2007) approach cannot be applied in the standard DiD setting with two groups and time periods, there are reasons to question whether it is the proper way to proceed more generally.

Bertrand, Duflo, and Mullainathan, and Hansen focus on the alternative case with multiple (more than two) time periods.[30,31,32] In this case, one may be forced to relax the assumption that the V_{gt} component of the regression error is independent over time. With more than two time periods, these authors allow for an autoregressive structure on the C_{gt}. For example,

$$C_{gt} = \rho C_{g,t-1} + r_{gt}, \qquad (B.10)$$

and $|\rho| = 1$ along with a serially uncorrelated error, r_{gt}. Using simulations and real data calculations based on data for 50 states and multiple time periods, the authors show that corrections to the conventional standard errors taking into account the clustering and autoregressive structure make a substantial difference. Hansen provides additional large-sample results under sequences where the number of time periods increase with the sample size.[33]

NOTES

1. Stratified, or block, sampling is also quite common in selecting a comparison group but is considered inferior to more flexible PS methods.

2. It is useful to know that if we are only interested in estimating the average treatment effect on individuals actually treated, we can assume a weaker version of both the unconfoundedness and overlap assumptions.

In particular, unconfoundedness requires only that W_i is conditionally independent of baseline or untreated outcomes but *not the gain* from treatment. The weaker overlap assumption allows some units in the population, based on x, to have zero chance of being treated. However, we still require that no units are treated with certainty.

3. Imbens, G., and D. Rubin, *Causal Inference for Statistics, Social, and Biomedical Sciences: An Introduction* (Cambridge, UK: Cambridge University Press, 2005), pp. I–IV, describe a stepwise procedure for adding explanatory variables to a logit or probit model when the explanatory variables come from the levels, squares, and cross products of elements of X.

4. Guido W. Imbens, and Jeffrey M. Wooldridge, "Recent Developments in the Econometrics of Program Evaluation," *Journal of Economic Literature, American Economic Association* 47 no. 1 (March 2009): 5–86.

5. Estimating the ATT assumes that data exist on intervention subjects regarding whether they were actually treated or not during the evaluation period. Many evaluations do not have information on whether subjects were actually contacted after being assigned, however, and even fewer have information on extent of contact, or dosage.

6. Rubin, Donald B. *Matched Sampling for Causal Effects* (New York: Cambridge University Press, 2006).

7. Crump, Richard K., V. Joseph Hotz, Guido W. Imbens, and Oscar A. Mitnik, "Dealing with Limited Overlap in Estimation of Average Treatment Effects," *Biometrika* 96 no. 1 (2009): 187–99.

8. Imbens and Wooldridge, 2009.

9. Abadie, A., and G. W Imbens. "Large Sample Properties of Matching Estimators for Average Treatment Effects," *Econometrica* 74 no. 1 (2006): 235–67.

10. Imbens and Wooldridge, 2009.

11. Abadie and Imbens (2012) have established the asymptotic normality of estimators that use PS matching using Stata command match and have shown that the asymptotic variance formula that ignores estimation of the PS is conservative when obtaining standard errors. Abadie, Alberto, and Guido W. Imbens, "A Martingale Representation for Matching

Estimators," *Journal of the American Statistical Association* 107 no. 498 (June 2012): 833–43.

12. Heckman, James, Hidehiko Ichimura, and Petra E. Todd, "Matching as an Econometric Evaluation Estimator: Evidence from Evaluating a Job Training Programme," *Review of Economic Studies* 64 no. 4 (1997): 605–54.

13. Imbens and Wooldridge, 2009.

14. Paul R. Rosenbaum, and Donald B. Rubin. "The Central Role of the Propensity Score in Observational Studies for Causal Effects" *Biometrika* 70 no. 1 (1983): 41–55. doi:10.1093/biomet/70.1.41.

15. Imbens, G. W., and D. B. Rubin. *Causal Inference in Statistics, Social, and Biomedical Sciences* (New York: Cambridge University Press, 2015).

16. Ibid.

17. Bootstrapping standard errors cannot be used in this case.

18. Imbens and Rubin, 2015.

19. Stephen G. Donald, and Kevin Lang, "Inference with Difference-in-Differences and Other Panel Data," *The Review of Economics and Statistics* 89 no. 2 (2007, May): 221–33.

20. Bloom (2005) provides simulations of the effects of group clustering on standard errors. Even small intraclass correlation, or the ratio of between to total population variance, can raise standard errors significantly. Bloom, H., *Learning More from Social Experiments* (New York: Russell Sage Foundation, 2005), Chapter 4.

21. Wooldridge, Jeffrey M. "Cluster-Sample Methods in Applied Econometrics." *The American Economic Review* 93 no. 2 (2003): 133–38.

22. Moulton, Brent R., "An Illustration of a Pitfall in Estimating the Effects of Aggregate Variables on Micro Unit," *The Review of Economics and Statistics* 72 no. 2 (1990, May): 334–38.

23. Moulton, Brent R., and William C. Randolph, "Alternative Tests of the Error Components

Model," *Econometrica, Econometric Society* 57 no. 3 (1989, May): 685–93.

24. Wooldridge, 2003.

25. Donald and Lang, 2007.

26. Bertrand, Marianne, Esther Duflo, and Sendhil Mullainathan, "How Much Should We Trust Differences-In-Differences Estimates?" *The Quarterly Journal of Economics* 119 no. 1 (2004): 249–75.

27. Christian B. Hansen, "Generalized Least Squares Inference in Panel and Multilevel Models with Serial Correlation and Fixed Effects." *Journal of Econometrics* 140 no. 2 (October 2007): 670–94.

28. Christian B. Hansen, "Asymptotic Properties of a Robust Variance Matrix Estimator for Panel Data When is Large," *Journal of Econometrics* 141 no. 2 (December 2007): 597–620.

29. Donald and Lang, 2007.

30. Bertrand, Duflo, and Mullainathan, 2004.

31. Hansen, 2007, October.

32. Hansen, 2007, December.

33. Ibid.

Index

Structural evaluation:
  defined, 30
  National Quality Strategy (NQS)
    measures, 278t
  value of, 30–31
Structured coding, 234–235
Summative evaluation:
  defined, 13–14
  evaluation framework development,
    13–14
  in impact evaluation, 13
  outcome evaluation in, 13
Surgical safety checklist (Ontario), 54 (box)
Surveillance, Epidemiology, and End
    Results-Medicare database, 38
Systematic analysis, 142, 150, 252

Target population, 19
TeamSTEPPS Teamwork Perceptions
    Questionnaire (T-TPQ), 160t, 161

Theory-driven evaluation, 12
Treatment effects. *See* Average treatment
    effect (ATE); Average treatment effect
    on the treated (ATT); Heterogeneity of
    treatment effects (HTE); Intent-to-treat
    effect (ITT)
Type I error, 58
Type II error, 58

Validity:
  construct validity, 60
  external validity, 55, 62
  internal validity, 60
  regression modeling and analysis, 127–129
  in statistical inference, 55, 59–62
  statistical validity, 60
Visual displays, 267, 268–269f

Within cluster effects, 130
Written reports, 273, 274 (box)